COMMUNICATION FOR THE HEARING HANDICAPPED

An International Perspective

Edited by

Herbert J. Oyer, Ph.D.

Professor of Audiology and Speech Sciences,
and Dean of the Graduate School, Michigan State University

University Park Press
Baltimore • London • Tokyo

UNIVERSITY PARK PRESS
International Publishers in Science and Medicine
Chamber of Commerce Building
Baltimore, Maryland 21202

Typeset by The Composing Room of Michigan, Inc.
Manufactured in the United States of America by Universal Lithographers, Inc., and The Maple Press Co.

Library of Congress Cataloging in Publication Data
Main entry under title:
Communication for the hearing handicapped.
Includes index.
1. Deaf–Rehabilitation–Addresses, essays, lectures. 2. Deaf–Means of communication–Addresses, essays, lectures. I. Oyer, Herbert J.
HV2390.C65 362.4'2 76-9081
ISBN 0-8391-0826-5

Contents

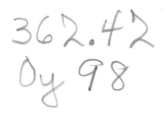

Contributors

Joseph Gisbert Alos, M.D., Director of Rehabilitation Center, Monteabrer de Godella, Valencia, Spain

Marie-Claire Barbera, M.D., Centres Médicaux de Phoniatrie, Université de Nice, Nice, France

Danuta Borkowski-Gaertig, M.D., Head, Children's Otolaryngological and Audiological Department, Institute of Mother and Child, Warsaw, Poland

Judith Borus, Ph.D., Associate Professor of Audiology and Speech Sciences, Department of Speech, Howard University, Washington, D.C.

Chua Tee Tee, M.S., Cert. Ed., Lecturer, Faculty of Education, University of Malaya, Kuala Lumpur, Malaysia

Bryan R. Clarke, Ph.D., Chairman, Department of Special Education, University of British Columbia, Vancouver, B.C., Canada

Edward J. Hardick, Ph.D., Professor and Head, Speech and Hearing Science Section, Department of Communication, The Ohio State University, Columbus, Ohio

Y. P. Kapur, M.D., Professor, Department of Audiology and Speech Sciences, Professor and Chief of Otolaryngology, Department of Surgery, Michigan State University, East Lansing, Michigan

David C. Kendall, Ph.D., Professor, Department of Education, University of British Columbia, Vancouver, B.C., Canada

Armin Löwe, Professor and Dean of Special Education, Heidelberg University, Heidelberg, West Germany

Tore Lundborg, M.D., Assistant Professor O.R.L., Director, Department of Audiology, Soderjukhuset, Stockholm, Sweden

Kevin P. Murphy, Ph.D., Director, The Audiology Unit, Royal Berkshire Hospital, Reading, England

Yoshitatsu Nakano, Ed.D., Associate Professor of Special Education, Department of Special Education, Hiroshima University, Hiroshima, Japan

Herbert J. Oyer, Ph.D., Professor of Audiology and Speech Sciences, and Dean of the Graduate School, Michigan State University East Lansing, Michigan

Guy Perdoncini, M.D., Professor, Centres Médicaux de Phoniatrie, Université de Nice, Nice, France

Jerome Reichstein, Ed.D., Director of Speech and Hearing Sciences, Tel Aviv School System, Tel Aviv, Israel

Salah M. Soliman, M.D., Sc.D., Assistant Professor of Otolaryngology and Audiology, Faculty of Medicine, Ain Shams University, Cairo, Egypt

Oscar Tosi, Ph.D., Professor, Department of Audiology and Speech Sciences, Director, Speech Sciences Laboratories, Michigan State University, East Lansing, Michigan

Jamil I. Toubbeh, Ph.D., Chief of Manpower Resources Branch, Division of Manpower Development, Rehabilitation Services Administration, Department of Health, Education and Welfare, Washington, D.C.

James T. Yates, Ph.D., Associate Professor and Director of Audiology, Texas Tech University, Lubbock, Texas

Preface

The central purpose of this book is to present to the reader a systematic comparative description of the manner in which habilitation-rehabilitation is carried out around the world for persons who sustain hearing loss with related communication handicaps. The input to the book is made by individuals who are working or have worked in some capacity in habilitation-rehabilitation of hearing handicapped people in each of the countries represented. In preparing their chapters they have followed a rather general outline provided them.

Rather than attempting to develop a book with contributions from every country having programs for the hearing handicapped, the effort was made to obtain a representative sample of countries. Thus, those included are as follows: Canada, the United Kingdom, Ireland, France, Spain, Federal Republic of Germany, Switzerland, Austria, India, Argentina, Sweden, the Arab World, Poland, Malaysia, Japan, Israel, and the United States. It will be up to the reader to determine the success to which the sample of countries chosen is representative.

It is the hope of the editor that students, teachers, clinicians, administrators, and researchers dealing with any facet of the habilitation-rehabilitation of hearing handicapped people around the world will find the material in this book helpful to them as they pursue their work. A further hope is that it will stimulate the thinking of some who will press on toward discovery of new facts concerning the habilitation-rehabilitation of the communication process of hearing handicapped children and adults.

H. J. O.

Foreword

That most unique human characteristic—communication—appears at times to have fostered as much enmity between nations as it has cooperation and harmony. The very act of expressing thoughts and attitudes to people whose language, culture, and thought processes are slightly to vastly different seems to have carried with it, throughout recorded human history, the risk that misunderstanding could invite catastrophe. Much of the fascination many of us find in studying cross-cultural communication is related to awareness of its consequences for improved relationships among the peoples of the world.

On a less global level, the communicatively impaired person, from any locale, is in some ways a microcosmic model of the larger universe; his problem sets him apart from his fellow citizens much as if he were outside his own society. This is particularly the case for the severely hearing impaired. It seems both necessary and fitting that a book such as this one should evolve, examining the problems of the hearing impaired from across the world and the way in which services are provided for them.

The universality of this concern can be deduced from a look at the list of the contributors in this volume. All around the globe we find this humanitarian concern not only for those within a given society in need of help but for their fellows in other countries as well. This in itself serves to help bridge the gap between nations. In sharing our problems, along with our solutions, we come better to understand each other and vastly increase our own knowledge at the same time.

From its first organized beginnings in the United States 50 years ago, the speech and hearing profession has tended to look inward as this field developed and paid little attention to the accomplishments of other countries. One of the persons in the United States who has been most concerned over this tendency—and has recognized its short-sightedness—has been Dr. Herbert Oyer. For many years an emissary to the profession all over the globe, he brings much of the world's greatest professional talent together in this volume in order that we may all share in the problems faced and the solutions rendered, thereby increasing in each of us the capability to serve those in need more effectively and more efficiently. The process of exchanging knowledge and viewpoints can contribute significantly to improved communication among citizens at all levels in their respective countries.

Sharing our concerns as well as our knowledge makes us all better citizens in the world we share.

Joseph L. Stewart, Ph.D.

Acknowledgments

The editor wishes to acknowledge the valuable assistance provided by Dr. Oscar Tosi, who gave unselfishly of his time and talents in translating several of the manuscripts.

Acknowledgment is also made of the expert secretarial services provided by Virginia McLeod, Marcia Foncannon, and Susan Forester.

To the millions of hearing-handicapped persons throughout the world and to all those who work in their behalf.

Communication for the Hearing Handicapped

PART I
Some Preliminary Observations

chapter 1

Habilitation-Rehabilitation of Hearing-handicapped People as an Area of Challenge

Herbert J. Oyer, Ph.D.

For centuries man has tried to find ways to help those individuals who are handicapped in communication because of loss of hearing. There was a time when the severely hard of hearing and deaf were considered unfit to hold citizenship but, fortunately, through the efforts of religious and educational institutions, the plight of hearing-handicapped persons was recognized and attempts were made to set up special programs first for children and later on for adults as well. The first structured programs were set up in France in the 17th century and later in Spain, Germany, and England. The emphasis was on teaching speech to the deaf. Since methods of testing hearing level were crude, there were probably some individuals classified as deaf whom today we might not classify as such but rather as severely hard of hearing.

Habilitation-rehabilitation of communication skills is considered by most professionals with whom this writer is acquainted as that area of endeavor which seeks to bring about self and social adjustment of the hearing handicapped, thus assisting them in overcoming the handicapping effects of hearing loss. This may mean to the medically trained professional, the use of medicines, or to the surgeon, the use of surgical procedures that reverse hearing loss. We know that only certain problems causing hearing loss can be treated successfully by medical or surgical approaches; thus, other procedures have been developed that are based upon audiological, psychosocial, and educational principles. These frequently include counseling, language and speech development through auditory training, lipreading, and manual methods, and also special approaches to the teaching of substantive materials so necessary for scholastic progress.

A CHALLENGE?

Habilitation-rehabilitation of hearing-handicapped people is truly a challenge, because one of the very most important things to strive for, i.e., effective communication, is often made very difficult by the hearing loss, and, in many instances, is not reversible through medical or surgical intervention or amplification. Thus, there must be other approaches used. These other approaches used by teacher, audiologist, counselor, etc., are often without a suitable scientific data base and there are identifiable reasons for this situation. Research has lagged in this area because the multiplicity of variables that must be considered are diverse and complex.

The difficulty of accurate measurement of the behavior of the auditorally handicapped makes the task a challenge. It is not enough by any means to measure auditory performance. This can be accomplished readily and, with the exception of very young children and the multiply handicapped, is frequently not a difficult job. However, the measurement of motivation, language (both expressive and receptive), the degree to which language is received via the visual channel, etc., present real challenges.

Habilitation-rehabilitation of communication is a challenge because there is no generally agreed upon framework for analyzing the process. As a result, there is no standard terminology for describing the problems with which we work or the objectives of our work.

Much is still being learned about the manner in which the normal ear responds to sound. This serves as background for studies made of the way in which hearing loss affects the processing of sound. Although we can make a reasonable estimate as to how sounds are perceived by those with various types of hearing losses, it is only an estimate. In order to design compensatory devices and programs we must be able to make the compensatory approaches more sensitive to the individual auditory handicap.

Although great strides have been made, a great challenge lies in the field of electronics. The development of this field has brought with it the refinement of instruments for testing auditory function. It has also provided for various types of group amplification units as well as the individual hearing aid. The latest development combines electronics with surgery in the cochlear implant procedure. What this will mean eventually for the hearing-handicapped person remains to be seen through further experimentation and evaluation.

The challenges of communication habilitation-rehabilitation of hearing-handicapped persons are great, for in-depth understanding of the process calls for knowledge of physical, neurophysiological, and psychosocial phenomena that can be measured. Additionally, it calls for clinical insights that might or might not be verifiable through measurement. To work successfully with communication problems of hearing-handicapped people calls for a blending of clinical arts and scientific procedures.

Perhaps the greatest single challenge is in the further development of a scientific data base upon which a prescriptive approach to communication habilitation-rehabilitation can be designed.

Part II of this book contains descriptions of what is being done for hearing-handicapped persons in the area of communication in various countries throughout the world. In some respects the approaches made by a number of countries are quite similar; however, the reader will note dissimilarities as well. It is heartening to learn that, in most countries, studies are being made to uncover new facts about the habilitation-rehabilitation process as related specifically to communication of those handicapped by hearing loss. In other words, there is, in some measure, an answer being made to the challenge of "communication for hearing-handicapped people."

chapter 2

Importance of an International Perspective

Herbert J. Oyer, Ph.D.

Over the past three centuries, hearing-handicapped individuals have been receiving special attention in many countries around the world. As programs and approaches have been developed and refined, they have, of course, reflected the value systems and cultural norms of a particular society. The communication of programs and approaches has been carried out largely through the occasional migration of professionals from one country to another. It has also occurred through recorded descriptions of help given to the hearing handicapped through writings which appear in journals and books and through international meetings.

The present work is the first known to this writer which attempts to provide a comparative view of philosophies, methods, techniques, programs, and research focused upon the hearing handicapped in selected countries around the world. The hope is, of course, that the cross-cultural comparative approach will broaden substantially the understanding of the multiplicity of problems related to communication and hearing loss. In addition to broadening one's view, the cross-cultural study of habilitation-rehabilitation of the hearing handicapped should help in achieving a number of other objectives.

OBJECTIVES

Develop Greater Objectivity

By learning of the approaches to habilitation-rehabilitation of communication of hearing-handicapped persons in other cultures, one should become more objective about the differences that characterize approaches other than our own. Moreover, objectivity highlights the fact that there are indeed multiple approaches to the problem.

Become More Analytical

When we view the approaches we are making in habilitation-rehabilitation against the backdrop of approaches made in other countries, we cannot help but become more analytical about our own approaches. Hopefully, the end result will be that of improved programs for the hearing handicapped.

Appreciate Common Needs

As one learns of the work taking place in other countries with the hearing handicapped, it soon becomes quite evident that, irrespective of the country, we share common needs. Pooled efforts toward working out strategies for meeting those needs could prove to be highly productive.

Help Us to Interpret Needs to a Wider Audience

One could reasonably expect that worldwide organizations such as the United Nations, the World Health Organization, and private agencies focused on health needs internationally would be interested in comparative cross-cultural data on the hearing impaired. An attempt has been made to provide this by describing programs of communication habilitation-rehabilitation systematically in the following chapters.

Share in Research Findings

Through cross-cultural efforts, it is possible to share and compare findings of research results carried out independently on common communication problems confronted by the hearing handicapped. This could lead to joint research projects in which a coordinated cross-cultural assault could be made on basic common problems.

Assist in Theory Development

Since well founded theory is yet to be developed in the area of communication habilitation-rehabilitation, a cross-cultural sharing of successful approaches could be useful in the development of hypotheses to be tested. Good theory development could enhance the further development of programs and should help all to be more economical in the use of resources.

In the field of habilitation-rehabilitation of hearing-handicapped persons, there are some universals with which professionals in all countries must contend. It serves us well to share our problems, experiences, and findings in order that those who sustain handicapping conditions associated with hearing loss might be helped even more effectively.

View Other Diagnostic Procedures

By making comparative analyses and evaluations of the diagnostic procedures employed in the various countries, we are able to make judgments as to those procedures which will be most useful in any given setting. Those engaged in the habilitation-rehabilitation of hearing-handicapped persons sustaining communication problems are aware that we are yet in need of further development of diagnostic tools for the measurement of hearing handicap. Audiometric tests give us useful clues as to the deficit, but there is need for other data in order to develop a profile of the performance of the hearing handicapped in many areas. It is not infrequent that individual teachers and clinicians will develop excellent diagnostic approaches and will not, because of one reason or another, communicate these to others. Cross-cultural descriptions of diagnostic procedures should be helpful in this regard.

With modern communication and transportation technologies so well developed, it is imperative that we no longer continue to work in relative isolation. For it is more possible than ever before to communicate quickly, either through the written word or through on-site visitation. With the many unanswered questions yet before us, it behooves us to search diligently not only within, but also across, national boundaries, in order that the communication needs of hearing-handicapped people might be served most effectively.

PART II
An International View of Philosophies, Programs, Methods, and Research

chapter 3

Communication for Hearing-handicapped People in the United States

Herbert J. Oyer, Ph.D.,
and Edward J. Hardick, Ph.D.

Hearing-handicapped children and adults in the United States have profited variously from developments of engineering technology, medical and surgical procedures, and educational programs that seek to ameliorate the effects of hearing loss. In some instances these developments have made the difference between being "tuned in" to environmental non-speech sounds and not being "tuned in." In other instances, these developments have meant the difference between being able to participate in oral communication and not being able to do so. In still other instances, these developments have made the difference between a handicapped individual's being able to hold a job and not being able to succeed vocationally.

Concern for education and rehabilitation of hearing-handicapped persons in the United States has its roots in the very early efforts made in Europe to educate the deaf and particularly in efforts to teach them to speak. Hearing loss, being an invisible disorder, has not attracted the attention of the general public as have some of the more readily visible disorders such as cerebral palsy, blindness, and so on. Although schools for the deaf were set up early in the development of the country, special programs in schools and clinics for the hard of hearing were established much later on.

One of the notable characteristics of a civilized society is in the provisions it makes for its members who sustain handicapping conditions. Cognizant of the effects certain handicaps have on the ability to relate to others, ability to learn, and the ability to achieve independence through self-support, a sensitive society plans in special ways to help the handicapped to cope with their problems more successfully. In the United States an attempt to accomplish this is being made through the efforts of private and community organizations as well as through government at local, state, and federal levels.

To educate, train, and counsel the hearing handicapped is the first great step toward preparing them to become self-supporting citizens. However, another important aspect of preparing the hearing handicapped for successful interpersonal interaction is in the counseling and education of parents, peers, and significant others with whom the handicapped child or adult must live, learn, play, or work.

The object of habilitative and rehabilitative programs for the hearing handicapped is focused primarily upon improving their skills in the area of communication. For it is communication with others that provides the humanizing element of existence. Self and social development are immutably linked with successful communication experiences.

There have been strides made in the United States toward the development of a scientific data base which is beginning to provide a foundation for aural rehabilitation procedures (Oyer and Frankmann, 1975). Most noteworthy in this regard are the data which form the substrate for the measurement of hearing level. Although considerable effort has been made to understand the importance of the visual pathway to communication, there yet remains the task of designing a valid test of visual communication. Tactile stimulation has been viewed as a possible communication aid, but as yet no viable system has been developed to make it so. Substantial efforts have been made to understand the effects of auditory stimulus input to those with normal and those with abnormal hearing. However, there is an outstanding need for thoroughgoing investigations into the actual auditory training procedures themselves with the hearing handicapped.

An encouraging sign in the United States is a growing awareness of the need for scientifically derived rehabilitation procedures by many who are responsible for programs of aural rehabilitation. Evidence of this fact is made manifest in the development of the Academy of Aural Rehabilitation in 1966. Perhaps one day when there is greater scientific underpinning for aural rehabilitation, we will be able to proceed with a much more highly refined "prescriptive" approach to the rehabilitation of hearing-handicapped persons.

DEFINITION OF AURAL REHABILITATION

One of the hazards of attempting to define anything is the risk one runs of not being comprehensive enough in the definition. When one attaches the "is" of identity to an object, state of being, or a process, one "excludes" as well as "includes." With this in mind then, let us examine the concept of aural rehabilitation.

Aural rehabilitation is best conceptualized as a process characterized by a series of related events. The process includes the identification of hearing handicap in the individual and motivation on the part of someone to do something about it. Following adequate motivation, there is the matter of obtaining evaluations by an otologist and an audiologist of the deficit and the handicap(s) after which specialized treatment is given. Upon completion of a treatment regimen, there is then the matter of determining the extent to which the treatment has brought about a change in the client's communication skills and related behaviors.

Research dealing with normal processes of audition and clinical measurement contributes greatly to the work of the audiologist who is involved in a rehabilitative relationship with the client in an attempt to help him overcome handicap(s) created by hearing loss. For it is essential that the audiologist directly involved in the rehabilitation process knows the capabilities of the normal auditory system and also knows the extent to which the client's responses to sound differ from responses of those with normal hearing.

The process of aural rehabilitation is psychosocial in nature and, as such, is characterized by procedures that aim at modification of communication behavior. Little has been accomplished by way of rehabilitation if changes in behavior as regards adjustment and/or learning are not enhanced through learning to communicate more successfully. The alert clinician will determine the extent to which changes have been brought about.

Perhaps other audiologists whose principal concern is in the area of habilitation and/or rehabilitation might choose to define aural rehabilitation in a way different from that given in this chapter. However, it is likely that many of the components of the process would be defined similarly.

HISTORICAL OVERVIEW

The following paragraphs present a brief overview of the development of programs in the United States that have had as their central purpose the habilitation-rehabilitation of hearing-handicapped individuals. In keeping with the thought that this section should present a brief overview, no attempt is made to name each program developed or to give detailed accounts of program developments. The objective is to provide readers who are somewhat unfamiliar with programs for the hearing handicapped in the United States the type of information that will help them appreciate those factors that led to the creation of programs.

For purposes of discussion, it serves well to think of three categories in which programs developed: (1) schools for the deaf, (2) special programs and classes for the hearing handicapped in schools, and (3) special programs for the hearing handicapped in clinics.

Schools for the Deaf

Schools for the deaf in the United States were most heavily influenced in the beginning by work that was taking place in England, France, Germany, and Spain. An Englishman, John Braidwood, came to the United States and through the help of local individuals in Virginia set up a small school for the deaf in Cobbs, Virginia (Rae, 1851).

Shortly thereafter, Thomas Gallaudet, a young graduate of Yale University and an ordained minister, undertook study with the Braidwoods of England but soon left them to study the methods of Sicard in Paris. Sicard was advocating the manual approach (Peet, 1852). This approach was subsequently brought back to the United States by Gallaudet and Laurent Clerc, a deaf teacher from Paris. They left France and started a school for the deaf in Hartford, Connecticut. The school progressed well and received federal support and became known as the American Asylum for the Deaf, which is now the American School for the Deaf.

Other schools were established and all employed the manual method until educators began to take cognizance of the success of the oral approach being utilized in England and Germany. It was in 1867, however, that John Clarke supported the construction of the Clarke School for the Deaf in Northampton, Massachusetts. In 1869, a day school for the deaf was established in Boston that emphasized use of the visual channel in teaching the deaf.

Through the years more schools developed throughout the United States. Today, there are 63 public residential schools for the deaf, and 12 private residential schools (American Annals of the Deaf, 1974).

There are approximately 65 public day schools throughout the country serving deaf children. There are 22 private day schools and 61 private day classes.

Special Programs in Schools

Rather than depending solely upon the residential and day schools to carry the burden for educating deaf children, a new pattern has developed which utilizes existing school systems. In the United States there are approximately 525 special programs for hearing-handicapped children that are integrated with regular classroom work. This is truly an important innovative approach and places the child within the mainstream of events along with all other children in the community. It offers the services of the multidisciplinary team that serves the normal school population and calls for a cooperative, understanding working relationship between the special educator and the regular classroom teacher.

A splendid treatment of the topic of integration of the hearing-handicapped child in the regular classroom is presented by Northcott (1973). This multiauthored book focuses upon improvement of the delivery of education and related services to hearing-handicapped children. It answers through its multiple authorship many questions regarding characteristics of hearing-impaired children who make successful adjustment in regular classes, age at which integration should be made, guidelines for initiating and maintaining integration, predictors of success, relevance of special support personnel, etc.

According to the latest statistics of the U. S. Office of Education (Annual Survey of Hearing Impaired Children and Youth, United States: 1973), there are 3 in every 4,000 children aged 5–19 years in the United States who are deaf (91 dB ISO hearing loss or greater in the better ear) and 1 in every 200 who are hard of hearing. These figures might suggest, at first glance, that probably most of the education of those with less severe handicaps would take place in regular schools. This is not so, for the survey figures of 1973 show that, of the 41,109 hearing-impaired (deaf and hard of hearing) students in the United States, 10.6% were being educated in integrated settings. By far the majority were being educated in residential schools for the deaf (45.5%). Those in day schools for the deaf were 7.2%, or in self-contained classes for hearing impaired, 30.8%.

Special Programs in Clinics

The advent of audiological clinics in the United States came about somewhat later. They have experienced their greatest growth over the past 25 years. Clinics are most frequently located in university or college training settings, in hospitals, in community-sponsored centers, and in schools. Some, however, are also located in private practice settings.

The latest figures show that there are presently 551 clinics in the U.S.A. providing audiological services. Of these, 450 have interim accreditation and 101 have regular accreditation by the Professional Services Board of the American Board of Examiners in Speech Pathology and Audiology. There are approximately 50 clinics that have been accredited by the Commission on Accrediting of Rehabilitation Facilities.

At present, there are approximately 2,500 audiologists who hold the Certificate of Clinical Competence in Audiology awarded by the American Speech and Hearing Association. This certificate signifies successful completion of prescribed amounts of coursework and clinical practicum as well as the successful completion of a supervised Clinical Fellowship Year after attaining a master's degree in addition to passing a national board examination. Holders of the Certificate of Clinical Competence in Audiology are able to work independently as practicing audiologists.

GENERAL DESCRIPTION OF PRESENT PROGRAMS OF AURAL HABILITATION AND REHABILITATION

Professional Involvement in Aural Habilitation and Rehabilitation Programs

Services to hearing-impaired children and adults are delivered by an assortment of professionally trained individuals in the U.S.A., whose training qualifies them to deliver specific services not rendered by others. In some cases, their areas of expertise overlap, which sometimes results in friction between professions and confusion for the hearing impaired, but if these individuals work together as a team, maximum services in identification, diagnosis, medical treatment, rehabilitation, and education can be delivered.

Some or all of the following professionals may be involved in the delivery of services to the hearing impaired: audiologists; teachers of the hearing impaired; speech and language pathologists; psychologists; various specialties of medicine including otologists, neurologists, and pediatricians. This list is not intended to be all inclusive with respect to medical or nonmedical professionals. It is not unusual for other medical specialists, including nurses, to be involved in the identification, referral, and counseling of hearing-impaired individuals or their families, and for nonmedical specialists such as social workers, regular classroom teachers, or special education teachers to be involved in rendering services. Hearing aid dealers, while usually not professionally trained at the present time, are also involved in the delivery of products and/or services.

The professionals most closely involved in the delivery of aural habilitation and rehabilitation services are audiologists, otologists, teachers of the hearing impaired, and speech and language pathologists. The audiologist is an individual who holds the Certificate of Clinical Competence in Audiology from the American Speech and Hearing Association. The audiologist is a nonmedical specialist who is highly trained in the function of the normal ear, the identification and measurement of hearing loss, and the habilitation or rehabilitation of those with hearing impairments. Teachers of the hearing impaired hold undergraduate or graduate degrees in elementary or secondary education with academic background and practice teaching experience that familiarize them with the communication problems of the hearing impaired, methods of teaching subject matter, and methods of developing receptive and expressive communication. There are approximately 10,400 teachers of the hearing impaired and administrators of programs for the hearing impaired in the United States of which 3,465 are certified by the Council on Education of the Deaf (CED) or the Conference of Executives of American Schools for the Deaf (CEASD) (Craig and Craig, 1974). The speech pathologist holds a graduate degree in speech pathology and the Certificate of Clinical Competence in Speech Pathology from the American Speech and Hearing Association. There are approximately 12,400 speech pathologists in the United States (American Speech and Hearing Association, 1975). Otologists are physicians who have completed the necessary medical residency in otology, although usually the residency is in otorhinolaryngology. In addition, these medical specialists have met the requirements and have, or are eligible for, Board Certification by the American Academy of Ophthalmology and Otolaryngology.

Delivery of Aural Habilitation and Rehabilitation Services

The services necessary for the identification, diagnosis, and treatment of hearing problems are delivered in a variety of organizational settings. Hearing testing, medical attention, habilitative-rehabilitative services, and educational programs may be obtained through community agencies, university clinics, hospitals, public schools, residential schools, or from private practitioners. While some communities in the United States may provide services through all of the organizational structures mentioned, many communities have limited services available. However, except in the less populated or remote areas of the country, the services of relevant professionals are readily accessible.

Since the end of World War II, the number of professionals and facilities offering services has increased tremendously. While many programs for the hearing impaired are available, one of the problems at present is educating the public about the availability of these services and the appropriate points of entry. While agencies of federal and state governments and professional organizations have attempted to remedy the situation through a variety of publicity programs, there is need for systematic, coordinated public education.

Professional organizations maintain lists of facilities offering services to the hearing impaired. These lists are published and are available in most public libraries. The American Speech and Hearing Association, for example, publishes a directory of clinical facilities (American Speech and Hearing Association, 1973) showing the type of services offered by these facilities. In addition, professional societies or associations provide lists of qualified practitioners meeting certification standards of their respective professions.

Community Speech and Hearing Centers

Many cities with a population exceeding 50,000 support a center providing diagnostic, habilitative-rehabilitative, and social services for those with communication impairments. In many cases these centers evolved out of hearing societies that were formed around the turn of the century for purposes of providing social and emotional support for the hearing impaired. Lipreading classes were also popular in the hearing society program, largely because of the attention focused on this area by Nitchie, Bruhn, and the Kinzie sisters. Present day community centers frequently receive considerable financial support from the Community Chest or United Fund. The additional money necessary to operate these centers is derived from direct contributions, endowments, and fees for service. Because these are community-funded centers, they provide services to all communicatively impaired people of the locality, irrespective of age, condition, or ability to pay. Fees for services in these nonprofit centers are usually based upon ability to pay. The modern center is often staffed by appropriate professionals from diverse disciplines. The director of the center is responsible to a board of directors that is made up of community leaders.

College or University Clinics

Colleges and universities that have academic and training programs in audiology and speech pathology offer diagnostic and habilitative-rehabilitative services through clinical facilities operated as an adjunct to their training programs. The services of these clinics are rendered by undergraduate or graduate students under the direct supervision of clinical supervisors or faculty members. These university training programs may be found in a variety of administrative organizational structures, either as subdivisions of a larger department or as separate departments of audiology and speech pathology.

Hospitals

An increased number of hospitals offers diagnostic and habilitative-rehabilitative audiology services. If the full range of audiology services is not available in a specific hospital, it is usually diagnostic audiological services that are offered as an adjunct to medical diagnosis of auditory disorders. An audiology clinic performing these services, however, serves as a very important referral agency to other community programs offering habilitation-rehabilitation services. Although statistics are not available, most hospital audiology programs offer rehabilitative as well as diagnostic services. While the first clinical audiology programs appeared in the large metropolitan hospitals associated with medical schools, there has been an increasing number developed in other types of hospitals, even in relatively small communities. Audiological services have been available in many Veterans Administration Hospitals since World War II. At the present time, complete audiological programs, including evaluation services, compensation claims, hearing aid evaluations, and dispensing of hearing aids including all associated services, are available in 37 V.A. hospitals and three contract clinics (Veterans Administration, 1974) located around the United States serving the needs of veterans living in those regions. In addition, audiological services are available to individuals presently in the military service. The Army and Air Force, in particular, provide audiological services through military medical facilities (Northern, 1968). Several state hospitals and training centers for the mentally retarded offer a full range of audiological services.

Public Schools

Aural habilitation-rehabilitation services have been available in many public schools for school-age children. The variety and quality of these services have varied considerably depending upon the availability of qualified people and the existence of outside clinical facilities offering these services. Unfortunately, at the present time, there are very few audiologists employed in the public schools and, in those cases where there are audiologists, the services offered are usually limited to screening evaluation and obtaining amplification. While these are important components of a habilitation-rehabilitation program, there is need for audiologists to assume greater responsibility in monitoring the adequacy and use of individual hearing aids and auditory training units, in counseling children and parents and advising teachers, and in participating directly in the development of receptive and expressive communication. Typically the services beyond testing hearing and recommending hearing aids are delivered by teachers of the hearing impaired and also speech pathologists. Because the primary focus of the teachers of the hearing impaired is to develop language and speech and teach academic subjects to the hearing impaired, there is usually little time for them to deliver comprehensive habilitation-rehabilitation services. The group of children receiving the least attention in the public schools are those with mild, moderate, and perhaps severe hearing impairment who have sufficient language and speech development to preclude their placement in the typical classroom for the deaf. Few schools have classes for the hard of hearing, so these children are likely to be found in regular classes with normal hearing children or in classes for the slow learner, retarded, etc. They are likely to receive no special attention from relevant professionals beyond periodic hearing tests and articulation therapy by a speech pathologist. Evidence would seem to indicate the need for habilitative-rehabilitative programs to help these children achieve full potential. There is great need for improvement of all habilitative-rehabilitative audiological services in the public schools. Whether or not this will be accomplished will be determined, in part, by the ability of public schools to afford these services and will depend upon audiology training programs producing rehabilitation-oriented audiologists (perhaps called educational audiologists) or by modifying the training of teachers of the hearing impaired and speech pathologists. Many states have enacted mandatory special education legislation which requires public schools to make available evaluative, placement, and training programs for those children who require "special" educational services. In Michigan this legislation affects people from birth to 25 years of age. It is hoped that, through this type of legislation, habilitative-rehabilitative audiological services might be made available to all hearing-impaired children in the public school setting.

Residential Schools

As stated previously, there are approximately 75 residential schools for hearing-impaired children in the United States (Craig and Craig, 1974). Residential schools may be state or public institutions funded by tax money or private schools funded by tuition and endowment. Approximately 80% of these schools are public. Many of the private residential schools for the deaf are associated with religious organizations. Most residential schools offer audiological services delivered by an American Speech and Hearing Association (ASHA) certified audiologist. In most cases, however, these audiology services fall short of the ideal in terms of aural rehabilitation. Mention should be made of Gallaudet College and the National Technical Institute for the Deaf. These two schools are the only degree-granting institutions of higher learning specifically for the deaf. Gallaudet College is located in Washington, D.C. and National Technical Institute for the Deaf is located in Rochester, New York. Both are funded by the United States Congress. They both have fully equipped hearing clinics and a staff of audiologists engaged in delivering diagnostic and habilitative-rehabilitative services and active research programs.

Private Practice

Reliable statistics on the number of audiologists engaged in private practice are not available, but it is believed that very few, if any, audiologists are engaged in private practice in the "pure" sense. In general, the audiologist in private practice is usually associated with an otologist or otological group. He may be an employee or hold some form of partnership in the organization. It would appear that the number of audiologists working in this type of setting has increased substantially over the past few years, and eventually all otologists, and perhaps pediatricians, may have audiological services available within their offices. In the metropolitan Detroit area there are approximately 10 audiologists in this type of practice, most of whom hold a Ph.D. degree. The aural habilitation-rehabilitation services are generally limited to the evaluation and recommendation of hearing aids. Unfortunately, most otologists in the United States do not employ the services of an audiologist to perform diagnostic and pre- and post-treatment testing or hearing aid evaluations. They either perform the diagnostic testing themselves, have a nurse, receptionist, or technician do it under their supervision, or refer the patient to an audiology center. While it is preferable for patients with residual hearing loss to be referred to audiology centers for habilitative-rehabilitative services, many do not receive appropriate counseling and are referred directly to the hearing aid dealer.

Types of Services Available for Children and Adults

The specific services offered by an audiologist may vary according to the clinical setting in which he is employed. That is, his services may be restricted to certain segments of the population; for example, an audiologist working in a public school will be concerned with the problems of hearing-handicapped children whereas the audiologist working in the Veterans Administration Hospital will see a preponderance of adult males. In addition, the number of services the audiologist offers may also be restricted by his employment setting. The purpose here is to give a panoramic view of the services the audiologist may provide in a center offering a comprehensive audiological program to all segments of the community.

Identification The audiologist may be involved directly, or indirectly through supervision of audiometric technicians, in the screening of segments of the population for identification of those with hearing impairment.

Diagnosis He will provide assistance to the physician in the diagnosis of hearing disorders by providing necessary audiological data and careful interpretation of case history information and test results.

Assessment of Communication Impairment The audiologist may be involved in complete assessment of the receptive and expressive impairment for purposes of educational, vocational, and habilitation-rehabilitation planning.

Hearing Aids The audiologist may be involved in the evaluation and recommendation of hearing aids for both children and adults. If involved in these activities, the audiologist should have instrumentation necessary for electroacoustic measurement of hearing aid performance and this testing should be an integral part of the hearing aid activities including periodic checking of the hearing aid following purchase. In many settings, the audiologist is directly involved in the dispensing of third-party-purchased hearing aids. A recent interpretation of the Code of Ethics of the American Speech and Hearing Association (Subcommittee on Hearing Aids, 1974) would allow audiologists to be involved in the direct dispensing of hearing aids to the hearing impaired providing the hearing aid was delivered at manufacturer's cost. The audiologist may also make impressions of the ear for the purpose of fabricating an earmold. The audiologist's involvement with hearing aids would not be complete without some type of program in hearing aid orientation. This might consist minimally of pre- and postfitting counseling, but many facilities offer more extensive orientation services.

Educational Services The audiologist may be involved in the planning of an educational program for a child, evaluating the effects of specific educational programs, or participating directly in the educational management of the child. Many hearing clinics provide speech and language development and educational programs for the preschool child, if not for older children. The audiologist working the school setting may be very much involved in the educational planning and management of hearing-impaired children.

Habilitation and Rehabilitation The audiologist may be involved in rendering additional services to the hearing impaired. These activities might include individual as well as group sessions to improve lipreading skills, to provide auditory training for improving auditory and listening performance or to conserve or improve speech, and to provide emotional support for adjustment.

Vocational The audiologist may assist the hearing-impaired person in vocational planning or aid in the resolution of vocational problems. Usually this aspect of rehabilitation would be done in cooperation with counselors of the state vocational rehabilitation service.

Counseling Counseling of various types is a very important part of the audiologist's role in the habilitation-rehabilitation of the hearing impaired. Interpretation of test results, counseling of parents of the hearing-impaired child, counseling children of geriatric patients, and counseling as to the benefits and limitations of amplification are integral parts of the audiologist's responsibility.

Financing Programs and Payment for Services

The aural habilitation-rehabilitation services provided by audiologists in hearing centers are financed in several ways. Funds are sometimes derived through organized community charity, such as United Fund campaigns; fee for service; third party payment through allocated federal and state taxes or private insurance companies; contributions from local charitable groups; gifts and donations; and subsidizing activities through other more profitable aspects of the program. Hearing centers or clinics associated with university training programs in audiology also receive support through the educational budget and through research, training, or service grants awarded by governments or philanthropic organizations. In addition, students sometimes receive financial support through scholarships, assistantships, or traineeships.

Programs in Veterans Administration Hospitals, military hospitals, and state institutions including public schools are funded entirely by federal, state, or local tax revenues, and the services offered by these programs are available at no cost to those individuals eligible under appropriate legal or administrative rules.

Federal and state funds are also available to purchase aural habilitation-rehabilitation services for many children, employable or underemployed adults, and for many people at any age who are on welfare. Each state has some mechanism for determining eligibility of individuals to receive necessary services under these programs. The funds and services for children have their origin in the Social Security Act of 1936. Michigan has had a federally funded program for hearing-impaired children since 1942. The program is administered by the Hearing and Speech Section and

Division of Services to Crippled Children of the Department of Public Health. Funds for working age adults are available through state vocational rehabilitation programs, which originated principally as a result of Public Law 236 passed by Congress in 1930 (Obermann, 1965). The services to individuals on welfare are available through local welfare agencies or through the Medicaid program. Medicaid is the public assistance medical care program under Title 19 of the Social Security Act of 1965, and is a series of separate state welfare programs funded jointly by federal and state tax revenues (Somers, 1971).

In Michigan all three of these programs require otological and audiological services if available, while it is required for crippled children. In addition, all three programs will pay for reasonable rehabilitation services beyond the evaluation and recommendation of hearing aids. Audiological involvement in hearing aid recommendations is not universally required in all parts of the country. Legislative attempts have been made recently to have hearing aids made available to recipients of Social Security funds, but to date this has not been accomplished. This means, at the present time, aural habilitation-rehabilitation services, including hearing aids, are unavailable to retired individuals under any third-party-payment system, unless the person qualifies for assistance under Medicaid, or Workmen's Compensation laws or industrial insurance benefits if the hearing loss is work related. Diagnostic services performed by audiologists may be paid for by health insurance companies if ordered by physicians to aid them in the diagnostic process, or in cases of litigation, although most services generally offered by audiologists are not reimbursed by the private insurance industry. It is possible that most, if not all, audiological services including aural habilitation-rehabilitation may be paid for by the private health industry when audiology achieves the status of a licensed profession (Brantman, 1973).

Methods of Obtaining Services

Mass hearing screening programs are generally not available on a statewide or national basis for purposes of identifying individuals of any age who have a hearing impairment. A notable exception to this statement would be the hearing screening programs that exist in the public schools, although these efforts are largely concentrated at the lower elementary level. With the passage of the Occupational Safety and Health Act of 1970 and the resultant development of hearing conservation programs in industry, it would appear that an effective detection program would eventually be available to all employees covered by the act. However, at the present time, such hearing screening and monitoring are not mandatory. Recent legislation requiring early and periodic screening, diagnosis, and treatment programs (EPSDTP), which required states to set up health programs for people on welfare, will eventually provide a means for the early detection of hearing disorders among people eligible for the Medicaid program.

Aside from these emerging screening programs on a nationwide basis, the availability of screening and referral agencies varies considerably from locality to locality. A small number of audiologists is involved in neonatal hearing testing programs that exist in some hospitals. Many community hearing centers offer hearing screening services either in their own facilities or through mobile testing units. In Michigan there is a statewide hearing and speech agency (Michigan Association for Better Hearing and Speech) funded, in part, by United Fund contributions. This agency maintains a mobile unit service program for the less populated areas of the state that do not have the availability of hearing testing and aural habilitation-rehabilitation services. The program consists of hearing screening, public education, diagnostic testing, industrial services, and hearing aid evaluations and recommendations. In addition, the program helps organize otological clinics for those individuals identified as having hearing impairments. Some other states may have programs similar to this; however, it by no means could be said that these services are available in the rural areas in all parts of the country.

The previously mentioned hearing screening programs provide one means of directing the hearing impaired to the services of audiologists and otologists. Another common means of obtaining services is through direct referral from other medical specialists, nurses, teachers, rehabilitation counselors, etc. Some clinics, particularly those in hospitals, may accept patients only on the basis of physician referral. Many other facilities, however, provide services to all individuals who express concern about their hearing. Significant numbers of hearing-impaired people learn of these community resources by word of mouth. The availability of aural habilitation-rehabilitation services in a community can usually be ascertained by contacting a physician, the local health department, or the local school system.

There certainly is need for better public education related to the availability of audiological services. In addition, there is also need for increased awareness by physicians and other professionals of aural habilitation-rehabilitation services and the benefits to be derived by the hearing impaired.

Accreditation of Clinical Services and Training Programs in Audiology

The American Boards of Examiners in Speech Pathology and Audiology (ABESPA) was established in 1959 by the American Speech and Hearing Association. At the present time there are three boards accrediting individuals and programs in speech pathology and audiology. The Educational Training Board (ETB) accredits academic programs providing a master's degree in speech pathology or audiology. There are 53 accredited training programs in audiology located in 28 of the 50 states including the District of Columbia (American Boards of Examiners in Speech Pathology and Audiology, 1975). There were a total of 94 programs certified either in speech pathology or audiology. There are many more unaccredited programs in existence and it should be kept in mind that there is no ABESPA accreditation of Ph.D. programs. The Professional Services Board (PSB) accredits clinical programs in speech pathology or audiology. It was established for the purpose of formulating standards and examining and issuing certificates to those clinical programs meeting the minimal criteria.

DIAGNOSTIC PROCEDURE

Diagnostic audiological procedures are obviously important because of the implications of cause, amount, site of malfunction, and auditory discrimination performance for the habilitative-rehabilitative program and prognosis. If the audiologist is to assume a central role in the habilitation-rehabilitation of hearing impairment, he must be willing to assume the responsibility for obtaining the necessary audiological, otological, and other pertinent data necessary in order to assure himself and the patient that the most appropriate steps to resolve the problem are taken. Whether the audiologist assumes this central position in the management of the patient, or whether the physician does, is perhaps academic; however, it is imperative that the audiologist have this information before him as he plans a habilitative-rehabilitative program. It is, therefore, important for the audiologist to be familiar with a wide range of audiological tests and their interpretation.

It is difficult to give a precise description of how audiological diagnostic services are delivered because of variations in the organizational structure of hearing centers. As we have seen, these centers may or may not be integral parts of a medical complex and the patient load may be restricted to either children or adults. In any given setting, the various audiological tests might be administered by audiologists, otologists, technicians, or some combination of these specialists. All diagnostic procedures might be accomplished in one facility while some might require outside referral. In any case, the most acceptable situation in terms of the utilization of professional expertise will be presented, wherein audiological tests and communication evaluations are administered and interpreted by individuals certified in audiology by the American Speech and Hearing Association and physical, chemical, and x-ray exams, etc., are performed or ordered by the physician. The final diagnosis and medical or surgical treatment would be determined and performed by appropriate medical specialists.

The otological examination may precede audiological testing, the reverse might be true, or the audiologist and otologist may interact throughout the examinations. There may be some areas of overlap; for example, both the otologist and the audiologist may obtain case history information. No matter what the medical-audiological interaction might be, the following aspects of audiological management of diagnostic procedures are involved, keeping in mind that, at this point in the habilitative-rehabilitative process, an accurate description of the hearing mechanism and its function leading to accurate diagnosis is the goal.

Hearing Test Environment, Equipment, and Calibration

Certification of an individual as an audiologist assumes knowledge of the importance of performing hearing tests in a suitable acoustic environment, that adequate equipment for performing the tests is available, that the audiologist is familiar with the function of this equipment, and that the audiologist has made certain that his instrumentation is in proper calibration. In addition, the Professional Services Board (of the American Boards of Examiners in Speech Pathology and Audiology) certification of clinical programs implies that the facility has appropriate acoustic environments, equipment, and calibration routines that insure the highest standards of accuracy consistent with the scope of the hearing center. All hearing clinics in the U.S.A. should have test rooms that meet current standards for conducting threshold tests (American National Standards Institute, S3.1-1960). Many of these are dual room arrangements, wherein the audiologist and all audiometric equipment are located in one room and the subject and appropriate transducers are in the other room. It is not deemed necessary to place the audiometric instrumentation in a sound room if "live voice" testing is not done or if the ambient noise is not sufficient to cause variations in test results obtained via microphone.

A hearing center will have the necessary instrumentation to perform a battery of pure tone and speech audiometric tests with necessary masking where indicated and will be capable of delivering these signals to the patient by way of earphones or loud speakers. This is most commonly accomplished through a clinical audiometer which consists of numerous input sources, such as pure tone oscillators, noise generators, microphone, tape recorder, and phonograph. The output of the audiometer can be channeled to earphones, bone oscillators, soundfield speakers, or some combination of these. This type of clinical audiometer is usually a two-channel system which gives the instrument the flexibility necessary for the more complex pure tone and speech tests. In addition, the hearing center will typically have a Bekesy type audiometer which may be a separate instrument or a component of the clinical audiometer. The greatest flexibility in Bekesy type audiometers for clinical and research purposes is obtained with a separate self-contained unit which is capable of discrete or continuous frequency presentation and is equipped with continuously variable narrow-band masking. The well equipped clinic will also have the necessary instrumentation for impedance testing and tympanometry. Hearing centers may have the capability of performing "brief tone" audiometry, evoked response audiometry, and the necessary instrumentation for electronystagmography, although this would probably be the exception rather than the rule. Some hearing centers specialize in testing difficult-to-manage children through positive reinforcement to auditory stimuli. Most hearing centers will have one or more portable audiometers that can be utilized for pure tone air conduction and bone conduction testing. These audiometers are frequently used with difficult-to-test patients where it is necessary for the audiologist to be in the same room with the patient to control behavior or where modified procedures, such as play audiometry, have to be used to elicit valid responses.

Although it is not at the moment required by the American Speech and Hearing Association (1975) in its Minimum Requirements for Hearing Programs Offering Guidance in Selection of Hearing Aids, we feel that all centers that engage in hearing aid activities should be equipped with the necessary instrumentation for electroacoustic evaluation of hearing aid performance. Within the past year there have been significant developments in the design and manufacture of suitable instrumentation for these purposes at reasonable prices. All centers have some plan for periodic calibration of the instrumentation used in hearing or hearing aid testing.

While all centers might not have an oscilloscope, VTVM, spectrometer, graphic level recorder, or an electronic counter necessary for complete calibration, they should have a sound level meter with appropriate filters and a 6-cc coupler necessary for checking the intensity and linearity of pure tone, speech, and noise circuits. Not all aspects of audiometer or ancillary equipment performance have been specified by American or international organizations concerned with standards.

Interview and Case History

Normally the first step in the diagnostic procedure is to obtain case history information through an interview with the patient or with some authority figure responsible for the patient. The skillful interviewer can obtain information very helpful in the diagnostic process. The information obtained leads to the development of one or more hypotheses concerning type, amount, and causation and, thus, aids the audiologist in determining the necessary auditory and communication tests needed to describe the problem adequately and to provide appropriate diagnostic data. Interviews are conducted utilizing an informal conversational approach, an authoritarian approach, or some combination of the two (Rosenberg, 1972). When interviewing adults and perhaps children with adventitious hearing loss, the interviewer will try to obtain information within the following categories.

Reason for Appointment Whether the patient has been referred by a physician or initiated the appointment himself, it is important to determine from the patient's point of view the reason for the appointment.

Hearing Loss History Information on the onset and duration of the hearing loss, family incidence, presence of tinnitus and vertigo, previous otological exams, and medical and surgical treatment is obtained.

General Medical History Any previous or present health conditions, including medications taken, are noted.

Receptive and Expressive Communication Problems The amount of difficulty of communicating in the interview situation is noted. In addition, questions are asked to determine the amount of difficulty hearing and understanding speech in a variety of settings. The skillful interviewer will also obtain some impression of lipreading ability. Any noticeable speech or language problems are also noted.

Educational Status In the case of school age children or young adults, information on school progress and adjustment is obtained.

Employment Status In the case of working age adults, information regarding the work history is obtained since it may be of primary or secondary importance in determining etiology or may be of significant concern to the patient because of communication demands. Communication requirements of employment may be a significant factor of concern in the satisfactory rehabilitation of the individual.

Previous Nonmedical Treatment Information concerning previous hearing tests, use of hearing aids, and therapy is noted.

In the case of diagnostic testing of young children, or in the planning of a habilitation program for the prelingual deaf child, it is important that a more detailed case history be obtained. Detailed case history forms, such as those presented by Myklebust (1954) or Katz and Struckman (1972), are useful.

Since interviewing, case history taking, and counseling are essential in the diagnostic and habilitative-rehabilitative process, it is important that the audiologist and physician give considerable attention to the development of these skills (Garrett, 1942; Enelow and Swisher, 1972).

Pure Tone Hearing Tests

Hearing tests employing pure tones as stimuli may be divided into two categories labeled "routine" and "special." This classification of tests infers something of their frequency of use as well as the fact that they may provide additional information as to the site of malfunction in the auditory system. The administration and interpretation of these tests will not be discussed here since they are more than adequately covered in other texts or papers. The intent here is merely to discuss current diagnostic procedures employed by audiologists in the practice of their profession in the United States.

The most commonly employed "routine" test of hearing is the pure tone threshold. Air and bone conduction thresholds are obtained with masking when indicated through the frequency range from 125–8,000 Hz. While threshold finding procedures have not been standardized, it is safe to say that the "ascending" or "modified Hugheson-Westlake" (Carhart and Jerger, 1959) is the most commonly accepted threshold finding procedure, that the "plateau" method outlined by Hood (1960) perhaps in conjunction with the initial use of "effective masking levels" (Sanders, 1972) is employed when masking is necessary, and that the symbols used on the pure tone audiogram are those recommended by the ASHA Committee on Audiometric Evaluation (1974). These symbols are presented in Table 1. The pure tone air and bone conduction audiogram gives basic information as to the amount of hearing loss present in the peripheral auditory mechanism. Peripheral mechanism is here defined as that portion of the auditory system from the external auditory meatus through the conductive and sensory mechanism to, and including, the

Table 1. Recommended symbols for pure tone threshold audiometry[a]

Test	Right ear	Left ear	Both
Air conduction–earphones			
Unmasked			
Masked			
Bone conduction–masked			
Unmasked			
Masked			
Bone conduction–forehead			
Unmasked			
Masked			
Air conduction–sound field			

[a]The same symbols may be used for other stimuli if so noted on audiogram. "No response" is indicated by placing appropriate symbol at maximum decibel limit of audiometer and drawing an arrow downward from the lower outside corner of the symbol.

integrity of the hair cells along the basilar membrane. Thus, information is obtained regarding the amount of hearing loss and the extent to which the sensory mechanism of the cochlea is involved.

Another test that is becoming increasingly routine is tympanometry and the measurement of the middle ear muscle reflex through measurements of acoustic impedance at the ear drum. While these tests have not replaced traditional pure tone audiometry, they do offer certain advantages in obtaining diagnostic information from difficult-to-test patients, about the presence and nature of middle ear conditions, and some information as to the integrity of the auditory system contained within the stapedius muscle's reflex arc. It is anticipated that all hearing clinics, otologists' offices, and perhaps pediatricians' offices will eventually have the capability of impedance measuring instrumentation.

Pure tone tests that are referred to as "special" tests would include Bekesy audiometry, Stenger, Short Increment Sensitivity Index (SISI), Alternate Binaural Loudness Balance (ABLB) test, Monaural Loudness Balance test, tests of threshold tone decay, brief tone audiometry, and evoked response audiometry. These tests are referred to as "special" tests because they are not necessarily part of the routine analysis of hearing function. One or more of them may be utilized to supplement pure tone audiometric results, but they do not enjoy the status of routine tests because some of them can only be given under certain hearing loss circumstances, some of them are difficult and time-consuming tasks for patients, or because they are best used as parts of a battery and cannot be meaningfully interpreted independently. Hearing clinics have the instrumentation and audiological expertise to administer and interpret all or most of these tests. The availability of brief tone and evoked response audiometry is not as widespread because of the amount and cost of instrumentation and the incomplete evidence of their importance in routine testing or their significant contribution to differential diagnosis.

Since conventional pure tone testing requires a certain degree of maturity, ability to attend to a difficult and inherently meaningless task, and requires the full cooperation of the subject, special modifications of test procedures or other forms of testing are necessary with infants, young children, the immature, or the retarded individual. A variety of "play audiometry" procedures, which consist of modifications of conventional test procedures to ensure the interest and cooperation of children, have been developed. There has been significant work done in the development of operant conditioning audiometry utilizing tangible reinforcers for purpose of eliciting responses from difficult-to-test subjects (Fulton and Lloyd, 1969). Procedures for evaluating the hearing of neonates and the very young child are presented by Northern and Downs (1974). Through the use of careful case history taking, observation of subject behavior, and the application of conventional pure tone tests or variations of them, it is possible for the clinical audiologist to obtain valid and reliable measures of the amount and type of hearing loss. In addition, through the use of selected special tests, the audiologist may be able to provide further information on the function of the peripheral auditory mechanism. It should be pointed out that many of the special tests, excluding tympanometry and evoked response audiometry, are not utilized with the very young or the difficult-to-test child.

Speech Audiometry

Audiometric tests using speech as the stimulus are an important part of diagnostic audiology. While playing a significant role in determining the validity of the pure tone threshold, a complex stimulus such as speech presents a whole set of problems that compromises its precision as a diagnostic tool. Nevertheless, speech is commonly used for threshold determination, suprathreshold discrimination testing, including discrimination under varying amounts of redundancy, and can be used to determine the size of functional auditory vocabulary.

Usually the first speech audiometric test administered is the speech reception threshold (SRT). This threshold is obtained for each ear separately under earphones and in the soundfield. The most commonly used materials are the CID W-1 list of spondee words (Hirsh et al., 1952). The administration of this test is not as standardized as perhaps it should be in that different speakers may be used from clinic to clinic and even within clinics and the threshold finding procedure may vary. This testing may be done utilizing live voice, phonograph records, reel to reel tapes, or cassette cartridges. Research has indicated the importance of familiarizing the subject with an alphabetical list of the words to be used in order that measurement error might be minimized (Tillman and Jerger, 1959). In addition to its value in determining the validity of the pure tone threshold, it is a very useful procedure for those difficult-to-test children or adults as a preliminary test to determine the presence of a hearing loss or to determine whether a suspected hearing loss is sufficient to interfere with normal communication. Except in these cases, the speech reception threshold may be of little diagnostic value.

Testing of suprathreshold discrimination is most commonly accomplished through the use of phonetically balanced lists of monosyllabic words. There are many problems in the use of speech units for discrimination testing that have not been satisfactorily resolved and, therefore, there is a plethora of monosyllabic word lists, sentence lists, test formats, and recommended sensation levels for presentation. Part of the problem arises from the fact that discrimination tests are used for at least two purposes that may be somewhat independent of one another. For example, they are used in the diagnostic process to aid the differential diagnosis of auditory disorders, while at the same time they are used to estimate impairment, to predict handicap, and to evaluate rehabilitation. Clinical experience would seem to indicate that there is no single set of materials and administrative procedures that can be utilized to serve both purposes. There is lack of standardization relative to materials used, presentation level, response format, or whether a full 50 word list or half list is used. The most commonly used materials for discrimination testing are the CID W-22 word lists (Hirsh et al., 1952). Probably the most popular closed response set test is the Modified Rhyme Test (House et al., 1965). The suprathreshold discrimination test is usually administered monaurally under earphones at sensation levels between 26 and 40 dB or at a most comfortable loudness level (MCL). In addition, a soundfield discrimination score may be obtained to determine whether a binaural effect is present, and many audiologists also obtain a discrimination score for materials presented at a normal conversational loudness. Discrimination scores: (1) are a very important method of describing the function of the auditory system, (2) may be of critical importance in differential diagnosis especially in cases involving VIIIth nerve lesions, (3) are useful to the physician to help him determine the suitability of surgery and to help him evaluate the success of his treatments, (4) are useful in medicolegal situations, and, (5) finally, provide some indication of the need for nonmedical rehabilitation services.

A considerable amount of research attention has been directed toward the use of speech materials as a means of detecting and differentiating lesions in the central auditory system. The audiological evaluation of patients with suspected lesions between the cochlear nucleus and the temporal lobe consists of using speech in which redundancy has been decreased in one of several ways. This has been accomplished by presenting the stimuli at low sensation levels, through low pass filtering, by accelerating the presentation, by periodic interruption of the message, by simultaneous dichotic messages, and by presenting the primary speech message against some competing message (Calearo and Lazzaroni, 1957; Matzker, 1959; Quiros, 1964; Brunt, 1974; Hodgson, 1974). While much work remains to be done related to the differential diagnosis of brain stem and cortical lesions and the refinement of tests for these purposes, the use of speech audiometry in the hands of a skillful audiologist may be of considerable importance in medical diagnosis and treatment. It should be pointed out that, at this time, standardized tests for these purposes are not available and, furthermore, not all hearing clinics would have the necessary instrumentation for producing or administering them.

Use of speech audiometry with children presents some problems in addition to those related to establishing rapport and securing cooperation for the length of time required. Such factors as the level of language development, maturity, and the ability of the youngster to repeat words intelligibly, in addition to the effects that amount and duration of hearing impairment have on speech handling capacity, have led to modifications of test materials and procedures. Estimates of speech reception threshold may be obtained by employing selected spondaic words, using picture or object identification materials or, if need be, using words, questions, and directions chosen from the child's receptive vocabulary. Suprathreshold discrimination testing may be accomplished using the same materials as used with adults or the kindergarten lists (PBK) developed by Haskins (1949). These monosyllabic word lists can be used only if the child has sufficient language and intelligible speech to provide meaningful responses; otherwise, picture discrimination tests using multiple choice picture formats developed by Myatt and Landes (1963) and by Siegenthaler and Haspiel (1966) may be employed.

Coordination of Otological and Audiological Test Results

The results of audiological testing and their interpretation are provided to the physician so that he might combine them with other information he has collected for purposes of making a diagnosis and determining the need for medical and surgical treatment. Following the completion of medical services, the hearing-impaired person should be re-evaluated by appropriate audiological procedures to determine the amount of improvement in hearing, the amount of residual hearing loss, and the need for nonmedical rehabilitation procedures. In those cases where medical or surgical treatment is not indicated, or where the patient chooses not to elect those treatments, the otologist ideally would refer the person to a hearing clinic for aural habilitation-rehabilitation services. In all honesty, it must be said that in many cases this ideal situation does not exist and the hearing-impaired person is referred to or in some way finds himself in the hearing aid dealer's office.

REHABILITATIVE PROCEDURES

It is difficult to define precisely when the habilitative-rehabilitative program begins. If the diagnostic procedures are performed by a rehabilitation-oriented audiologist, the program will begin to take shape in his mind as the hearing loss is described by the history and hearing test results. If this is the situation and the audiologist develops good rapport with the patient and his family, the habilitation-rehabilitation program outlined will be more readily accepted and completed. If the audiologist is not rehabilitation oriented and is primarily concerned with the diagnostic aspects of clinical practice, there is the great possibility that the patient may not be given appropriate counseling about the services he needs and their availability in the community. Even referral to another agency often leads to a breakdown in the delivery of needed services because of the discontinuity of professional contact, in addition to various other logistical problems that visiting other facilities might present. Obviously, any audiology program that has the best interest of the hearing impaired as its primary concern would provide all diagnostic and habilitative-rehabilitative services in the same facility, if not by the same person. Many hearing clinics in the United States offer comprehensive habilitative-rehabilitative programs as well as diagnostic testing, but there are not enough audiologists with the necessary commitment to say that they are among the outstanding services they render. The purpose of this section is to review: (1) procedures audiologists employ in assessing the receptive communication problem of the hearing impaired, (2) procedures commonly employed to improve communication status, (3) current procedures in teaching hearing-impaired children, and (4) the present status of hearing aid delivery services in the United States. While all of these services might not be delivered by U.S. audiologists in a hearing clinic (such as teaching the hearing-impaired school age children), they will be discussed because most of them are services that should be delivered by audiologists and are delivered in enough clinical settings to be considered the expected rather than the exception.

Evaluation of Language Development or Status

Since hearing impairment can have a profound effect on language development and on the oral expressive aspects of communication, the habilitative-rehabilitative audiologist will be interested in evaluating language and speech function. While there are not a large number of tests available and standardized for use with hearing-impaired children and adults, it is nevertheless possible to obtain information through the careful taking of case history data and observation through the interview process. Not only should auditory and visual performance be observed, but careful attention should also be directed toward the hearing-impaired person's ability to express himself either through speech or through meaningful gestures.

Administration of the Peabody Picture Vocabulary Test (Dunn, 1959) to hearing-impaired children will give the clinician a good idea of the size of the receptive vocabulary. Obviously, scores on this test or other tests mentioned should not serve as a basis for making statements about intelligence, but may be very useful in delineating the size of functional auditory or visual vocabulary.

The Illinois Test of Psycholinguistic Ability (ITPA) (McCarthy and Kirk, 1961) may provide useful information in other areas of language competence. The Peabody Individual Achievement Test (Dunn and Markwardt, 1970) has been found useful as a screening device. In addition, vocabulary and reading comprehension subtests of commonly accepted intelligence tests or tests of achievement are sometimes used to describe and summarize the language handling performance of the hearing-impaired individual.

The ability of the audiologist to evaluate the expressive communication of those hearing-impaired persons who communicate manually is obviously an advantage. The ability to communicate through writing is investigated by having the person write a paragraph about himself or about an interesting picture. Myklebust (1965) has devoted some attention to the use of such a procedure for evaluating the language disorders of several groups including the deaf. Careful attention is paid to articulatory, rhythm, and quality aspects of oral communication. Since the goal of aural habilitation-rehabilitation is to improve expressive communication as well as receptive, it is important that careful attention be directed toward the level of language development and expressive communication. In the case of hearing-impaired children with language and speech deficits, obtaining these facts provides the clinician with the information necessary to develop a habilitative program designed to build upon present competencies.

Evaluation of Auditory and Visual Reception of Speech

An important determinant of the need for aural habilitation-rehabilitation services, in addition to the recommendation of a hearing aid, is the degree to which the individual becomes effective in communication. The possibility of amplification accomplishing this is dependent upon many factors, including the amount of hearing loss, auditory discrimination, duration of loss, the communication needs of the hearing-impaired person, and his success in adjusting to wearing amplification devices. Habilitation-rehabilitation services supplementing the recommendation of a hearing aid should be available to all persons, but particularly those that could be predicted to have residual communication deficits and adjustment problems. Auditory discrimination testing, accomplished during the diagnostic phase combined with discrimination performance during the hearing aid evaluation process, gives considerable information about problems that will be encountered in most communication situations. Discrimination testing with the hearing aid in background noise or against competing speech gives additional information as to the auditory deficit. The contributions of visual cues to the understanding of speech are investigated. Although no tests have been standardized for this purpose, it is possible to employ the word or sentence lists used for auditory discrimination testing and permitting the subject to view the face of the speaker (Dodds and Harford, 1968).

Evaluating Lipreading Performance

Observing the speaker's face enables the hearing-impaired person to understand more. Clinical experience also indicates that the hearing-impaired person feels more confident when auditory cues can be reinforced by visual cues. One of the problems in aural habilitation-rehabilitation, however, is the fact that there is no test of lipreading or test of combined auditory and visual performance that has acceptable validity. Since the early part of this century, many attempts have been made to develop valid and reliable tests of lipreading performance (Conklin, 1917; Nitchie, 1917; Mason, 1943; Utley, 1946; Morkovin, 1947; Reid, 1947; Lowell, 1957; Moser et al., 1960). A review of tests is presented by O'Neill and Oyer (1961). Many of these tests use sentences as test items, some use words, some consist of two or more people in conversation, some are intended for face-to-face presentation while others have been filmed, some were developed for use with children, while others were developed for adults. In addition, a few of them have equivalent forms, and some of them were standardized on substantial numbers of subjects. However, none of them has achieved the status of an acceptable test of lipreading performance for several reasons: validity has not been established; only limited efforts have been made to sample variations in lipreadability that are known to exist from speaker to speaker; and, most of these tests do not take into account environmental, contextual, and gestural cues that are known to be important in the lipreading process. Another problem related to the evaluation of lipreading performance is that these tests were developed for use as "pure" measures of visual input only. While it is true that individuals with severe to profound hearing losses may be denied auditory cues, this is generally not true for most hearing-impaired people and is probably not true for those with severe to profound hearing losses who wear amplification. At the present time, there is no satisfactory test of lipreading performance that takes into account the factors mentioned. Furthermore, there is no test of lipreading performance with sufficient alternate forms to provide the necessary means of evaluating the habilitative-rehabilitative process. And last, there is no acceptable means of evaluating the effects of combined auditory and visual cues.

While there is great need for research and test development in this area, it does not mean that audiologists ignore measurements of lipreading and combined lipreading and hearing performance. It is the feeling of the authors that all tests of "lipreading" should be administered with sound at a normal conversational level, and that there is nothing to be gained by presenting these materials without voice or through the presentation of silent film. If a variety of speakers and materials is employed in measuring the contribution of visual cues to the understanding of speech, the audiologist is better able to predict performance outside the clinic.

Hearing Aid Evaluation Procedures

The evaluation and recommendation of hearing aids is a central part of the habilitation-rehabilitation program of audiological facilities. In most cases, the greatest gains in understanding the speech of others are realized through careful and thoughtful attention to the use of amplification.

An aural habilitation-rehabilitation program outlined by the Committee on Rehabilitative Audiology (ASHA Committee on Rehabilitative Audiology, 1974) mandates that audiologists be involved in the determination of need for amplification and the evaluation and recommendation of hearing aids as component parts of a total program whose goal is helping the hearing-impaired individual develop his communication potential to the maximum. From the audiologist's point of view, it is imperative to exercise control over this aspect of the habilitative-rehabilitative process. From the point of view of the hearing-impaired individual or his family, it is imperative that there be a continuity of service to minimize obstacles and confusion. If other aspects of the habilitative-rehabilitative program are to be effectively delivered, it is essential that the audiologist be involved in the hearing aid recommending process. Audiologists differ in their opinions as to how this is best accomplished and, therefore, it is not an easy task to describe hearing aid evaluation and recommendation procedures in the United States. While, at the present time, audiologists may disagree over test procedures and materials to use in the evaluation of hearing aids and the process by which hearing aids should be obtained for the hearing impaired, nevertheless, they are committed to this involvement because they realize that amplification is a critical component of habilitation-rehabilitation. They are also committed to this involvement because of the stimulation it provides for research into new methodologies and program development.

Probably the most commonly used procedure for evaluating hearing aids is the comparison method, wherein several hearing aids of similar characteristics are systematically placed on the individual and performance is observed using standardized speech tests. Since this process at the present time is less than an exact science, many variations in procedures exist. Proponents of the comparison method feel that actual use of several hearing aids maximizes the probability of the patient obtaining a hearing aid that provides optimal benefit. The various tests performed with each hearing aid on the individual tend to be patterned after those proposed by Carhart (1946). Minimal testing consists of noting improvement in SRT and obtaining an auditory discrimination score with each hearing aid. Other tests involving the dynamic range, testing discrimination in noise or against competing speech, obtaining aided pure tone thresholds, and obtaining discrimination scores at several hearing levels are also given. Whatever the type of test employed, materials used, or criterion employed in differentiating benefit to the hearing impaired, this process is culminated in the recommendation of a specific make and model of hearing aid and the ear to which it should be fitted. Unless the audiologist has provided a custom-made earmold himself, a recommendation for earmold type may also be included. If there is no clear delineation of an appropriate hearing aid on the basis of behavioral tests, other factors, including personal preferences of the patient, will be taken into account, so that the final recommendation will be based upon benefit provided in understanding speech supplemented by personal preferences of the patient modified by the clinical experience and judgment of the audiologist. The comparison method is often used with children. In cases where the speech and language development of a child would prohibit such evaluation, such comparisons are often made on the basis of improvement in detection thresholds or aided pure tone audiograms. The comparison method in these situations, obviously, has low validity since it cannot account for some of the variations in hearing aid response characteristics that might influence discrimination in quiet or in noise. Many hearing clinics, especially if they have a close working relationship with a preschool program for hearing-impaired children, employ a comparison method that extends over a longer period of time and allows for observations of the child's performance with each hearing aid in learning situations.

Gengel, Pascoe, and Shore (1971) describe a method of evaluating and selecting hearing aids for severely hearing-impaired children which best accommodates the frequency-intensity area of average speech into the available sensation area of the child's residual hearing.

On the basis of the research of Shore, Bilger, and Hirsh (1960), Shore and Kramer (1963) described a new system for recommending hearing aids that was implemented at the Central Institute for the Deaf. While at least one hearing aid was evaluated on each patient to demonstrate the limitations for discrimination, no specific hearing aid was recommended. Instead, the time was spent in counseling the patient and giving advice on how to shop for a hearing aid. He was provided with a hearing aid recommendation form that specified general characteristics of an acceptable hearing aid, including the amount of gain, suggested maximum power output, and ear to be fitted. They reported that this procedure proved to be as effective as the comparison procedure; however, this approach to hearing aid recommendation has not gained wide popularity.

Zerlin (1962) developed a paired comparison method for comparing hearing aids. He recorded speech against a background of cafeteria noise through hearing aids and presented the results by tape in such a fashion that subjects could compare all pairs of hearing aids through subjective judgments of intelligibility. While this procedure seems to hold merit, in that it produced some discriminations between aids that were not apparent through conventional testing, it has not gained wide acceptance, probably because of the complexity of instrumentation requirements.

The use of a "master hearing aid" in hearing aid selections has been advocated by the hearing aid industry for many years in order to reduce the inventory of hearing aids in audiology centers while not sacrificing the comparison method. However, no satisfactory master hearing aid has been produced that simulates sufficiently the actual hearing aid performance, especially with respect to the various forms of distortion and output limiting that may influence patient performance. As a matter of fact, it is the day-by-day experience of audiologists with actual hearing aids that has led to research on such items as distortion, volume control taper, and frequency response irregularity (Jerger and Thelin, 1968) among others.

The audiologist is very much concerned about any hearing-impaired individual who expresses concern over his ability to function in educational, vocational, and social situations. This point is stressed in *Aging and Communication* by Oyer, Kapur, and Deal (Oyer, Kapur, and Deal, 1976). While he knows that amplification probably cannot be found that will resolve all of these problems, the audiologist is interested in any variations in test procedures or materials, the application of variations in traditional hearing aid arrangements, such as CROS and BICROS, the differential effects of methods of limiting output, the possible beneficial effects of directional microphones, and the effects of varying methods of coupling and hearing aid to the ear that provide maximum function and comfort.

In addition to evaluating the benefit derived from amplification and the recommendation of hearing aids by whatever system the hearing center employs, an essential part of the hearing aid evaluation procedure is the counseling that follows. This counseling usually consists of discussion of the limitations of amplification, suggestions for adjustment to the hearing aid, and discussion of the possible need for follow-up services. A return visit to the hearing center is often encouraged but left to the discretion of the client. A more aggressive procedure is sometimes followed to ensure the return of all clients followed by a program of hearing aid orientation and related activities for those in need.

Current Procedures in Teaching Hearing-impaired Children

At the present time in the United States, probably all well known methods for teaching severely hearing-impaired children are employed. There has been much controversy surrounding this topic since Gallaudet opened the American Asylum for the Deaf and Dumb at Hartford, Connecticut in 1817. Gallaudet had learned the manual method of teaching from Abbé

Sicard in Paris. Thus, the manual method became the primary system for educating severely hearing-imparied children and, by the time the first oral school was opened in the 1860's, there were at least 22 manual schools in existence. These schools, led by the American Asylum for the Deaf and Dumb, successfully fought the development of an oral school until 1867, when the Clarke School for the Deaf was opened in Northampton, Massachusetts. A conflict between these two methods continues to this day, with proponents of each presenting very eloquent and emotional arguments for the elimination or minimal use of the other. An excellent review of the growth and development of the manual and oral methods in Europe and in the United States is presented by DiCarlo (1964). Much work has been devoted to refining methods for teaching children by each of these methods. There also have been attempts to combine elements of manualism and oralism. This is exemplified by the development of the "Rochester System" of simultaneous fingerspelling and lipreading. The early oral methods employed in the United States were essentially nonauditory in that they relied upon lipreading for understanding the speech of others and the combination of visual imitation, tactile, and kinesthetic training for the production of speech. One of the earliest people to point out the importance of residual hearing to the oral method was Goldstein (1939). His acoustic method was first employed in the United States at the Central Institute for the Deaf. With the development of electronic means of amplification and the application of these systems to wearable hearing aids, has come the development of auditory methods for teaching the severely hearing impaired. The work of Guberina (1964), the acoupedic method espoused by Pollack (1970), and the approach of Robinson and Gaeth (1975) exemplify the benefits of a strong auditory training approach combined with appropriate amplification to the development of communication skills. While the oral and manual methods, along with their variants, have produced some outstanding successes with many children, there have been significant failures, and, in general, none of these methods alone has satisfied the desire for an adequate education and communication status for all severely hearing-impaired children. Part of the problem stems from zealous proponents of each method closing their eyes to any value of opposing methodologies. While it is recognized that there are very important factors that might be determinants of the most appropriate method for each child, there has been little cooperation exhibited by proponents of various methods from audiology, otology, deaf education, and psychology to resolve this matter in the best interest of the child and the family. Some of these factors are age of onset, amount of residual hearing loss, evidence that residual hearing can be developed to provide more than tactile cues, general intelligence, duration of hearing impairment before discovery, family history and dynamics, and special aptitudes. As a result of general dissatisfaction with the education and communication achievement of hearing-impaired children, a new philosophy called "total communication" has emerged. Its proponents are as zealous about its advantages as those who espouse manual, oral, or auditory approaches. The basic premise of this approach is that all means of communicating with the hearing-impaired child should be used simultaneously. American sign language, fingerspelling, and lipreading are all used, with speech heard through an auditory training unit or hearing aid. This "shotgun" approach to educating the severely hearing-impaired child is still in its infancy and, thus, there are little data to validate its advantages or disadvantages, but some critics argue that increased redundancy may turn out to be detrimental. The work of Gaeth (1967) would indicate that this might be so; however, it is possible that the hearing-impaired child may learn which type of cue he prefers and ignore the superfluous information.

Approximately two-thirds of the severely hearing-impaired children are educated in public day school programs offered in their own communities. The remaining one-third attend residential schools that are either state funded or are private schools funded by tuition and endowment. Most audiologists are proponents of the aural approach that stresses early identification, the use of amplification as early as possible, auditory training, early enrollment in preschool programs, and careful monitoring of the child and his amplification system. Such a program maximizes the development of a "listening" posture similar to that of the normal hearing child and would establish the ear as the primary means of learning language, supplemented by visual cues. Unfortunately, however, there is no nationwide early intervention system for determining the hearing status of newborn children or for ensuring that children suffering hearing impairments postnatally will be referred to appropriate facilities. Finding hearing-impaired children can be a hit-or-miss proposition involving the awareness of the parent, the availability of a concerned pediatrician or family physician, and his knowledge of the importance of early intervention and training. There is need for more programs to provide aural habilitation services for pre-nursery school children. There is great need for audiologists and teachers of the hearing impaired to communicate when these children are enrolled in school programs to assure continuity of the aural method if it has proved successful. If not successful, alternate methods of teaching could be explored. The degree of flexibility in programming necessary to accomplish this, however, is usually not available, partly because of the barriers that proponents of various methods have erected.

Status of Hearing Aid Delivery Services

The status of hearing aid delivery services in the United States is in some state of confusion at the present time. The traditional system has been scrutinized and has been found seriously lacking in many respects, but it has not become clear what alterations in the hearing aid dispensing system will occur.

The profession of audiology originated out of the experiences in military hospitals during World War II, as hundreds of hearing-impaired military personnel were returned to these hospitals for rehabilitation. It was created through the collaborative efforts of speech pathologists and otologists who were faced with the problem of rehabilitating these war veterans (Newby, 1972). A complete diagnostic and rehabilitative program which includes procedures for determining the need for amplification, principles of selection of hearing aids, measuring benefit from amplification, hearing aid orientation, lipreading, auditory training, speech conservation, and psychological and vocational counseling was developed. These programs were so successful that those individuals who had been involved in the development and delivery of these services felt that their experiences could be beneficially applied to a civilian population. In addition, many of the speech pathologists who had been involved in these programs returned to university campuses and developed courses and clinical programs which have evolved into the field of audiology as it is known today. Over the intervening years audiologists have devoted much time and research attention to the development and refinement of hearing tests and their application to identification, diagnosis, and rehabilitation. As a corollary, they have developed large clinical programs dedicated to training while at the same time providing services to hearing-impaired people. These services have included the evaluation and recommendation of hearing aids and the delivery of other aural habilitation-rehabilitation services, but not the direct sale of hearing aids to the public.

Hearing aid sales organizations have been in existence in the United States since the second or third decade of this century; however, most of the growth in personnel engaged in sales has occurred since the end of World War II (Berger, 1970). From that beginning to the present time, no formal training has been required to prepare a person to engage in the business of selling hearing aids. While there have been attempts by the National Hearing Aid Society and interested people from the professions to upgrade the knowledge and competencies of hearing aid personnel, these efforts must be considered marginal at best. As electronic technology made possible the miniaturization of hearing aids, sales increased as did the number of sales personnel. By late 1969, there were some 1,550 members in the National Hearing Aid Society who had completed a correspondence course sponsored by the Society (Berger, 1970), although it is estimated that there are some 5,000 people engaged in sales. The overwhelming majority of this sales force, with no formal training in audiology or medicine, has been engaged in testing and examining procedures that imply professional training to the public. Recent statistics from the industry (Facts and Figures, 1973), for example, revealed that 69.5% of the people who purchased hearing aids in 1973 had not previously been seen by an otologist or an audiologist, Otology referrals accounted for 10.5% of sales, hearing centers accounted for 11.5% of sales, and governmental agencies purchased 8.5%. Statistics of this type have been stable over the past few years and indicate that over two-thirds of the hearing-impaired population obtain hearing aids without benefit of professional audiological examination or consultation. It is interesting to note that the industry apparently ceased publication of this information, since it does not appear in subsequent summaries. It has been obvious for some time that hearing aid dealers have been on a collision course with otology and audiology.

The traditional role of audiology with respect to hearing aids has consisted of the recommendation of one or more hearing aids for the hearing-impaired person to be purchased by that individual from a local hearing aid dealer. Whether the patient would actually obtain the aid recommended or even be seen again by the center for any follow-up service has been to some extent out of the control of the audiologist. There have been several notable exceptions to this traditional delivery system. Since World War II, the Veterans Administration has maintained an aural rehabilitation program which included, through many of its regional hospitals, a hearing aid evaluation, recommendation, and dispensing system (Anderman, 1970). Manufacturers volunteer to participate in the V.A. program by submitting hearing aid models to the V.A. for testing by the National Bureau of Standards. After extensive examination, the Veterans Administration determines the models it will purchase, based upon clinical need, performance, and cost (Veterans Administration, 1974). This dispensing system has made it possible for the hearing-impaired veteran to obtain the actual hearing aid that was used in the comparative evaluation. In addition, the veteran receives batteries and hearing aid repair services through the audiological facility. The other exception involves third party purchase of hearing aids for certain segments of the civilian population. The purchase program in several states has made it possible for the centers to order the specific hearing aid recommended and have it delivered to the center for verification of response characteristics and delivery to the individual. This procedure has been used in Michigan, although it may be undergoing some change because of extreme political pressure from the hearing aid industry. Whether or not it is required that hearing aids be delivered to the facility before fitting or payment to the vendor, it is possible in the Michigan system for the hearing center to be reimbursed for one or more follow-up visits after the hearing aid has been obtained. At least one follow-up visit is essential because of the importance of knowing the electroacoustical characteristics of the hearing aid at the time of dispensing or as soon after as possible. To attempt to render habilitation-rehabilitation services at this time or at any future time without being able to monitor variations in hearing aid performance characteristics is indefensible.

As early as 1966, it has been apparent to many audiologists that some significant changes in the hearing aid dispensing system were necessary. One of the recommendations of a panel participating in a conference on hearing aid evaluation procedures (American Speech and Hearing Association, 1967) recommended that audiologists be permitted, through appropriate changes in the Code of Ethics of the American Speech and Hearing Association, to be involved in the dispensing of commercial products. This recommendation and variations of it have been discussed since that time with a growing feeling among the audiology community that, whether or not that recommendation is accepted, some drastic change in the system is necessary in order that the hearing impaired receive appropriate habilitation-rehabilitation services including optimal benefits of amplification.

Many otologists have also been concerned about the quality of services rendered by the hearing aid industry, but have not necessarily agreed that audiological evaluation and recommendation are essential in all cases (Miller, 1973); however, they would agree that otological examination should be encouraged if not mandated before the sale of a hearing aid. In the meantime, consumerism has become a very important force in the American political and economic scene. The awakening of the consumer to the possibility that, through collective action, he might be able to influence government and business practices that affect him has been spearheaded by Ralph Nader. His activities have spurred the development of local, state, and national consumer groups that have made government and business aware of their concerns about a myriad of matters. Through studies and subsequent reports (IMPIRG, 1972; PIRGIM, 1973; RPAG,

1973), government has become aware of the need to exert control over the manufacture and distribution of hearing aids and the role of the hearing aid dealer in American society. While some audiologists and otologists are contemplating dispensing hearing aids in order to assure themselves and their patients the highest quality professional services and products, many of the consumer groups along with numbers of audiologists and otologists are recommending some form of "prescription" of hearing aids by audiologists and otologists. While these discussions and debates go on, the National Hearing Aid Society is trying to upgrade the competence of its members, to mount an aggressive public relations program, and to convince consumer groups and legislators that, with minimum modifications, the present delivery system is an excellent one and in the best tradition of American free enterprise. Hovering in the background is an anticipated national health program that, among other things, would probably involve delivery of services by audiologists and otologists to the hearing impaired and the delivery of hearing aids for significant numbers of Americans. The eventual role of the otologist, the audiologist, and the hearing aid dealer in the delivery of services and products might not be decided on the basis of relative professional expertise of the three groups, or in the best interest of the hearing impaired, but rather on the basis of political and economic power.

Rehabilitation Services for the Adventitiously Hearing Impaired

Except for the program of the Veterans Administration, there is no community or nationwide delivery of comprehensive aural rehabilitation services to this segment of the population. In addition to the fact that the audiologist may not be involved in the dispensing of hearing aids and the resultant problems in securing return to the hearing center for follow-up services if needed, is the problem of scheduling aural rehabilitation services at convenient times for working age people. Many centers, however, through commitment to the need for and value of aural rehabilitation, do manage to provide such programs and services to certain elements of the population at least. Most community hearing centers maintain comprehensive aural rehabilitation service programs, not only because they are needed, but also because it is in their tradition to do so. University hearing clinics frequently have organized aural rehabilitation programs for specific groups of people, for example, the elderly residing in nursing homes (Kasten and Goldstein, 1970; Harless and Rupp, 1972; Hull and Traynor, 1975).

While it cannot be said that aural rehabilitation services beyond the recommendation of hearing aids are routinely available to the hearing-impaired adult or that they avail themselves of these services when offered, there is evidence of commitment by many audiologists and centers and, where there is commitment, aural rehabilitation programs exist.

INTERPROFESSIONAL RELATIONSHIPS

The age of specialization, while increasing the competencies of the practitioner within the narrow scope of his specialty and, thus, improving the quality of services delivered, complicates relationships with other fields of specialty and leads to problems in serving the total person. With the proliferation of professions and areas of specializations within these professions, the possibility exists that a hearing-impaired child or adult might have to interact with a dozen or more specialists who will be looking at this problem from different frames of reference. For example, the hearing-impaired person is likely to come in contact with one or more physicians, including the family doctor, pediatrician, otologist, neurologist, industrial physician, and physiatrist, to name a few. He is likely to require or seek out the services of audiologists, teachers of the hearing impaired, regular classroom teachers, speech pathologists, psychologists, social workers, and vocational counselors. Ideally, all of these professionals should have sufficient knowledge of the total needs of the hearing impaired, an awareness of the limitations of their own specialty in meeting these needs, and knowledge of the contributions that other professionals can provide. Obviously these conditions usually are not met and, thus, discontinuity of service to the hearing impaired occurs which leads to the development of irritation among professions.

Members of these groups possess at least some surface knowledge of the other professional fields. There is the possibility that the old maxim "a little bit of knowledge is dangerous" might be true, because each professional group to some extent possesses unrealistic expectations of what the others can or should accomplish. In addition, individuals of each discipline are often too prone to offer advice or make recommendations outside their area of expertise that inappropriately influence the behavior of the hearing impaired and produce irritation among the other professional groups. Unfortunately all professional groups seem to be somewhat guilty of this behavior, partly because the lines of demarcation between professions are not clearly delineated and, in some cases, there is considerable overlap. The best solution to these problems lies in closer communication between professions at the state and national level and a better utilization of an organized team approach. Interprofessional problems tend to be minimal in those facilities where otologists, audiologists, speech pathologists, teachers of the hearing impaired, social workers, and psychologists work together to habilitate or rehabilitate the hearing impaired. Unfortunately, the number of facilities that function in this manner is relatively small.

Another current problem has to do with whether the services provided by audiologists and speech pathologists, in particular, shall be prescribed by the physician or whether these professionals will be defined as independent colleagues of the physician. This conflict occurs in some instances on the level of individual interactions with respect to specific patients and to some extent exists nationally between professional groups. The issue reveals itself as medical insurance policies are written that include payments for services rendered by audiologists and speech pathologists and is apparent as legislation concerning national health insurance is being written. This matter has not been resolved as yet, but it is quite evident that audiologists and speech pathologists have traditionally functioned as professional colleagues of the physician and are resistive of attempts to make their services prescriptive. The final resolution of this problem will obviously have significant implications for the role of audiologists in the future.

A 2-year study on the interprofessional relationships of audiology and education of the deaf, which included a conference attended by leaders of each discipline, resulted in some significant conclusions (Joint Committee on Audiology and Education of the Deaf, 1965). The conference concluded that audiologists needed greater knowledge of the educational management of hearing-impaired children, that they needed greater exposure to educational and language problems imposed by deafness, that audiological services offered to severely hearing-impaired clients needed to be improved, that teachers of the hearing impaired were not making adequate use of audiology services, that teachers needed better training in utilizing audiological information in planning an educational program, that the role of the speech pathologist working with the deaf needed to be reevaluated, and that interprofessional relationships needed to be improved. While it cannot be said that the problems highlighted by these conclusions have been resolved, there have been small but significant steps taken that will eventually improve the situation and lead to improved and better coordinated services to the severely hearing impaired. For example, the Michigan Speech and Hearing Association through by-law revision has created an Education of the Hearing Impaired Committee, chaired by a Vice President for Education of the Hearing Impaired. This vice president and a majority of the committee must be teachers of the hearing impaired.

Much of the work in aural habilitation-rehabilitation is performed by speech pathologists working in the public school setting, although to a lesser extent they may be involved in delivering these services in other employment settings. While speech pathologists have considerable training in speech and language disorders, they tend to have inadequate preparation for working with speech and language disorders associated with hearing loss. The field of audiology, at the training level and at the delivery of service level, must assume responsibility for this unfortunate situation. Improved training of the speech pathologist to render these services will only occur through the leadership of habilitation-rehabilitation oriented audiologists, if indeed, it is decided that aural habilitation-rehabilitation services are to be delivered by the speech pathologist. Audiologists also must assume a greater responsibility in rendering aural habilitation-rehabilitation services in their employment settings, and increased pressure must be exerted on public and private schools for the hearing impaired to employ audiologists to provide habilitative-rehabilitative services.

There is need for a closer working relationship with social workers and psychologists. A few hearing centers have staff positions for these individuals; however, this situation is by no means nationwide. Social workers and psychologists who are knowledgeable about the impact of hearing loss on speech and language development, educational and vocational planning, and family and social interactions, are seen to be of tremendous benefit to the habilitation-rehabilitation process.

FAMILY INVOLVEMENTS

Children

One of the most important functions of the family is providing for socialization of its young. As Kenkel (1973) comments, the question is not whether the young should be socialized but rather how and by whom this task should be performed. Socialization is education in its broadest sense and involves a learning of the mores and standards of the group as well as its traditions. This might take place formally or informally and, when accomplished, facilitates adjustment to the group and fosters a sense of belonging.

When there is deprivation of sensory input, as in hearing impairment, the learning process is short circuited and, thus, the socialization process is affected. One can see readily the counseling implications of this for parents of children who are hearing handicapped. During the preschool years, they might have worked out very satisfactory adjustments to the family as a social unit; however, upon entry into school, whether it be a school for the deaf or a regular classroom, there is an additional socialization process that must get underway quickly, for the child must learn what the role expectancies are of him.

In the United States, provisions have been made in numerous ways for involving families of hearing handicapped in helping to bring about psychosocial adjustment of children to the demands of the formal school experience. This is accomplished through programs of counseling carried out by trained counselors who seek to interpret to parents the psychosocial expectancies of the school system. It is also accomplished by social workers, hearing clinicians, and, of course, by teachers themselves through parent interviews. "Time devoted to counseling the family of the hard-of-hearing person serves a valuable purpose" (Oyer, 1966).

Some clinics include counseling and education sessions into their programs of habilitation-rehabilitation for their hearing-handicapped clients. This may involve parents, the family members of clients, and/or the clients themselves. The objective is to provide for a greater understanding of what a hearing problem means to the hearing handicapped and also to those in the immediate environment. By so doing, the probability of eliciting supportive behavior from "important others" is enhanced.

A very important step was taken by the Alexander Graham Bell Association in the development of a section of its organization called the International Parents Association. This association attempts to relate to parents of deaf children not only throughout the United States but also the entire world in an effort to promote understanding of the multiple problems associated with deafness and to elicit cooperation for developing better programs for the hearing-handicapped child.

Parents have been active in many places throughout the United States in establishing local groups that focus upon the various needs of their hearing-handicapped children. An example of this is in the religious education classes organized in Cincinnati for hearing-impaired children (Huston, 1969). A need felt by parents for providing basic religious concepts to their hearing-handicapped children led to the establishment of religious education classes. Many other examples of parent involvement in moving forward the learning, recreational, and other opportunities of hearing handicapped in the United States could also be cited.

Adults

The early emphasis in aural rehabilitation in the United States was focused upon children. Not until the decade of the 1890's was much done for adults who sustained hearing handicaps. It was at this time that Lillie Warren, who had devoted her time to teaching lipreading to children, became interested in helping adults. In her book, *Defective Speech and Deafness,* she included a chapter on "How the Hard of Hearing Adult May Enjoy Conversation" (Warren, 1895). Following her initial attempts, the hearing-handicapped adult in the United States received more attention. Today there are many audiology clinics and special programs carried out by the National Association for Hearing and Speech Action, as well as other local units sponsored through programs of continuing education, that focus upon problems encountered by the hearing-handicapped adult. Federal and state programs of vocational rehabilitation have made great contributions in training, research, and direct service to the hearing-handicapped adult.

The effects on the family of hearing handicaps sustained by adult members were recently investigated by Oyer and Paolucci (1970). Their study was designed to answer some basic questions concerning the relationship of homemakers' hearing losses to family integration. They found the husbands' marital tension increased significantly as a function of the severity of the hearing loss of the wife. They also found that family members tended to provide hearing-handicapped homemakers with significantly more help in the home than did family members of the comparison group.

In a pilot study of the family and mental health problems of a deaf community in New York (Rainer et al., 1963), it was shown that marriage rates among the deaf population were somewhat lower than for the population in general; however, the divorce rate was somewhat higher. This comprehensive study also revealed that almost 25% of deaf parents have at least one deaf child. Deaf children were granted a higher degree of self-determination as regards education than were hearing siblings; however, parents were found to exert greater influence upon the choice of vocational goals for the deaf children than for their hearing sisters and brothers.

At this time in the history of the development of aural rehabilitation, it is fair to say that as regards the effects on the family of hearing-handicapped persons there is a great deal to be known. Emphasis has been placed generally upon doing something by way of habilitation or rehabilitation of the hearing-handicapped person, and rightfully so. To measure the effects of what is being done, as it affects the family as a social unit, remains a challenge of no small magnitude.

TRAINING OF PROFESSIONALS FOR THE FIELD OF HABILITATIVE-REHABILITATIVE AUDIOLOGY

Audiology in the United States came into existence as a result of the need to rehabilitate large numbers of hearing-impaired military personnel. This was a multifaceted venture that required the development and application of precise testing procedures utilizing electronic instrumentation and the development and application of therapeutic and counseling techniques to supplement the less than ideal rehabilitation provided by hearing aids. Certain aspects of hearing loss yielded readily to measurement and quantification while others presented more formidable obstacles to such definition. In some sense it can be said that, until recently, the efforts of audiology during the post-World War II period have been sidetracked from the main goal of the pioneer work which was the maximal rehabilitation of the hearing impaired. The intervening years have been filled with the refinement of diagnostic procedures, the development of new procedures for evaluating the more subtle aspects of malfunction of the auditory system, the development of new training programs, and the establishment of audiology as a respected profession working with the medical and educational communities. This is not to imply that audiologists have not contributed to the habilitation-rehabilitation of hearing-impaired persons during this period, but it must be said that the same commitment of time and energy has not been devoted to the development of habilitation-rehabilitation procedures or in preparing students for this role. This has probably been a very normal evolutionary process with those problems most readily yielding to scientific inquiry being accomplished first. These developments, along with parallel developments in otology, always hold the promise of new discoveries that will preclude the use of amplification as we know it today and the need for ancillary habilitation-rehabilitation services. An increased number of audiologists have become aware that the tremendous strides audiology and otology have made over the years, however, have not significantly altered the need for habilitative-rehabilitative programs or the need for audiologists interested in pushing back the frontiers in this area. Despite technological advances in the hearing aid industry, the benefits of amplification for the understanding of speech are not much different today from what they were 25 years ago. Children are still born with profound hearing losses and other children develop postnatal sensorineural hearing losses. Our noisy industrial society increases the number of hearing-impaired adults, and increasing lifespan produces greater numbers of elderly people with auditory impairments. The communication problems of the elderly that are related to hearing loss are addressed in detail in a book that focuses on the aging person (Oyer and Oyer, 1976). Audiologists in the United States seem to be increasingly aware of the shortcomings of their professional training and orientation with respect to the delivery of adequate habilitative-rehabilitative services to these children and adults. Some examples of the shortcomings might be listed as follows:

1. Many hearing-impaired children do not develop auditory skills to their maximum potential.
2. Too many hearing-impaired people are wearing amplification systems that are malfunctioning in some significant way.
3. Many parents of hearing-impaired children do not receive sufficient or appropriate counseling so as to participate maximally in their child's development.
4. Audiologists make few significant contributions to the adult deaf community.
5. Research attention has been lacking in areas of auditory training, lipreading, development of tests of everyday listening efficiency, or multimodality receptive communication. As a consequence, many of the habilitative-rehabilitative procedures, if employed, remain unchanged from those employed in the Veterans Hospitals during World War II, and do not enjoy the same level of respect as other aspects of audiology.
6. Audiologists, by and large, are ill prepared to participate in the language and speech learning of hearing-impaired preschool children, even though they are the most appropriate professionals to provide that service because of their early contacts with these children and their competencies with respect to hearing loss and amplification.

Before discussing the qualifications of the ideal habilitative-rehabilitative audiologist, it might be of interest to review the certification requirements for teachers of the hearing impaired, audiologists, and speech pathologists, and to comment on the training of otologists. Teachers of hearing-impaired children may be provisionally certified by the Council on Education of the Deaf with a core program of 30 semester hours, 3 of which must be in speech science and audiology. In part, full certification requires an additional 20 semester hours, but course work in audiology and acoustics is not mandatory although they are listed as possible alternatives (Craig and Craig, 1974). Thus, it is possible for certified teachers of the hearing impaired to have very minimal training in audiology, amplification systems, and auditory learning. The American Speech and Hearing Association requires a total of 60 semester hours in areas relevant to the management of the communicatively handicapped. Twelve of these semester hours must be in courses pertaining to normal development. Thirty semester hours must be in courses having to do with the communication disorders, with 24 of the hours in the major professional area (audiology or speech pathology) and the remaining 6 in the other area. For the Certificate of Clinical Competence in Audiology, the applicant must demonstrate no less than 6 semester hours in habilitation-rehabilitation of hearing impairment. The Certificate of Clinical Competence in Speech Pathology requires that a minimum of 3 semester hours must be in habilitative-rehabilitative procedures associated with hearing impairment. In addition to the formal course work, there is the additional requirement of 300 hours of supervised clinical practice. For audiologists, no fewer than 50 of these hours must be obtained in habilitative-rehabilitative procedures, but quite frequently that requirement is met through the evaluation and recommendation of hearing aids. The speech pathologist must also demonstrate some supervised clinical experience with hearing-impaired people, but the minimum requirement is 35 clock hours of which 15 must be in assessment and management of communication problems associated with hearing loss. While many programs provide more than the minimal academic and clinical training for the certificates in audiology or speech pathology, it can be seen that the potential for audiologists and speech pathologists to be ill prepared to deliver the highest quality habilitative-rehabilitative services is possible.

While many otologists in the United States have made significant contributions to aural habilitation-rehabilitation, and many others are supportive of services rendered by audiologists, it must be said that this interest in general does not come as a result of the formal training in audiology, hearing aid technology, or other aspects of nonmedical habilitation-rehabilitation. Otology in most medical schools is categorized as a surgical specialty and, while the board examinations in otolaryngology presume some knowledge of audiological testing, noise, and noise-induced hearing loss, formal coursework in these and other relevant areas is not required. Recent developments in cochlear implant surgery (Merzenich, Schindler, and Sooy, 1974) perhaps hold promise of a significant contribution to habilitation-rehabilitation; however, at the present time, the technology and procedures are so crude that their widespread use has been discouraged. To date, the implantation of cochlear devices would not appear to decrease the continuing need for habilitative-rehabilitative procedures; indeed, it would appear to increase the need. Whether there will be changes in the future in the training of otologists, to include the content of diagnostic and rehabilitative audiology, is not known, but the fact that there is a relative shortage of otologists in the United States and a large and growing number of well trained audiologists would seem to indicate that these two professions will not change their roles relative to one another.

The soul searching that audiologists have been undergoing has led to some suggested changes in traditional services and training of future audiologists. The fact that many audiologists view traditional hearing aid dispensing systems as deterrents to the delivery of high quality habilitative-rehabilitative services is one indication of this commitment. In addition, the Joint Committee on Audiology and Education of the Deaf (1975), which consists of representatives from the American Speech and Hearing Association and the Conference of Executives of American Schools for the Deaf, has prepared a proposed set of guidelines for audiology programs in educational settings. These proposed guidelines discuss the need for more audiologists in school settings and suggest that one certified audiologist be available for every 75 hearing-impaired children. They made further suggestions about necessary facilities and equipment and the necessity for an electronics technician to be available. Under these guidelines the audiologist would be responsible for: (1) periodically assessing the hearing of all children involved in the program and those being considered for admission; (2) completely assessing the suprathreshold hearing capabilities of the children by known or newly developed procedures; (3) evaluating and recommending hearing aids and monitoring the performance of them and the children wearing them; (4) assuming responsibility for the acoustic environment and the use and function of all amplifying equipment; (5) conducting auditory training programs, speech and language development programs utilizing an auditory approach; (6) conducting in-service workshops for teachers; (7) making earmold impressions; and (8) participating in parent counseling programs. While this is not a complete list of job responsibilities as proposed by this committee, it does serve the purpose of familiarizing the reader with the orientation and competencies proposed as necessary for the audiologist in the United States who works in an educational facility. The present American Speech and Hearing Association certification requirements, while being somewhat general in terms of the specific knowledges and skills required in habilitative-rehabilitative audiology, are sufficient to supply professionals for educational programs for the hearing-impaired people who could perform these responsibilities.

O'Neill (1974) has discussed the need for a school or educational audiologist. He discusses the goals for such a program and presents a possible curriculum to prepare audiologists for that role. While the curriculum he presents prepares the individual for American Speech and Hearing Association certification, and indeed requires it, there are some additional requirements in education and psychology. The focus of his proposed program is to prepare audiologists to work with the hearing-impaired child who is educated outside of the usual "deaf education" program. Typically this is the child with a mild to moderately severe hearing impairment who has some language and speech proficiency and is found in his neighborhood school in a regular classroom or in some "nondeaf" special education classroom.

Berg (1974) reviewed the educational audiology training program at Utah State University. This is a rather marked departure from the traditional training of audiologists and represents a blend of audiology and deaf education. The following list is the quarter-by-quarter class registration in educational audiology spanning 10 quarters of undergraduate and graduate study (Berg, 1974, p. 46). Additional course work in psychology, general professional education, and special education is also included in addition to the courses listed.

1. Introduction to Communicative Disorders
   Phonetics
   Fundamentals ofAnatomy for Speech and Hearing
2. Fundamentals of Communication Science
   Language, Hearing, and Speech Development
   Clinical Processes and Behavior
   Apprenticeship in Communicative Disorders
3. Basic Audiometry
   Hearing and Speech Management
   Disorders of Articulation
   Apprenticeship
4. Speech Audiometry
   Advanced Hearing and Speech Management
   Language Disorders and Hearing Impairment
   Internship
5. Structure, Function, and Dysfunction of the Hearing Mechanism
   Teaching Language to the Hearing Impaired
   Education of the Hearing impaired
   Internship
6. Pediatric Audiology
   Introduction to Research in Communicative Disorders
   Teaching Reading to the Hearing Impaired
   Internship
7. Hearing Aids
   The Young Hearing-Impaired Child
   Thesis
   Internship
8. Differential Diagnosis of Auditory Disorders
   Curriculum for the Hearing Impaired
   Dactylology
   Seminar in Educational Audiology
   Internship
9. Externship

10. Medical Backgrounds in Communicative Disorders
    Internship
    Thesis

The graduate of this program might or might not meet the certification requirements of the American Speech and Hearing Association in audiology or the certification requirements of the Council on Education of the Deaf. Nevertheless, Berg reports that they have achieved outstanding success in placing their graduates in educational settings either as a school audiologist, resource room specialist, classroom teacher of the hearing impaired, or as a preschool clinician-educator.

While the same amount of attention has not been devoted to the competencies, role, and methods of delivering habilitative-rehabilitative services to the adult, we would conclude that it is forthcoming and that the satisfactory resolution of the hearing aid dispensing issue is of critical importance. This is not to say that habilitative-rehabilitative services of audiologists are not being delivered presently to hearing-impaired adults. To do so, however, requires the energetic work of the audiologist and cooperation from audiologists, physicians, speech pathologists, hearing aid manufacturers, and hearing aid dealers.

RESEARCH

Areas of Research

The area of aural rehabilitation has substantially less research to point to than has the general area of measurement of hearing. Programs of research have in the main been carried out in academic settings. The Rehabilitation Services Administration and the Bureau of Education for the Handicapped, both within the U.S. Department of Health, Education, and Welfare, have largely been the source of financial support for government-sponsored research projects in this area.

Rather than attempting to enumerate isolated efforts made to carry out programs of research, the writers shall attempt to state succinctly the areas in which research has taken place and to follow with research needs yet unmet.

Measurement of hearing deficit has by far commanded the greatest research attention. Procedures have been carefully spelled out for determination of air and bone condition thresholds. Standardization of tests for speech reception and speech discrimination is at hand. Additionally, there are special tests for determining site of lesion in the auditory pathway. Tests for recruitment are also constructed. Also there are procedures for measuring hearing thresholds of children which are based upon research. Beginning attempts have been made to describe the language deficit that accompanies hearing loss.

Considerable research work has been directed toward the lipreading process, but only too little directly focused upon lipreading as related to rehabilitation measures. There has been examination of the code, the speaker, the transmission mode, and the receiver. Most attention, as one might expect, has been directed toward the receiver.

Manual language has received some research attention; however, most effort has been put toward understanding the combined manual methods.

Auditory training research has shown that both speech intelligibility and discrimination can be improved in those sustaining hearing losses. Research has shown that the slope of the loss is a determining factor in the extent to which auditory training is a viable approach to rehabilitation.

Substantial work has taken place in the area of amplification and procedures by which hearing aids should be selected. Several tests—Synthetic Sentence Identification, Speech Sound Comparison Test, and Intermodulation Distortion Test—are useful in the hearing aid evaluation selection procedure. It has been shown that binaural hearing aids and CROS hearing aids are best for some persons who sustain communication handicaps, particularly in adverse listening conditions.

Tactile stimulation has received some attention by researchers interested in exploring the desirability of this channel with the hearing handicapped. The work is still in the beginning stages and does not as yet present a body of data that indicates that this will be a useful input mode.

Even though there is some evidence which indicates that the multisensory approach is not desirable, there seems to be a real interest in the use of the multisensory approach in aural rehabilitation. Because of this, work continues that is aimed at determining the relative effects of multiple sensory input on aural rehabilitation.

Considerable effort has been directed toward investigation of the effects of hearing deficit upon academic achievement. Additionally, research has been carried out that is aimed at the effects of hearing loss upon self and social adjustment. Deaf children have been found to be considerably below normal hearing children in school achievement. There are studies that show, however, that hearing-handicapped individuals do have realistic attitudes toward their handicaps.

There has been some effort to learn about attitudes of employers toward hiring of minimally trained deaf job seekers. It seems that the most significant barriers to the employment of deaf persons are those of language inability and lack of skills in responding to the interview situation.

Research Needs

The need for research in aural rehabilitation is great. For example, further description of the handicaps accompanying hearing loss is needed. This should be examined in relation to age, sex, attitude, and vocational adjustment. Self-recognition of hearing handicap in relation to recognition by others needs further study in relation to the success or lack of success in the rehabilitation process.

Effects of hearing handicaps on self-concept and the subsequent effects on academic and vocational success need examination. Thorough researching of compensatory behavior of those failing in social situations because of hearing handicap is needed. Social class as related to success in aural rehabilitation needs scrutiny as well.

A careful study should also be made of those factors that are relevant as regards the identification and use of professional assistance by those who are hearing handicapped. Help can be obtained from a variety of persons who play some part in the rehabilitation process. Who is chosen, and why?

The whole area of measurement of handicaps brought about by hearing deficits is in dire need of full and complete exploration. So much attention has been paid to the measurement of deficit–so little to the measurement of the accompanying handicaps. The whole area of language needs in-depth study. Determining the effects of amplification on the deficit-handicap relationship needs probing.

Research which would lead to scientific construction of materials for rehabilitative sessions is needed, as well as research on the effects of specified training or retraining procedures on eventual communication performance.

Also the broad area of counseling with the hearing-handicapped individual or the parents or spouse needs rigorous scientific study. To date we have paid all too little attention to the effects of hearing handicap on the basic unit of society, the family.

The above suggestions are but a few of the many that could be cited as critical needs for research. In a recent book, which analyzes the aural rehabilitation process within a conceptual framework, Oyer and Frankmann (1975) point up over 120 specific topics in the area of aural rehabilitation that need research.

More research is needed so that more standardized approaches can be made in the rehabilitative process. With this accomplished, we shall be able to do a better job of predicting outcomes of rehabilitative efforts and, thus, be more accountable to the clients and/or to those who support their programs of habilitation-rehabilitation.

ORGANIZATIONS AND ASSOCIATIONS RESPONSIBLE FOR THE HEARING HANDICAPPED

There are numerous associations that have been set up for purposes of helping along the cause of the hearing handicapped in the United States. At the national level, the professional associations are the Convention of the American Instructors of the Deaf, Convention of Executives of American Schools for the Dcaf, American Speech and Hearing Association, the Academy of Rehabilitative Audiology, and the American Academy of Ophthalmology and Otolaryngology.

Conference of Executives of American Schools for the Deaf

This organization was founded in 1868 with H. P. Peet serving as its first president. It has a membership of 225 persons, limited to the executive leadership of schools for the deaf. The purpose of the conference is "to promote the management and operation of schools for the deaf along the broadest and most efficient lines and to further and promote the general welfare of the deaf." It participates in the certification of teachers of the hearing impaired. Its national office is located at 5034 Wisconsin Avenue, N.W., Washington, D.C. 20016.

Convention of the American Instructors of the Deaf

The members of this group have been meeting since 1850, at which time the first meeting was held in New York City on August 28–30, with Christopher Mogan as its first president. It was incorporated by an enactment of the Senate and House of Representatives of the United States of America on January 26, 1897 for purposes of ". . . the promotion of the education of the deaf on the broadest, most advanced, and practical lines . . ." (Report of the Proceedings of the 42nd Meeting of the Convention of the American Instructors of the Deaf, 1965). The group is composed of educators of the deaf and has at present a membership of approximately 4,700 individuals. The address of this organization is: Convention of the American Instructors of the Deaf, 5034 Wisconsin Avenue, N.W., Washington, D.C. 20016.

American Speech and Hearing Association

This group was begun as the American Academy of Speech Correction and has been meeting annually since 1925, with Robert W. West as the first president. It was incorporated in 1925 in Kansas. Its principal concerns are "... to encourage basic scientific study of the processes of individual human communication, with special reference to speech, hearing, and language, promote investigation of disorders of human communication, and foster improvement of clinical procedures with such disorders; to stimulate exchange of information among persons and organizations thus engaged; and to disseminate such information" (American Speech and Hearing Association Directory, 1973). The association has a membership of approximately 20,000 individuals and is composed of audiologists, speech pathologists, and related professionals. The address of this association is: American Speech and Hearing Association, 9030 Old Georgetown Road, Washington, D.C. 20014.

Academy of Rehabilitative Audiology

This academy was founded in 1966 with Herbert J. Oyer serving as its first president. It meets twice each year. It was incorporated in Michigan as "... an organization of professionals dedicated to foster and stimulate professional education, research and interest in habilitative and rehabilitative programs for hearing handicapped persons" (Journal of the Academy of Rehabilitative Audiology, 1973). It has a membership of approximately 100 individuals composed of audiologists, otologists, educators of the deaf, and related professionals. Dr. Edward J. Hardick is the current president.

The address of this association changes with the election of a new president but is currently: Academy of Rehabilitative Audiology, Department of Audiology, 261 Mack Building, Wayne State University, Detroit, Michigan 48201.

American Academy of Ophthalmology and Otolaryngology

This academy was founded in 1896, with Adolph Alt serving as its first president. It meets on an annual basis and has a membership of approximately 4,150 persons composed of medical specialists in eye, ear, nose, and throat, and also associated professionals in related fields. Its statement of purpose is "... to promote and advance the science and art of medicine pertaining to the eye, ear, nose, and throat; and to encourage the study of the relationship of these specialties to surgery, general medicine, and hygiene" (American Academy of Ophthalmology and Otolaryngology Directory, 1963). The address of this association is: American Academy of Ophthalmology and Otolaryngology, 15 Second Street, S.W., Rochester, Minnesota 55901.

In addition to the national associations and organizations set up specifically to assist in the study and rehabilitation of the hearing handicapped, there are also state and local associations of audiologists, otolaryngologists, and educators of the deaf.

The principal national level groups involving the laity who are active in the affairs of the hearing handicapped are the Alexander Graham Bell Association, the National Association of Hearing and Speech Action, and the National Association of the Deaf.

Alexander Graham Bell Association

This association was first called the American Association for the Promotion of Teaching Speech to the Deaf and was set up in 1890 with Alexander Graham Bell serving as its first president, and the Volta Bureau in 1893, with the purpose of serving as a center ". . . for the increase and diffusion of knowledge relating to the deaf" (Association Report, 1974). The membership of the Alexander Graham Bell Association is diverse, including not only laity but also audiologists, educators of the deaf, otologists, and related professionals. Total members number approximately 7,000. The address of this association is: Alexander Graham Bell Association for the Deaf, Inc., 3417 Volta Place, N.W., Washington, D.C. 20007.

National Association for Speech and Hearing Action

This organization began in 1919 with Wendell C. Phillips serving as its first president. It was then called the American Association for the Hard of Hearing. Its membership is mixed with professionals and laity. Its centeral purpose ". . . is to promote the interests of persons with speech and hearing handicaps–including deafness–by means of enlightened public understanding. Stimulation of consumer advocacy, direct assistance to hearing and speech agencies, extension and upgrading of services, fostering needed social action, and launching a program of prevention" (Nation Association for Speech and Hearing Action's New Look, no date). The address of this association is: National Association for Speech and Hearing Action, 814 Thayer Avenue, Silver Spring, Maryland 20910.

National Association of the Deaf

This group consists of approximately 17,000 adult deaf individuals from various walks of life. It was started in 1925 with Robert P. McGregor serving as its first president. The objectives of this group are ". . . to serve the deaf and promote their unique needs in legislation, education, communication, health, research, taxes, rehabilitation, information on personal and family counseling and fighting discrimination in insurance and employment" (National Association of the Deaf, no date). The address of the headquarters office is: National Association of the Deaf, 814 Thayer Avenue, Silver Spring, Maryland 20910.

Some other organizations that also are related to questions concerned with hearing and/or hearing impairment are listed as follows: (1) American Board of Otolaryngology, 1301 E. Ann Street, Ann Arbor, Michigan 48104; (2) American Otological Society, Marshall-Taylor Doctors Building, Jacksonville, Florida 32200; (3) Acoustical Society of America, 335 E. 45th Street, New York, New York 10017; (4) Deafness Research Foundation, 366 Madison Avenue, New York, New York 10017; (5) National Society for Crippled Children and Adults, Inc., 2023 W. Ogden Avenue, Chicago, Illinois 60612; (6) Information Center for Hearing, Speech, and Disorders of Human Communication, 310 Harriet Lane Home, The Johns Hopkins Medical Institutions, Baltimore, Maryland 21205; and (7) The Hearing Aid Industry Conference, Suite 628, 1001 Connecticut Avenue, Washington, D.C. 20036.

PERIODICALS OF HEARING PUBLISHED IN U.S.A.

1. dsh Abstracts (Deafness Speech and Hearing Publications).
2. Journal of Speech and Hearing Disorders.
3. Journal of Speech and Hearing Research.
4. ASHA.
5. Language Speech and Hearing Services in the Schools. American Speech and Hearing Association, 9030 Old Georgetown Road, Washington, D. C. 20014.
6. Journal of the Academy of Rehabilitative Audiology, Department of Audiology, 261 Mack Building, Wayne State University, Detroit, Michigan 48201.
7. The Journal of Auditory Research, C. W. Shilling Auditory Research Center, Inc., Box N, Groton, Connecticut 06340.
8. Hearing and Speech News.
9. Washington Sounds, National Association for Hearing and Speech Action, 814 Thayer Avenue, Silver Spring, Maryland 20910.
10. The Volta Review, A. G. Bell Association, 3417 Volta Place, N. W., Washington, D. C. 20007.
11. Transactions, American Academy of Ophthalmology and Otolaryngology, 15 Second Street, S. W., Rochester, Minnesota 55901.
12. Archives of Otolaryngology. American Medical Association, 535 North Dearborn Street, Chicago, Illinois 60610.
13. American Annals of the Deaf, Convention of the American Instructors of the Deaf, Conference of Executives of American Schools of the Deaf, 5034 Wisconsin Ave., Washington, D. C. 20016.

14. The Silent Worker, National Association of the Deaf, 814 Thayer Avenue, Silver Spring, Maryland 20910.
15. Journal of American Audiology Society, The Williams & Wilkins Co., 428 E. Preston St., Baltimore, Md. 21202.

LITERATURE CITED

American Academy of Ophthalmology and Otolaryngology. 1974. Directory. Rochester, Minn.

American Annals of the Deaf. April, 1974. p. 159.

American Boards of Examiners in Speech Pathology and Audiology. 1975. Accredited training programs, education, and training board. Asha 17: 59–60.

American National Standards Institute. 1960. Criteria for background noise in audiometer rooms (S3.1-1960, R-71). New York.

American Speech and Hearing Association. 1967. A conference on hearing aid evaluation procedures. Asha Rep. No. 2: 71 p.

American Speech and Hearing Association Committee on Audiometric Evaluations, 1974.

American Speech and Hearing Association. 1973. Directory. p. VII.

American Speech and Hearing Association. 1973. Guide to clinical services in speech pathology and audiology. Author. Washington, D. C. 120 p.

American Speech and Hearing Association. 1975. Directory. Washington, D. C. 600 p.

American Speech and Hearing Association Committee on Rehabilitative Audiology, 1974.

Anderman, B. M. 1970. The Veterans Administration audiology program. *In* H. Davis and S. R. Silverman (eds.), Hearing and Deafness, pp. 449–456. 3rd Ed. Holt, Rinehart, and Winston, Inc., New York. 522 p.

Annual Survey of Hearing Impaired Children and Youth, United States. 1970–1971. March 1973. Office of Demographic Studies, Gallaudet College, Washington, D. C.

ASHA Committee on Audiometric Evaluation. 1974. Guidelines for audiometric symbols. Asha 16: 260–264.

ASHA Committee on Rehabilitative Audiology. 1974. The audiologist: Responsibilities in the habilitation of auditorily handicapped. Asha 16: 68–70.

Association Report. 1974. Volta Rev. 76: 9, 518.

Berg, F. S. 1974. Educational audiology at Utah State University. J. Acad. Rehab. Audiol. 7: 40–49.

Berger, K. W. 1970. The hearing aid: Its operation and development. National Hearing Aid Society, Detroit. 212 p.

Brantman, M. 1973. The status and outlook for commercial health insurance coverage of speech and hearing services. Asha 15: 183–187.

Brunt, M. A. 1974. The staggered spondaic work (SSW) test. *In* J. Katz (ed.), Handbook of Clinical Audiology, pp. 334–356. The Williams & Wilkins Co., Baltimore. 842 p.

Calearo, C., and A. Lazzaroni. Speech intelligibility in relation to speech of the message. Laryngoscope 67: 410–419.

Carhart, R. 1946. Tests for selection of hearing aids. Laryngoscope 56: 780–794.

Carhart, R., and J. Jerger. 1959. Preferred method for clinical determination of pure tone thresholds. J. Speech Hearing Disord. 24: 330–345.

Conklin, E. S. 1917. A method for the determination of relative skill in lipreading. Volta Rev. 19: 216–220.

Craig, W. N., and H. B. Craig. 1974. Directory of programs and services for the deaf in the United States. Am. Ann. Deaf 119: 60–285.

DiCarlo, L. M. 1964. The Deaf. Prentice-Hall, Inc., Englewood Cliffs, N.J. 149 p.

Dodds, E., and E. Harford. 1968. Application of a lipreading test in a hearing aid evaluation. J. Speech & Hearing Disorders 33: 167–173.

Dunn, L. M. 1959. Peabody Picture Vocabulary Test. American Guidance Service, Inc. Nashville, Tenn.

Dunn, L. M., and F. C. Markwardt. 1970. Peabody Individual Achievement Tests. American Guidance Service. Circle Pines, Minn.

Enelow, A., and S. Swisher. 1972. Interviewing and Patient Care. Oxford University Press, New York. 229 p.

Facts and Figures. 1973. Hearing Aid J. 27: 4.

Fulton, R., and L. Lloyd (ed.). 1969. Audiometry for the retarded. The Williams and Wilkins Co., Baltimore. 276 p.

Gaeth, J. H. 1967. Deafness in children. *In* F. McConnell and P. H. Ward (eds.), National Symposium on Deafness in Childhood, pp. 279–292. Vanderbilt University Press, Nashville. 333 p.

Garrett, A. 1942. Interviewing: Its Principles and Methods. Family Service Association of America, New York. 123 p.

Gengel, R. W., D. Pascoe, and I. Shore. 1971. A frequency response procedure for evaluating and selecting hearing aids for severely hearing impaired children. J. Speech Hear. Disord. 36: 341–353.

Goldstein, M. A. 1939. The acoustic method. The Laryngoscope Press, St. Louis. 246 p.

Guberina, P. 1964. Verbo-tonal method and its application to the rehabilitation of the deaf. Report of the Proceedings of the International Congress on Education of the Deaf and the 41st Meeting of the Convention of American Instructors of the Deaf. U. S. Document No. 106, pp. 279–293. U. S. Government Printing Office, Washington, D. C.

Harless, E. L., and R. R. Rupp. 1972. Aural rehabilitation of the elderly. J. Speech Hear. Disord. 37: 267–273.

Haskins, H. 1949. A phonetically balanced test of speech discrimination for children. Unpublished Master's thesis, Northwestern University.

Hirsh, I., H. Davis, S. R. Silverman, E. P. Reynolds, E. P. Eldert, and R. W. Benson. 1952. Development of materials for speech audiometry. J. Speech Hear. Disord. 17: 321–337.

Hodgson, W. R. 1974. Filtered speech tests. *In* J. Katz (ed.), Handbook of Clinical Audiology, pp. 313–324. The Williams and Wilkins Co., Baltimore. 842 p.

Hood, J. D. 1960. Principles and practice of bone conduction audiometry. Laryngoscope 70: 1211–1228.

House, A. S., C. E. Williams, M. H. L. Hecker, and K. D. Kryter. 1965. Articulation testing methods: Consonantal differentiation with a closed response set. J. Acoust. Soc. Am. 37: 158–166.

Hull, R. H., and R. M. Traynor. 1975. A community wide program in geriatric aural rehabilitation. Asha 17: 33–34.

Huston, N. 1969. Parents groups organize Cincinnati religious education classes for hearing impaired children. Volta Rev. 71: 2, 115–117.

Jerger, J., and J. Thelin. 1968. Effects of electroacoustic characteristics of hearing aids on speech understanding. Bull. Prosthetic Res. 11: 159–197.

Joint Committee on Audiology and Education of the Deaf. 1965. Audiology and education of the deaf. Vocational Rehabilitation Administration, Department of Health, Education, and Welfare, Washington, D. C. 171 p.

Joint Committee on Audiology and Education of the Deaf. 1975. Guidelines for audiology programs in educational settings for hearing impaired children. Asha 17: 17–20.

J. Acad. Rehab. Audiol. 1973. Back of front cover.

Kasten, R. N., and D. P. Goldstein. 1970. Present barriers to aural rehabilitation of the elderly. ARA Newsletter 3: 11–17.

Katz, J., and S. Struckman. 1972. A case history for children. *In* J. Katz (ed.), Handbook of Clinical Audiology, pp. 486–497. The Williams & Wilkins Co., Baltimore. 842 p.

Kenkel, W. F. 1973. The Family in Perspective. Prentice-Hall, Inc., Englewood Cliffs, N. J. p. 232.

Lowell, E. L. 1957. A film test of lipreading. John Tracy Research Papers. II. John Tracy Clinic, Los Angeles.

Mason, M. K. 1943. A cinematographic technique for testing visual speech comprehension. J. Speech Disord. 8: 271–278.

Matzker, J. 1959. Two new methods for the assessment of central auditory function in cases of brain disease. Ann. Otol. Rhin. Laryng. 68: 1185–1196.

McCarthy, J., and S. A. Kirk. 1961. Illinois Test of Psycholinguistic Abilities. University of Illinois Press, Urbana, Ill.

Merzenich, M. M., R. A. Schindler, and F. A. Sooy (eds.). 1974. Electrical Stimulation of the Acoustic Nerve in Man. Velo-Bend, Inc., San Francisco. 213 p.

Miller, M. H. 1973. The politics of hearing: Medicaid in New York City and the audiologist. Asha 15: 524–528.

Minnesota Public Interest Research Group. 1972. Hearing Aids and the Hearing Aid Industry in Minnesota. Minneapolis. 81 p.

Morkovin, B. V. 1947. Rehabilitation of the aurally handicapped through the study of speech reading in life situations. J. Speech Disord. 12: 363–368.

Moser, H. M., H. J. Oyer, J. J. O'Neill, and H. P. Gardner. 1960. Selection of Items for Testing Skill in Visual Recognition of One Syllable Words. The Ohio State University Development Fund Project No. 5818. Columbus.

Myatt, B. D., and B. A. Landes. 1963. Assessing discrimination loss in children. Arch. Otolaryng. 77: 359–362.
Myklebust, H. R. 1954. Auditory Disorders in Children: A Manual for Differential Diagnosis. Grune & Stratton, Inc., New York. 367 p.
Myklebust, H. R. 1965 Development and Disorders of Written Language. Vol. I. Grune & Stratton, Inc., New York. 278 p.
National Association for Speech and Hearing Action's New Look. (No date). p. 1.
National Association of the Deaf. (No date).
Newby, H. A. 1972. Audiology. 3rd Ed. Appleton-Century-Crofts, Inc., New York. 421 p.
Nitchie, E. B. 1917. Tests for determining skill in lipreading. Volta Rev. 19: 222–223.
Northcott, W. H. (ed.). 1973. The Hearing Impaired Child in a Regular Classroom: Preschool, Elementary, and Secondary Years. The Alexander Graham Bell Association for the Deaf, Inc., Washington, D. C. 301 p.
Northern, J. L. 1968. Military opportunities in speech pathology and audiology. Asha 10: 325–330.
Northern, J. L., and M. P. Downs. 1974. Hearing in Children. The Williams & Wilkins Co., Baltimore. 341 p.
Obermann, C. 1965. A History of Vocational Rehabilitation in America. T. S. Denison, Inc., Minneapolis. 389 p.
O'Neill, J. J. 1974. The school-educational audiologist. J. Acad. Rehab. Audiol. 7: 31–39.
O'Neill, J. J., and H. J. Oyer. 1961. Visual Communication for the Hard of Hearing. Prentice-Hall, Inc., Englewood Cliffs, N. J. 163 p.
Oyer, E. J., and B. Paolucci. 1970. Homemaker's hearing losses and family integration. J. Home Econ. 62: 3, 257–262.
Oyer, H. J. 1966. Auditory Communication for the Hard-of-Hearing. Prentice-Hall, Inc., Englewood Cliffs, N.J.
Oyer, H. J., and J. P. Frankmann. 1975. The Aural Rehabilitation Process, A Conceptual Framework Analysis. Holt, Rinehart, and Winston, New York. 260 p.
Oyer, H. J., Y. P. Kapur, and L. V. Deal. 1976. Hearing Disorders in the Aging: Effects upon Communication. *In* H. J. Oyer and E. J. Oyer (eds.), Aging and Communication. University Park Press, Baltimore.
Oyer, H. J., and E. J. Oyer (eds.). 1976. Aging and Communication. University Park Press, Baltimore.
Peet, H. P. 1852. Tribute to the memory of the late Thomas Gallaudet. Am. Ann. Deaf 4: 65–67.
Pollack, D. 1970. Educational Audiology for the Limited Hearing Infant. Charles C Thomas, Publisher, Springfield, Ill. 237 p.
Public Interest Research Group in Michigan. 1973. You Know I Can't Hear You When the Cash Register's Running: The Hearing Aid Industry in Michigan. Lansing, Mich. 59 p.
Quiros, J. B. 1964. Accelerated speech audiometry. Trans. Beltone Instit. Hearing Res. 17: 5–40.
Rae, L. 1851. Thomas Braidwood. Am. Ann. Deaf 3: 255–256.

Rainer, J. D., K. Z. Altshuler, F. J. Kallman, W. E. Deming (eds.). 1963. Family and Mental Health Problems in a Deaf Population, pp. 14–15. New York State Psychiatric Institute, Columbia University, New York.
Reid, G. 1947. A preliminary investigation in the testing of lipreading achievement. J. Speech Disord. 12: 77–82.
Report of the Proceedings of the 42nd Meeting of the Convention of the American Instructors of the Deaf. 1965. P. VI, Washington, D.C.
Retired Professional Action Group. 1973. Paying through the Ear: A Report on Hearing Health Care Problems. Public Citizen, Inc., Washington, D. C.
Robinson, D. O., and J. H. Gaeth. 1975. A procedure for testing and training pre-linguistic hearing-impaired children. Volta Rev. 77: 249–254.
Rosenberg, P. E. 1972. Case history: The first test. *In* J. Katz (ed.), Handbook of Clinical Audiology, pp. 60–66. The Williams & Wilkins Co., Baltimore. 842 p.
Sanders, J. W. 1972. Masking. *In* J. Katz (ed.), Handbook of Clinical Audiology, pp. 111–142. The Williams & Wilkins Co., Baltimore. 842 p.
Shore, I., R. C. Bilger, and I. Hirsh. 1960. Hearing aid evaluation: Reliability of repeated measurements. J. Speech Hear. Disord. 25: 152–170.
Shore, I., and J. C. Kramer. 1963. A comparison of two procedures for hearing aid evaluation. J. Speech Hear. Disord. 28: 159–170.
Siegenthaler, B., and G. Haspiel. 1966. Development of Two Standardized Measures of Hearing for Speech by Children. Penn State University Press, University Park, Pa.
Somers, A. R. 1971. Health Care Transition: Directions for the Future. Hospital Research and Educational Trust, Chicago. 176 p.
Subcommittee on Hearing Aids, ASHA Ethical Practices Board. 1974. EPB statement concerning hearing aid dispensing as related to the ASHA Code of Ethics. Asha 16: 618–624.
Tillman, T. W., and J. Jerger. 1959. Some factors affecting the spondee threshold in normal hearing subjects. J. Speech Hear. Res. 2: 141–146.
Utley, J. 1946. Factors involved in the teaching and testing of lipreading ability through the use of motion pictures. Volta Rev. 48: 657–659.
Veterans Administration. 1974. Hearing aid performance measurement data and hearing aid selection procedure. U. S. Government Printing Office, Washington. 432 p.
Warren, L. E. 1895. Defective Speech and Deafness. Edgar Werner, New York.
Zerlin, S. 1962. A new approach to hearing aid selection. J. Speech Hear. Res. 5: 370–376.

chapter 4

Communication for Hearing-handicapped People in Canada

Bryan R. Clarke, Ph.D.,
and David C. Kendall, Ph.D.

Canada is a large country (3,851,809 square miles; second only in size to the U.S.S.R.) with a small population currently estimated at 22,446,000 (Statistics Canada, 1974). It is bilingual, with both French and English as official languages. Although the majority of the almost 6,000,000 French-speaking Canadians live in the Province of Quebec, there are sizable Francophone minorities in Ontario, Manitoba, and New Brunswick. Since World War II, immigration has contributed significantly to the increase in the total population, with immigrants coming from all over the world, especially from Europe and the Far East. In Metropolitan areas such as Toronto and Vancouver there are now large numbers of families for whom neither English nor French is their mother tongue.

Canada was first settled by the French in 1605 and by the English in Newfoundland, then a separate colony, in 1610. The first citizens of the country, the Canadian Indians, though decimated by war, disease, and other civilizing influences of the white man's culture, have survived, along with the Eskimos, to add yet another dimension to the country's cultural melange. The rights of some Canadian Indians are protected by treaty and through the establishment of land reserved for their sole use and services provided by the government.

With its vast natural resources, Canada is a rich country, but dependent to a large extent upon its export of raw materials. In its development of secondary and tertiary industries, it has tended to become closely related to, and heavily dependent upon, the United States. Economically the two countries are, thus, very closely linked.

Politically and administratively there are three levels of government—federal, provincial, and local, with elected assemblies or parliaments at the federal and provincial levels and elected councils and boards at the local level. At the federal level, the parliamentary system resembles the English model, with an upper (appointed) house and a lower (elected) house. The government is usually formed from the majority party in the elected house. There is also an elected assembly in each of the 10 provinces; their governments are formed in much the same way. In addition, there are two territories (Yukon and Northwest Territories) where the administrative arrangements are somewhat different.

Very broadly speaking, the federal government has the right to impose taxation on all the country's inhabitants, goods, and services, and has the responsibility for foreign affairs, defense, communications, and certain aspects of programs in health, welfare, manpower, etc. The provincial governments have responsibility for education and justice and for the administration of health and welfare services. They also have the right to impose direct and indirect taxation. In many areas, apart from education, where provincial responsibility is practically absolute, the effective administration of services requires a close working relationship between the various levels of government; while this does not always occur, and there are many areas of disagreement, there are provisions for consultation and discussion at all levels.

In relation to services for the hearing impaired (e.g., education, health, and welfare) and to the control of professionals working with the hearing impaired, much of the responsibility of government, as we shall see, has to be exercised at the provincial level; apart from the federal research-granting agencies and manpower services, there are few areas in this field where the federal government has any direct responsibility. However, it should be noted that many programs operated by provincial governments (e.g., day care) are in part federally funded and depend for their support upon a cost-sharing formula between the two or even three levels of government.

It is not, therefore, surprising to find that there are very great differences between provinces in respect of what is being done for the hearing impaired by provincial governments. Much the same applies to voluntary organizations serving the handicapped which, in the past, have tended to be weak or nonexistent at the national level, but to be much stronger at the provincial or, in some cases, at the local level.

PERSONAL STATEMENT BY THE AUTHORS

The writers of this chapter combine training in clinical and educational psychology, audiology, and education of the hearing impaired with experience of working in clinics, schools, and classes, and with teacher training in the United Kingdom, Australia, and Canada. Although the bulk of our experience has been with hearing-impaired children, both of us have also been involved in services to organizations concerned with the adult hearing impaired.

Because of our graduate training, our philosophical basis with respect to methods of communication might well have remained strongly aural-oral. However, we feel that it would be to deny reality if we were to ignore other methods which are employed widely and with some success in schools for the deaf and sometimes exclusively among the adult deaf. We have come to realize the importance of remaining open minded about methods of communication with and among a population as diverse as the hearing impaired, sharing as they do only one common identifying characteristic, that of difficulty in the reception and expression of spoken language.

No one would propose one method of teaching the "hearing" nor indeed one method of teaching in a subject area such as language arts and reading. We, therefore, find it difficult to see one method of communication as best suiting all hearing-impaired children and reject the notion that educational programs must be conducted on an exclusive basis. Similarly we believe that services for the adult hearing impaired must be conducted by means of the method of communication which best fits the individual's skills, needs, and wishes.

We have, therefore, tried to adopt an eclectic approach to aural rehabilitation and to give equal weight to the various approaches and techniques that may be required by the different needs and the unique development and background of each hearing-impaired individual. This has been the philosophy underlying our own development of a training program for teachers of the deaf at the University of British Columbia (see section entitled "The Training of Professionals and Paraprofessionals"). It is also our hope that the pressing need of the hearing impaired for emotional and intellectual security and socioeconomic emancipation will indeed direct the fuller study of all methods of communication and that hearing-impaired children especially will not continue to serve as pawns in the chess game of opposing methodologies.

DEFINITION OF AURAL REHABILITATION

It had escaped our attention until now that authors of articles and books on auditory rehabilitation appear to have avoided or met with difficulties in defining this term.

We see aural rehabilitation as the alleviation of the physiological and psychological problems associated with hearing impairment—in other words, the steps taken to ensure prevention and therapy of aural disability affecting the developmental, social, and occupational well being of a hearing-impaired individual. In this holistic yet multifaceted approach, we must consider the principles and procedures to improve receptive and expressive verbal and nonverbal communication. We must concern ourselves also with information processing, acoustic phonetics, linguistics, the acquisition of language, perception, and kinesics to name but a few. The tools we have to consider are appropriate utilization of residual hearing through amplification, speech, speechreading, fingerspelling, sign language, and language teaching. The personnel who must be consulted include educators, psychologists, physicians, psychiatrists, physical scientists, audiologists, speech pathologists, and the hearing impaired themselves. The settings would include the classroom, the clinic, the laboratory, the work field, the community, and the home.

Throughout this chapter we will refer to the "hearing impaired" as a generic term for all degrees of hearing loss. We do not wish to propose hard and fast educational or other criteria for "deaf" or "hard of hearing" because the many variables involved make this impractical as well as open to lengthy debate. For our purpose we have used a social criterion for "deaf," namely, that everyday auditory communication is impossible or nearly so and the individual relies on visual input and a manual or written form to express himself. The hard-of-hearing individual, on the other hand, obtains various amounts of benefit from audition and speechreading and communicates orally. The "deafened" refers to an individual who loses part or all of his hearing after the natural acquisition of speech and language.

EDUCATIONAL PROGRAMS FOR HEARING-IMPAIRED CHILDREN

Education in Canada is, as we have stated, a provincial, not a federal, responsibility. Each of the 10 provinces and two territories has its own school system, which in the provinces is based upon educational legislation. Apart from a few schools and institutions controlled directly by a provincial department (for example, the provincial schools for the deaf), the administration of schools is carried out through local school boards, each of which is responsible for a school district. These local districts are funded by a combination of property taxes and grants from the provincial government; the formula varies from province to province. There are important differences between provinces with respect to both legislation and organization, so that, although there are obvious commonalities, it is difficult to generalize about Canadian education. It is important to remember that Canada is officially and historically a bilingual country and that there are both French- and English-speaking schools for the deaf. The educational systems of the provinces have been differently affected by a variety of foreign influences—especially the school systems of France, Britain, and the United States—and these influences are apparent even in such a specialized field as education of the hearing impaired. In some provinces (e.g., Quebec), public education reflects not only the language spoken by the family, but also the family's religious affiliation; in both Newfoundland and Quebec, school districts may, thus, be organized on a denominational base. In other provinces support from the public purse for denominational schools varies considerably.

In recent years there has been a large influx of immigrants from a variety of countries and linguistic backgrounds. This has given a new dimension to bilingualism. In a recent survey in Vancouver, British Columbia, it was shown that almost 40% of elementary school children had some language other than English or French as their mother tongue. This extreme diversity in language is more common in the metropolitan areas; it poses problems not only for the general educator, but also, and perhaps especially, for the educator of hearing-impaired children.

The only areas of education in which there has been a tradition of federal responsibility are those pertaining to the children of personnel in the armed forces and to native Indian and Eskimo children. However, in neither case has this been extended to the operation of special education programs for the hearing impaired: the federal government does, however, pay fees in schools for the deaf for children under its jurisdiction. Recently the outline of administrative responsibilities has become more blurred, through federal funding of welfare programs which have brought nonteaching personnel into day care and, in some instances, school programs, including many preschools and special services for the handicapped.

All 10 provinces have some form of legislated responsibility for the education of deaf children and, in each province except for Prince Edward Island, there is now at least one school for the deaf, including the school shared by New Brunswick and Nova Scotia. In the past the pattern was for provinces with schools for the deaf to share this resource with provinces without such a school, largely by means of fee-paying agreements. There are still examples of this today; indeed the Atlantic Provinces (Nova Scotia, New Brunswick, Newfoundland, and Prince Edward Island) have recently established an Interprovincial Special Education Authority concerned with the development and operation of educational programs for the severely handicapped (including the hearing impaired) in the four provinces (Statutes of Nova Scotia, 1974).

Provincial responsibilities for the hard of hearing (as opposed to the deaf) are less clearly defined; Canadian provinces have not established separate and distinctive educational categories such as those found in the

English system. There are marked differences between provinces with respect to school programs for hearing-impaired children operated under the jurisdiction of school districts. In some provinces (e.g., British Columbia), it is possible to see over the past 15 years a gradual development of special classes for the hearing impaired and especially for the hard of hearing within the local school system that are independent of the provincial school for the deaf, whereas, in other provinces (e.g., Nova Scotia and New Brunswick), these local provisions have developed with direct funding and control from the Interprovincial School for the Deaf.

Early History: Nineteenth Century Developments

The first Canadian school for the deaf was founded in 1848 by Monseigneur I. Bourget in the community of Mile-End in Montreal. This school for French deaf boys, the Institution Catholique des Sourds-Muets, was under the jurisdiction of the Community of Clerics of St. Viator and was supported by this organization, as well as by fees and by charitable donations. At first the manual system was used for instruction, but, after the Milan Conference, this was replaced by the oral system. Instruction was normally in French, but boys with English-speaking parents could be taught in English. The curriculum followed that of the French schools in Quebec, with a strong vocational emphasis. In 1851 Sister Marie de Bonsecours started a small school for French deaf girls in the same city, financed by the Sisters of Charity of Providence and by fees and charitable donations. This school was also manual at first; oral methods were introduced toward the end of the 19th century, following a visit by the school's resident chaplain to schools for the deaf in Europe. A third Montreal school, the Protestant Institution for Deaf-Mutes, opened in 1869 with an enrollment of 16 pupils. The first principal, Thomas Widd, was a resident of Montreal who had taught deaf children in England. Teaching at this school (which, like the other Montreal schools, was residential) was exclusively manual. Although there was a demand for places, the school struggled for existence for several years until a local citizen, Joseph Mackay, came to its rescue by donating land, buildings, an endowment, and his own services to the Board of Management. The school was renamed the Mackay Institution for Protestant Deaf-Mutes after its re-opening in new buildings in 1877. Like the other Montreal schools, it was partially dependent upon fees and charitable donations for its support; it also received an educational grant from the Quebec government. Between 1884 and 1914 the school also admitted blind pupils; at various times in the present century it has admitted substantial groups of children from other provinces, notably Newfoundland, New Brunswick, and Alberta, and now also contains a program for crippled children.

Meanwhile, residential schools for the deaf had been opened in two other provinces. The School for the Deaf in Halifax, Nova Scotia, which had opened in 1856, grew out of the spare time teaching activities of a deaf man, William Gray. Up to this time, a few children from the Maritimes had been sent to the school for the deaf at Hartford, Connecticut. Gray, however, was concerned with trying to teach a small number of deaf children who had received no education. His efforts prompted support from influential citizens to start a school. The first principal of the Nova Scotia school, James Scott Hutton, was brought out from England to take charge of the new program; he was accompanied by his father, who worked without salary. Funds to support the school were raised in the community and were assisted by the efforts of the principal, who took selected students from the school on tour and displayed their talents at public meetings before passing a hat among the onlookers. Grants-in-aid were obtained from the provincial governments of Nova Scotia in 1857, New Brunswick in 1860, Prince Edward Island in 1866, and from the then Crown Colony of Newfoundland in 1877. The school, however, remained a private corporation, administered by a Board of Managers, until it was replaced more than 100 years later by the Interprovincial School for the Deaf. It moved into new buildings in 1895, at which time there were 80 pupils enrolled, at a fee of $150 per year per child.

The first class for deaf children in Ontario was established in Toronto in 1858 by J. B. McGann, an Irish grammar school teacher. Much interest was aroused by his efforts and, after some pressure from physicians and other professional people and by McGann himself, the Ontario Institution for the Education of the Deaf and Dumb was eventually opened in October 1870 in Belleville, on the north shore of the Bay of Quinte. The initial enrollment for this residential school was quite large—107 pupils; financial support was derived from fees, from the municipalities, and, in the case of indigent children, from the provincial government.

Apart from a fourth Quebec school for the deaf—the school at Ste. Marie, Beauce, which had a brief and poorly documented existence in the 1880's—the only other 19th century Canadian school for the deaf was the Manitoba School for the Deaf. This, the first school for the deaf to be operated by a provincial government, opened at Brampton in 1875, and was relocated at Tuxedo, near Winnipeg, in 1889. The Brampton school looked after deaf children from the Northwest Territories, as well as from Manitoba. Like other Canadian schools of this era, the methods of instruction were initially manual, but later changed to oral.

Seven schools for the deaf were thus opened in Canada between 1848 and 1885. Three of these were French-speaking schools. Only one school started with full government financial support; by the end of the century the six schools still in existence were all receiving some public financial support for their operation, although this took different forms in the four provinces. Both religious organizations and secular fund raising had played a significant part in initiating and maintaining the schools. They were all predominantly residential schools; yet all, except for one, were situated in or near large centers of population. Instructional methods in all schools were manual at first, but, by the end of the century, most of them had become wholly or partially oral. A few teachers of the deaf had been imported from other countries; in a country as vast, as undeveloped, and as isolated as Canada, a great deal of responsibility for the development of these early programs must have been laid on the shoulders of the few experienced teachers. Actual records are sparse and poorly documented and are mostly in the form of statistics of attendance interspersed with anecdotal comments. It is interesting to note that five of these seven schools are still in operation today.

BACKGROUND OF CURRENT EDUCATIONAL PROGRAMS FOR THE HEARING IMPAIRED

Later Developments in Residential Schools

No new schools for the deaf in Canada were constructed for almost 50 years after the opening of the Manitoba school. As the railways spanned the prairies and eventually crossed the Rockies, the population of the country west of Winnipeg began to expand, and the provinces of Saskatchewan, Alberta, and British Columbia were established. However, it was not until 1915 that the Vancouver School Board established its first day class for deaf children at Mount Pleasant School and not until 1920 that the British Columbia provincial school for the deaf was opened in the city of Vancouver under the superintendency of C. H. Lawrence. The day classes operated by the school board had been taught orally under the direction of Mr. Hobson, a teacher of the deaf trained in England. When Lawrence came from the Halifax School for the Deaf, he brought with him the methods currently used in Halifax—oral teaching in the classrooms, fingerspelling and signs after school hours. The new school for the deaf accepted pupils from outside the city, but, because of shortage of residential accommodation, these pupils were placed in foster homes. In 1922 buildings became available at the former Boy's Industrial Home on what were then the outskirts of Vancouver; the school for the deaf, together with the school for the blind, was moved into this site, both schools coming under the superintendency of Lawrence.

Before the opening of the Vancouver classes and the British Columbia school, the deaf children from British Columbia had been sent to the Manitoba school for the deaf, where they had been taught manually. For the benefit of readers unfamiliar with the geography of Canada, some of these children had to travel more than 1,500 miles to go to school. Children from Alberta and Saskatchewan were also sent to the Manitoba school, although, when the Manitoba government increased the fees in 1914, the Saskatchewan government decided to start a school of its own and opened this the following year in the old legislative buildings, under the superintendency of Thomas Rodwell, who had taught at Belleville before moving to the school for the deaf in Faribault, Minnesota. The school quickly became overcrowded and closed in 1916, with its pupils returning to Manitoba. It was not until 1932 that the Saskatchewan provincial school for the deaf was finally built in Saskatoon, largely as a result of the efforts of two men, R. J. D. Williams, a deaf resident, and G. M. Donald, Chief of Police in Saskatoon, the father of two deaf daughters. This new school, established under the superintendency of E. G. Peterson, who had been trained in the United States, had some oral and some manual classes and used the combined system of communication out of school hours. The staff included some deaf teachers and supervisors. During the 1940's, however, there was a determined effort to make the school purely oral. As a result, the deaf teachers and supervisors left. The size of the school had been considerably increased by the closing, during World War II, of the Manitoba School for the Deaf. Some Manitoba children, and eventually many Alberta children (who had for a while attended the Mackay School in Montreal, another formidable journey), helped to fill the Saskatoon school. Alberta children remained at the Saskatchewan school until 1956 when, after long agitation by the Calgary and Edmonton Association for the Deaf, a new provincial school was opened in Edmonton.

Meanwhile in Manitoba the buildings of the provincial school at Tuxedo had been taken over by the Air Force at the outbreak of war in 1939. Children from the towns and rural Manitoba were placed in the Saskatoon school, while children from Winnipeg were sent to day classes for the deaf instituted by the Manitoba government in one of the public schools in Winnipeg. By the end of the war, the number of these classes had grown but they were still occupying space in the school system. The Tuxedo site had been reclaimed, but was immediately turned into a teacher training college. So the residential children continued in the Saskatoon school and the day classes remained in Winnipeg, eventually being located in a separate, oral day school in 1958. The Manitoba school for the deaf has only recently been reestablished at its original Tuxedo site.

The Belleville school buildings also suffered the inroads of the military during World War II, and the pupils were scattered throughout the city community at this time. During the period of the war many day classes for the deaf had been set up in several of the larger population centers of Ontario, and, in view of their success, the Ontario government considered closing the Belleville school and replacing it with a day class system. This proposal brought a storm of protest, especially from organizations of the adult deaf, but also from a number of professionals in the field. As a result, the government's proposal was modified, and the school was re-opened and substantially reorganized. Subsequently, a second residential school for the deaf was opened at Milton in 1963 and a third school at London in 1972.

In the Atlantic provinces, children from Prince Edward Island and Newfoundland had for a long time been sent to the Halifax School for the Deaf. However, in 1958, the Newfoundland government withdrew its deaf children from the old, crowded Halifax school and arranged to send them to the Mackay School in Montreal, with the Newfoundland Kinsmen Club at first paying the school fees, although later the government took over this responsibility. This arrangement was initially planned for at least 3 years while a decision was being made about establishing a school for the deaf in Newfoundland. Eventually this school was started in temporary ex-Air Force buildings at Torbay, St. John's, where it remains today; until it was opened, some Newfoundland children continued at the Mackay School, and others were placed in the new Interprovincial School at Amherst, Nova Scotia. The Interprovincial School was opened in 1961 by the two provinces of Nova Scotia and New Brunswick by means of legislation covering a cost-sharing agreement, joint participation in the board of management, and the winding up of the old Halifax School for the Deaf (Nova Scotia Laws, 1960).

Finally, deaf children from Prince Edward Island were accommodated in a small day program in Charlottetown, attached to an ordinary school. Children who could not travel daily to this school were boarded in foster homes during the week.

By the early 1970's, there were, therefore, 14 schools for the deaf in Canada, offering some kind of residential program in every province, including the Interprovincial School serving Nova Scotia and New Brunswick and the small program in Charlottetown, P.E.I. Apart from the Interprovincial School, which represented a deliberate effort at regional planning, there was, thus, an end of the wholesale practice of shipping children from one province to another according to the availability of places, although this still occurs in individual cases and at a tertiary level. The only exceptions were the Northwest Territories and the Yukon, neither of which had a school for the deaf and both of which were still forced to send children to the British Columbia School (renamed the Jericho Hill School in 1956) and to the new school in Edmonton. Five of these 14 schools could trace their history back for 100 years or more. During this time there had been many changes, not only in the development of the provincial school systems but also in the theory and practice of teaching deaf children and in the acceptance of public responsibility for the education of the handicapped. Except for the Quebec schools, which were largely government supported, all schools for the deaf were fully controlled by their provincial governments. As was noted in the section entitled "Educational Programs for Hearing-Impaired Children," the older schools were all originally manual, but gradually adopted an oral approach, at least in most classrooms, while maintaining a strong tradition of manual communication outside the classroom or, in some schools, in the senior classes. For the most part, the newer schools adopted the same pattern. Undoubtedly there were significant differences between schools–some employed deaf teachers and supervisory staff; others did not. Some were more aggressively oral; others, in practice, relied more on manual communication. The ratio of day students to residential students also varied widely. There is no point in detailing these interschool differences, except to point out that the documentary evidence suggests that, up to the mid-1960s at least, official policies and attitudes in virtually all schools reflected a kind of double standard, in which oralism and oral teaching were encouraged officially and practiced in most classrooms while manualism was permitted in some classrooms and in out-of-school activities.

Alternatives to Residential Schools

Not everyone was satisfied with this kind of compromise. Moreover, not every parent wanted to send his child to a residential school, nor to a segregated school, nor to a school where there was little distinction between the needs of deaf children and those of the hard of hearing. Some parents felt strongly that their hearing-impaired child should have an exclusively oral education and were dissatisfied with what the traditional schools had to offer. These parents were often encouraged by the views of other professionals, such as otologists, audiologists, speech and hearing therapists, and psychologists, who had become involved with clinical, diagnostic, and parent counseling services, and with programs directed toward preschool children. Technical advances in communication science brought about during World War II had begun to revolutionize hearing aids and had brought far greater sophistication to the accurate measurement of hearing. Armed with these tools, a small army of "new" professionals began to encroach on the hitherto esoteric and remote world of education of the deaf, often with very different ideas about what needed to be done.

One of the sticks with which the new professionals belabored the schools was the comparative failure of the traditional residential school for the deaf to produce adequate standards of speech communication in its pupils. Another was the comparative neglect by many schools of the children's residual hearing. Signing and fingerspelling were often seen as unnatural, abnormal, and objectionable modes of communication, and their acquisition was viewed as a fate from which hearing-impaired children must, if at all possible, be saved. By contrast, there was optimism about the chances of successful acquisition of speech and oral communication skills, provided that auditory stimulation was begun early enough and provided that hearing-impaired children were given frequent opportunities to mix with hearing, talking children.

Ironically, schools for the deaf, as they struggled to accommodate to these new ideas, came under increased fire from deaf adults, and from organizations concerned with the deaf, for failing to teach manual communication skills adequately or systematically to these same pupils. Organizations for the deaf had been expressing these concerns for a good many years. In Canada, as in other countries, it is probably true to say that, as long as they were the views of the deaf, they were ignored or undervalued by many teachers and other professionals. But when these same views began to be put forward by reputable professionals who were not deaf, they became not only easier to accept, but actually in vogue. Since about 1968, the emergence of total communication, that is, the use of all methods of communication in teaching deaf children, as a respectable educational philosophy, has been little less than dramatic: 10 years earlier its adoption would have seemed inconceivable.

In the brief review that follows, it is impossible to present a detailed discussion of all these influences and their implications. What we have tried to do is to pick out what have seemed to us to be some of the key developments affecting the education of hearing-impaired children in Canada. Many, but not all, of these have taken place outside the orbit of the traditional residential schools.

Day Schools and Classes

In the preceding section it was pointed out that from time to time circumstances had led to the adoption of a day school model in the provision of teaching programs for the deaf. In the first program in Vancouver, for example, the children lived in the city, as no residential accommodation was available. During the war years, the loss of residential accommodation forced the schools in Manitoba and Ontario to develop some day class services. Even during the nineteenth century, the first steps toward providing a school for the deaf were often taken through a small group gathered together for daily instruction. And in the period that was reviewed above, most but not all residential schools offered places to some day children, although in some schools this option seems to have been discouraged by school staff, especially for older children, on the grounds of the social advantages of recreational and extracurricular activities planned specifically for the deaf.

Ontario was the first province in Canada in which there were systematic and deliberate attempts to provide day classes or schools for the deaf (Toronto in 1924, Ottawa in 1928, Toronto again in 1943, and Hamilton in 1944). Eventually the Metropolitan Toronto Board established a large day school for deaf children, which opened in its present site (half of the Davisville Junior School) in 1964 and which was associated with a large number of classes in elementary and secondary schools for both deaf and hard-of-hearing children. This school emphasizes an oral approach and makes a deliberate attempt to integrate hearing-impaired children within ordinary school programs wherever practicable. The Toronto Board has also begun to follow a decentralized program of day services for the hearing impaired, thus keeping the numbers of pupils at the Metro Toronto School for the Deaf at a stable level.

During the 1960s, a number of school boards across Canada, faced with increasing parental pressure, began to assume some responsibility for the provision of educational services for hearing-impaired children. These services included not only special classes but also resource and itinerant teachers, preschool classes, speech therapists, and, in some instances, specialized facilities and hardware such as hearing aids and loop induction systems. At first these services were restricted to the metropolitan areas, but they have gradually—and in a piecemeal and uneven way—begun to spread to smaller communities.

It is difficult to collect accurate statistical information about these local programs. Even special classes are not always listed in provincial, let alone national, reports, and services such as those of itinerant teachers of the deaf tend to become lost altogether in statistical summaries. However, it would appear that at least three distinctive types of programs were developed in public school settings, mostly after 1960. These may be briefly characterized as follows:

1. Special classes for hard-of-hearing children, often organized on the basis of the partial or gradual integration of the hearing-impaired children into the ordinary school, operating predominantly at the elementary level, but sometimes extending to the secondary level. Teaching methods are mainly or exclusively oral.
2. Special classes for deaf children, functioning more as separate, detached special classes, although sometimes permitting a degree of integration; essentially an alternative to special school placement; teaching methods may be oral or combined.
3. Special services (lipreading, auditory training, speech therapy, speech teaching, tutoring, remediation, and counseling) made available to hearing-impaired children on an individual or small group basis.

Some special classes for deaf children (i.e., type 2), while located in a public school, are actually administered by a school for the deaf. Off campus classes of this type have been operated in the Vancouver Schools by the provincial school for the deaf since 1953 and in several Maritime communities by the Interprovincial School since 1969. In each case the school for the deaf controls entry into the program, supplies the teacher and the teaching materials (including the hardware), and provides supervision and supportive resources, while the school district provides the classroom and the physical facilities of the school. Sometimes the local school's part amounts to little more than this (Cory, 1959), although there are examples of a more dynamic relationship between host school and special class (Kendall, 1971). Cory and Kendall, in reviewing the Jericho Hill and Interprovincial School programs respectively, both draw attention to the delicate questions of divided administrative responsibilities and staff loyalties in this situation. It should be noted that the Jericho Hill School program is restricted to children at an intermediate level, and to classes situated at most only a few miles from the school, whereas the Interprovincial School program covers a wide age range, a large geographical area, and is part of a deliberate policy of decentralization. Over the past 3 years the out classes at the Interprovincial School have become more responsive to local administration and direction, again as part of the school's policy (Interprovincial School for the Deaf Annual Reports).

Much of the early impetus for these special classes in the public schools, including those operated by schools for the deaf (Cory, 1959), seems to have come from direct parental pressure on the local school districts or upon the institutions themselves rather than from a deliberate expression of policy on the part of the boards. Certainly there appears to have been a close relationship between the activity and attitude of the parent groups and the development of these services in particular areas. In the case of hard-of-hearing children, it is easy to understand why parents were reluctant to send their children to schools for the deaf where there was seldom specific provision for hard-of-hearing children. In the case of deaf children, the reasons advanced by parent groups in their briefs to school boards included the following: (1) to ensure that the child was taught orally; (2) to avoid having to send the child away from home; and (3) to give the deaf child access to hearing companions and a hearing society. Our personal experience of parent counseling suggests that some parents, at least, were readier to accept for their children a special class in an ordinary school than what seemed to be a more socially unacceptable placement in a special school and that, for a few parents (especially of severely or profoundly deaf children), this solution to the child's educational placement may have partly reflected their own denial of the severity of his disability. Since about 1970, and particularly since the publication of the report of the Commission on Emotional and Learning Disorders in Children (1970), the climate of opinion in most provinces has tended to support integrated rather than segregated placements for all handicapped children. The rapid growth in recent years of special arrangements for hearing-impaired children in ordinary schools probably reflects a significant change in official social policy rather than an increase in parental pressure.

One factor which may well have helped to delay the development of public school services for hearing-impaired children is an economic one. In all provinces provincial financial responsibility for the education of deaf children was mandated legislatively long before the moral (or mandatory) responsibility of the school district to provide special services was recognized. As we have seen, provincially funded services for hearing-impaired children were set up in many provinces in the 19th century. As long as provincial governments were willing to provide and pay for these, and taxpaying parents willing to accept provincially funded services, there was little incentive to school districts to take on this additional burden.

School district administrators have also argued against the creation of highly specialized services such as those required by the deaf on the grounds that there was no one on the district staff qualified to supervise a teacher of the deaf. Clearly this presents a more serious problem to systems with a rigid, vertical hierarchy than to those with a more flexible, lateral organization. This problem is compounded by the lack of universally accepted qualifications for a teacher of the deaf. In no province could these be said to be rigorous, and in most provinces there is no specialist requirement whatsoever. From the information available to us, it seems that at least one-third of those teaching the hearing impaired in provincial and school board programs in Canada are untrained and do not have specialist qualifications as teachers of the deaf. Once again, there are widespread interprovincial variations; for example, almost all Ontario teachers of the deaf are trained.

The total number of children in residential schools for the deaf in 1975 expressed as a percentage of the age-relevant population was 0.028%. This figure may be compared with the percentage in 1950 of 0.034%. The relative decline in enrollments in residential schools is uneven across the country. As might be expected, there are significant interprovincial variations. But taken in combination with the incomplete figures for children attending special classes in public schools and the unknown number of hearing-impaired children receiving other kinds of service in the public school, there is some evidence to support the growing importance of the public schools in providing educational services for the hearing impaired. We cannot, of course, show from these figures how many of the children who would have been in a school for the deaf are now in a public school program nor how many who are now being served by special programs would not have received help under the earlier provisions. Nor, for that matter, can we do more than speculate about the number of children now in schools for the deaf who, in earlier years, might have been excluded from school altogether (Bunch, 1973). It cannot then be argued purely from the statistics of enrollment that there has been a substantial move toward integration of hearing-impaired children within regular schools, although examination of the programs themselves suggests that this has begun to take place. Even if this has happened, we do not have a clear or comprehensive picture of the nature of this integration, nor of its quality. As Cory pointed out in 1959, with respect ot the Jericho Hill School program, merely housing a class of deaf children in a public school does not ensure their acceptance. This area cries out for careful evaluative research.

Oral Schools for the Deaf

Although all of the provincial schools had at one time or another declared themselves to be at least partially oral, none had found it possible to offer a totally oral program. Cory's description of Jericho Hill School in 1958 is probably representative of the situation at that period. She describes an elementary division where all teaching was oral, an intermediate division where fingerspelling was allowed, and a senior division "where signs and fingerspelling were needed" (Cory, 1959, p. 56). Some parents were dissatisfied with a situation where they felt that oral education was neither being prosecuted with sufficient vigor nor at a sufficiently early age. A group of 10 English-speaking parents of hearing-impaired children in Montreal formed an organization later known as Education for Hearing Handicapped Children Incorporated, gained some public and financial support, and in 1950 started a small oral preschool program with six deaf children and one teacher. In 1957 the school was renamed the Montreal Oral School and, in the following year, reported an enrolment of 32 pupils and four teachers. The school was by now receiving support from the Protestant School Board in the shape of classroom space and the salary of one teacher and was offering a program for both elementary and preschool children and a parent guidance program.

About 10 years after the opening of the Montreal Oral School, a rather similar development took place in Vancouver. The Society for Hearing Handicapped Children, a group consisting largely of parents of young hearing-impaired children, most of whom had been closely associated with the speech and hearing clinic at the Health Center for Children, took over the preschool which had been started by the clinic, and relocated it at the Sunny Hill Hospital, under the direction of a former teacher at Jericho Hill School. The small program quickly outgrew the space at the hospital and the funds available to operate it, despite assistance from the provincial department of education relayed through the Jericho Hill School budget. Eventually the preschool was located in new premises and renamed the Vancouver Oral Centre; classes for school age hearing-impaired children were organized in a nearby public school, and an extensive parent guidance program was continued. The teaching program at the Centre and in the public schools is fully supported by provincial grants. In the 1974–1975 year the enrollment had climbed to 29 in the preschool, seven in the school age classes, with 14 on a home training program, and eight school aged children being served by an itinerant teacher.

Preschool Services and Services to Parents

In recent years the movement toward providing educational services for very young hearing-impaired children has gained considerable momentum. Both the Montreal and Vancouver Oral Schools started as preschools and have continued to maintain active preschool classes and, along with these, counseling and guidance services to parents. A number of schools for the deaf, both day and residential has, for some time, operated preschool classes of their own, and in Ontario some school districts have also done this. At one time the only preschool classes for hearing-impaired children were to be found in the larger centers of population, but now they exist in several small towns and rural areas. Their development has, however, been sporadic and uneven across the country and seems to have reflected pressures from both parent groups and professionals. Most, but not all, of these preschools have been oral. For a short while the Western Institute for the Deaf operated a preschool in Vancouver for the deaf children of deaf parents in which both manual and oral communication were used (Clarke, 1974). The preschool at the Mackay Centre also uses combined methods of communication.

The movement toward services for younger children was given considerable impetus by the diagnostic clinics established in many children's hospitals after World War II. These clinics strongly espoused the cause of family involvement in the education of hearing-impaired children and were closely involved in the setting up of the programs in, for example, Montreal, Winnipeg, and Vancouver. Subsequently, there have been interesting developments of the functions of home visiting teachers and home school coordinators based on residential schools in Quebec, Nova Scotia, Ontario, and British Columbia, and on some school boards in Ontario. These provincially (or locally) funded peripatetic teachers provide regular parent guidance and instruction to help the family work with their deaf child. In some cases, they also play a consultative role with local programs and facilities so that the needs of an individual or a group may be met in the home community when necessary and practical.

Day school programs also offer parent guidance either in the home and/or at school (e.g., Montreal Oral, Vancouver Oral, Winnipeg Preschool, and Metro Toronto). The Winnipeg rural program offers guidance to out-of-town families and their hearing-impaired child by bringing them to Winnipeg during the spring and summer. As a follow-up procedure to reinforce the techniques taught to parents, the Winnipeg program has developed a series of kits which includes materials to facilitate language development, together with instructions and suggestions for their use. These are mailed to and collected from parents at periodic intervals.

The Jericho Hill Preschool Society (which, despite its name, is an organization independent of the Provincial School), apart from its involvement with preschools scattered throughout British Columbia, has arranged several workshops at the provincial school for out-of-town families who, during the workshop, live at the school.

Much more recently there has been a development of sign classes (and, in Vancouver and Victoria, cued speech classes) available for parents and interested members of the family or neighborhood. These classes are offered by community colleges, organizations serving the deaf, school board night school classes, schools for the deaf, and parent associations.

A recently announced research project in Vancouver has applied for funding to study an approach to the early education of deaf children in the family setting, utilizing considerable formal instruction in signs (Freeman, 1975).

Although school and provincial funding has thus been obtained for these preschool services, across the country there have been considerable interprovincial variations in the pattern of funding which supports the services and in the administrative arrangements under which they have been operated. Usually it is possible to recognize at the initial stage the same components described for the Montreal and Vancouver projects—an active, involved group of parents; professional support, usually from medical and paramedical personnel rather than from the traditional schools for the deaf; several sources of financial support (voluntary funds and donations, day care grants, Community Chest, school boards, provincial education grants, fees); and a cooperative school district. The complex and rather confused funding arrangements nicely illustrate the lack of clear-cut legislation and government responsibility and the important and sustaining contribution of voluntary organizations, as well as the Canadian genius for arriving at compromise solutions to problems in a peculiarly circuitous way.

Multihandicapped Hearing-impaired Children

Until Cory's study in 1959, information was sparse about multihandicapped children attending schools and classes for the hearing impaired. In her report, Cory mentions work being done with deaf-blind children in the Halifax School for the Deaf. She also quotes figures reported from the 1957 statistical report on schools for the deaf in Canada published in the American Annals of the Deaf. These showed, for the 10 schools reporting, a total enrollment of 1,778 pupils, 40 (or 2.25%) of whom were listed as multihandicapped. The breakdown into categories was as follows: aphasic (1); blind (4); orthopedic (1); cerebral palsy (20); mental retardation (10); and brain injury (4).

Cory comments that "at present schools do not have many of these multi-handicapped children, but numbers are increasing each year" (p. 58). From her discussion, it is clear that she saw the main educational problem presented by these children in terms of their difficulties in acquiring speech, language, and communication skills, and that what was needed was an extension of classes using manual methods and an adaptation of teaching methods used with slow learners.

Over the next 10 years, schools for the deaf found themselves under increasing pressure to admit hearing-impaired children with other handicaps. Since 1922 in British Columbia, the School for the Deaf had existed side by side on the same campus as the Provincial School for the Blind, and, in the early 1960's, admitted a few deaf-blind children to an experimental program housed in the school for the blind. Subsequently these children were transferred to the deaf-blind unit in the School for the Deaf, Vancouver, Washington. In Montreal, the Mackay School, in a reorganized program, included crippled children as well as the deaf and, thus, paved the way for the reception of multihandicapped hearing-impaired children. And it is clear from annual reports and sporadic surveys and from our first-hand knowledge that a significant, although undocumented, number of multihandicapped hearing-impaired children had been, and were continuing to be, placed in residential institutions and day schools for the mentally retarded and in special classes for educable mentally retarded and slow learning children.

The most recent major survey of this problem in Canadian schools for the deaf was carried out by Bunch in 1972 and reported by him the following year (Bunch, 1973). Bunch sent questionnaires to all 12 schools for the deaf and received detailed replies from nine of them. These revealed that five of the nine responding schools had developed specific programs for the multihandicapped, although for the most part these programs and those of the other four schools appeared to be of a stop-gap nature. No province had developed specific arrangements to provide thorough or comprehensive training of teachers of the deaf to work with multihandicapped children–hardly a surprising finding in view of the fact that so many teachers of the deaf outside the province of Ontario lack even basic training. The figures quoted by Bunch, however, showed that by 1972 the nine schools had total enrollments of 2,332 children, and that no fewer than 514 of them (22.3%) were reported to be multihandicapped. This figure, together with the categorical breakdown, may be compared with those reported by Cory only 15 years earlier: retarded (205); disturbed (122); orthopedic (29); cerebral palsy (64); visually impaired (22); learning disability (57); other (65).

It must, of course, be remembered that Cory's and Bunch's figures are derived from two different kinds of questionnaires, that some of the categories are different, and that the second largest category used by Bunch (disturbed) does not appear on Cory's list. However, it would certainly appear that there has been a sizable increase in the number of multihandicapped children identified as such in Canadian schools for the deaf, and that probably the actual number of these children in schools has increased also.

Two other recent reports give some information about specific programs in individual schools. Kysela and Masciuch (1972) give a descriptive report on the operation of a multidisciplinary unit for emotionally disturbed and multihandicapped children in operation at the Alberta School for the Deaf since 1970 and provide some details of the progress of three children during the 3½ months of the program. Buller (1973) gives a more general description of the special classes for multihandicapped hearing-impaired chidren at the Ontario School for the Deaf at Belleville. His report shows that 39 children (8.9% of the total school population) were placed in seven special classes and that, while many of the children were characterized by descriptive labels such as seriously emotionally disturbed (6), brain damaged (9), or cerebral palsied (5), 35 of the 39 children were reported to have intelligence quotients below 89, 22 of them in the 50–74 range. Buller's report also makes it clear that only the most severely multihandicapped children are involved in the special classes–others, who might fit particular descriptive categories, may still be provided for in the general program. As Buller points out, Canadian schools for the deaf seem to be faced with continuous expansion of their services for the multihandicapped, and this probably reflects the operation of several factors: (1) with the lowering of the infant mortality rates, an increase in the number of multihandicapped children; (2) an increase in the public school services for the hearing impaired, likely to "cream off" the more straightforward well functioning children; and (3) greater sophistication in detecting and diagnosing learning disabilities in deaf as well as in normally hearing children.

Language and Communication Skills: A Current Perspective

The topic of educational rehabilitation of hearing-impaired children is actually many topics because auditory deficits vary considerably with the age of onset, degree of impairment, etiological factors, previous management, socioeconomic, and family circumstances. It is for these reasons that educational opportunities for the hearing impaired in Canada are now beginning to be more flexible within the constraints of financc, facilitics, and trained personnel. We have noted earlier that the options range from totally integrated programs in regular schools, to special classes in regular schools, and to special day and/or residential schools. Within these options are a variety of methodologies or teaching strategies; namely, oral, oral-aural, visible English (fingerspelling), signing, and combined methods (recently renamed total communication).

Language An arbitrary and superficial categorization of the approaches to language teaching in Canadian schools for the deaf would divide them into two, the natural and formal methods. The former would follow Groht (1965), Ewing and Ewing (1967), Van Uden (1970), and Harris (1971); whereas the latter borrows from Fitzgerald (1965), Pugh (1965), Buell (1968), Peck (1969), Caniglia et al. (1972), Clarke School for the Deaf (1972), Streng (1972), and McCarr (1973), etc.

Bunch (1975) utilized a program evaluation model to investigate the possible differential effectiveness of the two mainstream language methodologies. His findings indicated that both methods are equally effective but that neither provides the average deaf child to age 16 with the ability to deal competently with basic grammatical principles. It was found in both schools involved in the study that "incongruencies existed betwen intended and observed situational, input, process and outcome factors while the contingencies imputed for these factors were highly suspect" (p. 121).

Auditory Training Although the importance of early auditory experiences has long been recognized, the extent to which auditory stimulation is combined with specific modes of visual input such as speechreading, gesture, fingerspelling, and sign varies from school to school and is the subject of much debate. In some instances, there is a deliberate unisensory approach–visual, auditory, or tactual; in others, a bimodal input audiovisual, audiotactile, and visual-tactile, and again there are multisensory approaches. The inhibitory and facilitative effects of these components remain at best a pervasive question among educators.

Speechreading and Speech There has been recent research (Ling and Clarke, 1975) on improving the efficacy of speechreading skills using Cornett's (1972) cued speech, which is being tried in several classrooms across the country. With the advent of modern auditory equipment, oscilloscopic tracings, visible speech patterns, visual-tactile systems, and pitch and loudness meters (all of which have received sporadic and intermittent attention from teachers), there has been a noticeable decline in the traditional methods of teaching speech, stressing as it did the articulation of phonemes.

Fingerspelling and Sign Fingerspelling is being combined with oral methods at three provincial schools in Ontario, but in other provinces (except for oral programs) both fingerspelling and sign are used. Historically sign language has been seen as a continuum; at the one end is a proper sign language where signs relate to meanings just as words do, and, at the other end, is English exactly represented in signs (Stokoe, 1974). Probably neither of these exists in pure form because when deaf people interact they use more or fewer rules of a proper sign language or more or fewer rules of English, depending on their linguistic competence. Recently, however, a series of sign-for-morpheme codes have proliferated.

These include *Linguistics of Visual English* (Wampler, 1971), *Seeing Essential English* (Anthony et al., 1972), *Signing Exact English* (Gustason,

1972), and *An Introduction to Manual English* (Washington State School, 1972). Stokoe also points out that many language systems, including English, combine parts into single words, but the new sign systems go contrary to our linguistic knowledge and take words apart and represent them in a string of discrete signs. Hearing children at an early age put out whole ideas in chunks of language ("Daddy work"; "Mummy go") and only later are the chunks broken down to include syntactical and morphological rules. However, in some of our total communication schools, these new sign-for-morpheme codes are introduced from the earliest years, and young deaf children are expected to break up their attempts at communication into English morphemes.

The fact that deaf children acquire language at a much slower rate than their hearing peers is well documented. The strength of this need and the felt responsibility and dedication of the teaching profession have inevitably led to the ready acceptance of any new method. The new signs are readily available in book form which appears to distract teachers and administrators alike from an evaluative study of these systems. Observations of the everyday communication of deaf children encourage our belief that the use of sign-English (a mingling of proper sign and sign codes) may lead the way for deaf children to learn in time to be bilingual to some extent in both proper sign and English. Some fear is expressed here that the impending controversy (Rhodes, 1972) concerning signs may become as acrimonious and as futile as the oral-manual debate.

Total Communication Total communication arrived on the Canadian scene in the early 1970's (Clarke, 1972). Those who immediately adopted the slogan (and not the philosophy) included untrained teachers of the deaf with some knowledge of a sign-for-morpheme and a sign-for-letter code but little, if any, skill as far as the teaching of speech, speechreading, and auditory training are concerned. Although several schools report a total communication philosophy which, more often than not, is manual, with no more than lipservice to the development of audition, speech, and speechreading, several alternate and viable programs are available to accommodate the differing needs of hearing-impaired children in many school systems.

Continuing Education

Although adult education classes are available in some centers, many capable deaf adults cannot participate because of their geographical isolation and, in some instances, a lack of support services.

In Ontario, courses are offered in London (Parents' Association), Milton (Sheridan College), Welland (Niagara Community College), and Toronto (Ontario Mission for the Deaf, Parkway Vocational, and Northern

Secondary). Red River College in Manitoba (which also serves Saskatchewan), Alberta College in Alberta, and Vancouver Community College in British Columbia also offer continuing education classes for the deaf and hard of hearing. Generally, these programs offer opportunities to complete academic and, in some instances, vocational training. Upgrading of communication skills, receptive and expressive language, and mathematics form the core academic curricula.

Other courses included "Social Living"–comprising practical aids to daily living which will assist interpersonal relationships and "World of Work" which will help students decide on realistic vocational goals. None of these programs offers a liberal arts education, and Canada relies heavily on American institutes–e.g., Gallaudet College, National Technological Institute of the Deaf, and Minneapolis-St. Paul–for undergraduate academic and technological studies for its deaf students.

Concluding Summary

It is clear from our survey that school services for hearing-impaired children in Canada have developed immeasurably if untidily from the time when a few residential schools, administratively, socially, and professionally isolated from the mainstream of public education, opened their doors to a selected group of deaf children and offered them instruction through the medium of signs and fingerspelling.

Subsequent developments show that there have been not only far reaching changes in administrative and public responsibility for the hearing impaired and in the numbers of children caught up in the network of special schools and classes, but also in the teaching methods utilized for their instruction. Admittedly the picture is a confused one: there are many fingers in a great number of pies, and many gaps and shortcomings continue to exist. Yet it is the very diversity of these services proliferating in a country with such a relatively small population that is perhaps its most striking feature. As we have seen, this diversity is partly attributable to the fact that there are 10 educationally autonomous provinces and many hundreds of school districts. But it also reflects, as it has always done, other factors and influences: the importation of talents and ideas from outside the country; the vitality of voluntary, consumer, and citizen groups; the flexibility (which some might see as lack of leadership) of the local and provincial authorities.

In this system, Canadian parents retain cherished rights as far as the educational placement of their children is concerned. Because of the homeowner tax structure which helps to support educational programs, parents expect to have a good deal of involvement in decision making. It is not difficult then to understand how they can generally enroll their hearing-impaired children in a program of their choice, regardless of whether the placement is the most appropriate one for the child. There are, thus, situations in educational planning where the rights of parents and children, internal and external evaluations of the programs, and the decisions of teachers and administrators are precariously balanced. Yet in this system there is also a good deal of openness to external influences and a readiness to change in response to these. This is both its strength and its weakness.

To conclude, we have thought it worthwhile to list, in point form and without discussion, those aspects of the current programs which seem to us to have the greatest importance for our understanding of the programs and the directions in which they appear to be developing.

1. The loosening of positions with respect to methodologies. There are welcome signs that fewer people are entrenched in extreme positions and that there is a greater willingness to experiment.
2. Provincial financial support is not now restricted to the established residential schools for the deaf but is made more freely available to a greater variety of programs.
3. Increasing opportunities for hearing-impaired children to be integrated in ordinary school programs.
4. Despite this, a continued need for residential services, especially for deaf children from remote areas, and for multihandicapped hearing-impaired children. The number of this last group seems to be increasing.
5. A comparative lack of good teaching facilities for hard-of-hearing children, particularly outside the metropolitan areas.
6. An increasing trend toward the use of schools for the deaf as resource centers and the deployment of their resources over larger geographical areas and in a greater variety of teaching situations.
7. In some areas—notably the Atlantic provinces—an attempt to regionalize the planning and funding of services on a broader population base while at the same time permitting a much greater degree of decentralization of the service delivery system. It is too early to see how well this is going to work. But in theory at least it should provide the structures for the better long term planning and coordination of services.

DIAGNOSTIC PROCEDURES AND INTERPROFESSIONAL RELATIONSHIPS

It would make tedious and repetitious reading, if we were to list both the well known and sophisticated array of auditory and other tests used in Canada, since this would duplicate much, if not all, of the material contained in the chapter on the United States of America. We, therefore, thought it more profitable to examine some of the broader problems, including community provisions for diagnostic procedures, interprofessional relationships, and the delivery of these services at a regional level.

Neonatal Screening

Because the neonate is a captive subject for the first few days of his life in the newborn nursery, early screening for deafness at this stage appears to be an attractive and worthwhile project. Programs often sponsored and funded by the Elks services clubs and patterned after the early work of Downs and Sterritt (1964; 1967) have been instituted in various hospitals across the country. Through these programs, it has become evident not only that the number of infants being screened out is small, but also that there is a relatively large number of false positives and false negatives. At McGill, Ling, Ling, and Doehring (1970) tested 12,000 newborn infants, but only four babies (one with bilateral congenital atresia and one with multiple abnormalities) were found to have hearing impairments. Seven who passed the screening test were later identified as deaf. A further experimental study of stimulus response and observer variables (Ling et al., 1970) suggested that the high proportion of invalid responses recorded would generally account for the failure of any applied neonatal screening program. It can be seen then that the number of false positives and the number of cases missed will be high, and this has serious repercussions. The former will cause unfounded anxiety and distress, and the latter will give a false sense of security to parents who, if they suspect a hearing loss, may dismiss it on the basis of what information they had been given. Because the results of mass screening programs here and in other countries lack proved reliability or validity, research is continuing with further examinations of stimuli, response patterns, observer behavior, status of neonate at time of testing, and other variables. In the meantime, many professionals are urging, as an alternative, the establishment of a high risk register and a follow-up program of testing in well baby clinics. This follow-up technique is not very expensive or time consuming and simple screening procedures (Ewing and Ewing, 1944) can be used by regular personnel in these settings. It must also be noted that there is no evidence that a delay of six months or so is critical to language development, and, furthermore, the postponement of diagnosis may be of psychological advantage to both parents and child. Certainly the chances of successful identification and accurate assessment increase dramatically at an age level of approximately eight months. A difficulty here, however, is that many congenitally deaf children would not be recorded in a high risk register (Budden et al., 1974).

School Age Screening

Most, but not all, provinces have personnel who routinely carry out audiometric screening of children of school age at various grade levels. These tests for pure tone and/or speech are carried out either by school board personnel specially hired for the purpose or through the Department of Health by the ubiquitous public health or school nurse. In other instances, school referrals are made to health units or to clinics.

Clinics

Over the last 20 years there has been a rapid growth in the number of speech and hearing clinics across the country. From Human Communication (No. 1, 1973; No. 2, 1973), a listing of Canadian clinics is available and presented in summary form in Table 1.

The clinics in this table do not include professionals working in government departments or agencies, schools for the deaf, and school boards, health units, or organizations serving the deaf. It should be noted that all of these are in urban centers (populations greater than 1,000) and that many of them are speech clinics. If one examines the descriptions in the listings, it is found that clinics which include services to the hearing impaired are reduced to the following: British Columbia (4), Alberta (8), Saskatchewan (5), Manitoba (3), Ontario (20), New Brunswick (1), Newfoundland (1), Nova Scotia, Prince Edward Island (1). (Listings, but not descriptions, were available for clinics in Quebec.) It is also interesting to observe that 19 of these clinics are hospital based: two in Vancouver, three in Alberta, one in Saskatchewan, two in Manitoba, 10 in Ontario, and four in mobile vans.

To illustrate the diagnostic procedures, the nature and examples of hearing tests and interprofessional relationships, two hospitals set an exemplary model.

At the Hospital for Sick Children in Toronto, the audiology facility is one of the largest pediatric units in North America and consists of eight audiometric test suites housed in a new wing of the hospital which is specially designed for a pediatric population. Complete instrumentation is available for routine pure tone and speech tests, impedance audiometry with conditioned orientating reflex audiometry (CORA), evoked response audiometry (ERA), and electrocochleography. The hospital's IBM 1800 computer will present stimuli as well as analyze results for more sophisticated ERAs and has a program which handles all audiological and ear, nose, and throat (ENT) records. The multidisciplinary team includes an otolaryngologist, psychiatrist, audiologist, neurologist, geneticist, speech pathologist, pediatrician, psychologist, neuroradiologist, teacher of the deaf, and representative from the local school board authority.

Table 1. Speech and hearing clinics in Canada

Location	Number of clinics
British Columbia	
Victoria	2
Vancouver	7
Surrey	1
Traveling van	1
Alberta	
Calgary	4
Edmonton	5
Lethbridge	1
Brooks	1
Traveling van	1
Saskatchewan	
Yorkton	1
Moose Jaw	1
Swift Current	1
Saskatoon	6
Regina	2
Traveling van	1
Manitoba	
Brandon	1
Winnipeg	5
Traveling van	1
Ontario	
Barrie	1
Brantford	1
Brockville	1
Chatham	1
Guelph	1
Hamilton	5
Kingston	4
Kitchener	1
London	3
Mississauga	1
Niagara Falls	1
Oshawa	2
Ottawa	4
Petersborough	1
St. Catherines	1
St. Thomas	1
Sarnia	2
Saulte Ste. Marie	1
Sudbury	1

Continued

Table 1—*Continued*

Location	Number of clinics
Toronto	26
Thunder Bay	2
Windsor	2
Newfoundland	
St. John's	1
Quebec	
Montreal	23
Verdun	1
Sherbrooke	3
St. Jerome	2
Trois Rivieres	2
Sillery	1
Chicoutimi	1
Riviere du Loup	1
Ste. Foy	2
St. Hyacinthe	1
Nova Scotia	
Halifax	2
Kentville	1
Digby	1
New Brunswick	
St. John	1
Fredricton	1
Prince Edward Island	
Charlottetown	1

In Vancouver, the Children's Hospital Diagnostic Centre has broadened its services to include multiple handicapping conditions. It not only aims to provide a flexible medical, social, and education assessment but also helps in planning a continuing program of rehabilitation and education which is to complement existing community services.

The services available include:

1. Coordination of assessment and help with continuing supervision of children with multiple complicated problems including: cleft palate; meningomyelocele; communication disorders, including hearing loss, language delay, and speech problems; developmental delay and neuroepileptic disorders; learning disorders; visual impairment, including blindness and other multiple handicap combinations.
2. Collaboration with school screening and assessment committees in evaluation of children with learning problems which will often be related to school admissions, accommodation, and progress.

3. Collaboration with treatment centers in assessment of children with the complicated problems listed above.
4. Parent education and home management programs for children with chronic diseases including: diabetes mellitus, dwarfism, epilepsy, muscular dystrophy, etc.
5. Assessment of emotional and social problems of handicapped children and their parents.
6. Genetic counseling and identification of rare syndromes.
7. A unit for continuing diagnostic observations of young children with communication disorders.

The staff includes physicians (pediatricians, psychiatrists, and surgeons) working in association with audiologists, speech pathologists, occupational and physiotherapists, public health nurses, social workers, special education consultants, dieticians, psychologists, dentists, and orthodontists. The armamentarium of the audiological team is not as sophisticated as that of the Hospital for Sick Children but, as in other Canadian clinics, pure tone, speech, and impedance audiometry are commonplace.

Both of these hospitals illustrate medical models of interprofessional relationships. Each individual has, of course, certain skills, which are applied when indicated, but it is only when the total needs of the client are examined and when each discipline contributes as part of a team to the overall rehabilitation of the individual that the full efficiency of each professional discipline is actualized. On financial grounds alone, it is difficult for other places to replicate these models, but in a number of smaller clinics there is a growing awareness of the need for cooperative efforts between professionals. It is true that the teacher of the deaf needs to know more about the competencies of a speech therapist and vice versa if meaningful dialogue and cooperative efforts are to result. One promising sign for the future is the number of speech pathologists, audiologists, psychologists, and medical consultants working in schools for the deaf and with school boards. One can also not help but notice the wide range of professional interactions at seminars, workshops, and conferences. In some instances, however, there is still a begrudging tolerance of education of the deaf and speech pathology toward their precocious offspring, audiology, while the parents themselves sleep in separate rooms.

Adult Testing

We think it true to say that, in the past, the clinical facilities and programs provided mainly for a deaf pediatric population and that by contrast both the hard of hearing and the deaf adult have been somewhat ignored. Rehabilitative facilities for adults are now increasing with a concurrent development of diagnostic facilities for these populations, but research in both these areas is rare. In the past (see the section entitled "Organizations and Associations Serving the Hearing Impaired"), many of the organizations serving the deaf have themselves developed badly needed adult auditory rehabilitation services. We must not forget that otologists in private practice have also long had an important role in diagnosis and therapy, including the fitting of hearing aids. Currently we find that many have availed themselves of the services of an audiometrist or audiologist and that they are kept one of the busiest medical specialists in the community.

Decentralization of Services for the Communicatively Impaired

There are also current moves to decentralize services. For example, Tonkin (1974) proposed to the government of British Columbia that Vancouver provide the principal secondary care and the only tertiary care in the province, and that provision be made for districts to be designated as secondary care centers following established procedures and standards and reporting to the tertiary center. The districts in turn are to be divided into local areas which will include space and facilities for the identification and evaluation of the communicatively impaired. The districts would include the following primary care:

Direct Services to People All preventive measures, all screening, referrals to central facilities, continuity of care within the community and its institutions, maintenance and supply of appliances and other devices, and the provision of educational and rehabilitation services to most communicatively impaired with the possible exception of some multiple handicaps.

Support Services Counseling (individual and family), social assistance and family support where required, work opportunities and vocational programs, interpreter services and transportation.

The recommendation was for a multidisciplinary approach with the program being funded, managed, and staffed by the Departments of Health, Human Resources (formerly Welfare) and Education. It would seem that the next move is to set up such a program in one of the regional centers and evaluate its effectiveness. The catch cry of "take the services to the people" may well become the practice of the late 1970's.

HEARING AIDS

In 1973 the Saskatchewan government broke new ground with an act respecting the Establishment of a Program to Provide Hearing Aids to

Certain Persons with Defective Hearing. Under this act, the Minister of Public Health was given the power to establish a program within his department for obtaining hearing aids and making provision for residents with defective hearing to acquire such hearing aids upon such terms and conditions as the Minister may consider advisable. To translate this legalese into practice, it is now possible to obtain a hearing aid from a collection of more than 20 different instruments from several different countries which range in price to the individual from $15 for a body aid to $275 for a binaural (stereo) aid. The average price is about $85. In provinces where provincial assistance is not provided, this was close to $600 (Interdepartmental Committee on Consumer Affairs, 1970).

Newfoundland also provides hearing aids to all persons in need of assistance up to the age of 17 (Wallace, 1973, p. 64).

One should also note the generosity of the many service clubs in Canada which, over the years, have readily made available funds for hearing aids to children whose parents are in financial difficulty.

In British Columbia, a report edited by Walsh et al. (1974) has recommended to the provincial government among other things that "The degree to which the government wishes to proceed with the provision of aids (free, subsidized or at cost) and services (for all or part of the aid) should be governed by the availability of services." A suggested procedure is: provision of aids and services first to the 0–5 age group; then, the 0–10 group; then, the 0–18 group; then, the over 65-year-old group.

It is assumed that, through the Workmen's Compensation Board and the Department of Human Resources, some consumers in the 18- to 65-year-old group will receive special consideration.

Because of delineation of powers of the federal and provincial governments, the participation of the former with respect to the provision of hearing aids is limited. Aids are provided free by the Federal War Veterans Administration to any veteran pensioned for a hearing problem or a veteran approved under The Treatment Eligibility War Veterans' Allowance Act. With respect to the native Indian population, the Medical Services Branch of Health and Welfare of Canada will also provide hearing aids free of charge.

Contrary to developments in England and Australia, it would appear that the federal government will apply mandatory legislation on the operating procedures of dealers, but it will be left to the provinces to legislate licensing and to provide funding for the general dispensing of aids. In this latter regard, Saskatchewan has set a precedent which is being closely examined, not only by other provincial governments, but also by pressure groups concerned with the welfare of the auditorally impaired. The future abounds with interesting prospects.

TRAINING OF PROFESSIONALS AND PARAPROFESSIONALS

Teacher Training in Education of the Deaf

Canada has never had a national policy regarding the training or certification of teachers of the deaf. Indeed, even in the provinces—with the possible exception of Ontario—there are no clearly defined standards for the selection of teachers in schools and programs for the hearing impaired. From the beginning, the approach that has been taken has depended largely upon the initiative and vision of individual superintendents and administrators and upon a pool of willing, but untrained, teachers. Until recently, in-service education in one or two schools, supplemented by summer courses, and the recruitment of trained, experienced teachers of the deaf from other countries, particularly the United States, the United Kingdom, and Australia, have supplied the schools with their cadre of more highly trained professionals.

The first formalized program in teacher training on staff basis began with Katherine Ford in 1919 at Belleville, Ontario. It was not until 1967 that the formalized 1-year training course was placed under a Principal of Teacher Training, independent of the Superintendent of the School but still responsible to the Ontario government.

Selection is based on the hiring by the provincial schools or school boards of personnel who have a basic Ontario Teaching Certificate or Letter of Standing. The program consists of 25 weeks of lectures and seminars and 13 weeks of practice. At the conclusion of the 1-year training period and 2 years of supervised teaching in the schools, a Specialist Certificate as a teacher of the deaf is issued. It is interesting to note that fingerspelling and signing were not introduced until 1972 and that, 2 years later, deaf candidates were acceptable without a Teaching Certificate if they had a college degree and were selected by the employing school or board as suitable to meet an anticipated vacancy on its staff.

The University of British Columbia offered the first full time course at a university level for teachers of the deaf in 1968. Applicants (either hearing or deaf) must have a degree from a recognized university. The program consists of 1 year full-time study involving theory and extensive practica. They take a core academic program in education of the deaf together with electives from other courses offered by the Department of Special Education. Students are expected to become proficient in all methods—aural, oral, manual, and combined. Successful candidates are awarded the university diploma in education of the deaf which may satisfy requirements for provincial teacher certification. The Provincial Department of Education does not issue specialist certificates.

The Université du Québec in Montreal began offering courses in education of the deaf in 1971. These courses can be applied to a program leading to a B.A. in special education (Neveu, 1974).

At the Interprovincial School for the Deaf in Amherst, Nova Scotia, a training program began in September 1972. This 1-year program for both French and English teachers enables them to become qualified to teach deaf children in all four Atlantic provinces. Applicants must be already qualified to teach in public schools or have a degree in related fields (social work, psychology, etc.). Associations with nearby universities have been developed—a course on exceptional children comes by video tape from Acadia, and students have been known to divide their time between the training program and the University of Moncton where they are working toward a degree in special education (Kennedy, 1972).

In 1973 the University of Manitoba offered a 1-year program in education of the deaf for trained teachers, but it was not offered in 1974 and the course outline does not appear in the current calendar. Each year one or two summer courses are also available at the University of Saskatchewan (Saskatoon).

At the School of Human Communication Disorders, McGill, a program is being planned to train oral rehabilitation workers at a master's level together with speech pathologists and audiologists, for whom programs have been available since 1962. In British Columbia, a Task Force (1974) recommended to the Ministers of Health, Education and Human Resources that a Faculty of Communication Sciences be established at the University of British Columbia to integrate the undergraduate and graduate training of all professionals and academics in the area of communicatively impaired. This proposal is currently being examined by a President's Committee.

Apart from these Canadian training centers, it must be pointed out that many Canadians have acquired teacher training either through full-time study at Manchester, Oxford, or London in England or Victoria in Australia. Others have attended full-time or summer school programs at the Clarke School for the Deaf, Central Institute at St. Louis, St. Joseph's, San Francisco State, Lexington, Minnesota, or other training centers in the United States. In some of these cases, financial support for study came from provincial governments and school districts.

The teacher training obtained in England, the United States, and other countries, and the immigration to Canada of many teachers of the deaf has brought an eclecticism to many Canadian schools which may have an advantage over the inherent dangers of inbreeding in a program or programs in which future teachers are trained by the same administrative organizations which employ them. There are, however, a number of teachers and administrators who have had little or no professional training in education of the deaf and, in all provinces except Ontario, there is no question but that the training facilities are inadequate to meet the demands of the school system.

The first national publication—"The Canadian Teacher of the Deaf"—was published in October 1971 as a learning experience by graphic arts students at the Interprovincial Vocational School, Amherst, Nova Scotia, as a federal interprovincial project. At the 1st National Conference of Canadian Teachers of the Deaf in Belleville, Ontario, August 23rd–25th, 1973, a national teachers' organization was founded and named "The Association of Canadian Educators of the Hearing Impaired." The journal was renamed the *ACEHI Journal–la Revue ACEDA* and produced its first issue under this new title in March 1974.

ACEHI (commonly referred to as ace-high) has national and regional directors. One of the association's subcommittees is engaged in investigating professional standards for teachers of the hearing impaired across Canada with a view to proposing a model for national certification. At present only two of the 10 provinces (namely, Ontario and Nova Scotia) possess regulations concerning certification of teachers of the deaf.

University Programs in Speech Pathology and Audiology

Canada has also arrived late with university-based programs in these areas, although today six universities offer professional training.

A master's program was established in 1962 at McGill University (Montreal, Quebec), and later a doctoral program was added. Courses are offered in the Faculty of Graduate Studies by the School of Human Communication Disorders. Students can enter either an M.Sc. program, which is required for doctorate studies, or an Applied M.Sc. program, which is a career prerequisite along with specific licencing measures. There are generally two M.Sc. students, 15 in the Applied M.Sc. course, and one or two on doctoral programs.

The Université de Montréal (Montreal, Quebec), Faculté des Études Superieures, École de Readaptation offers a graduate program in Audiology and Special Pathology. It was established in the early 1960s. The course leads to an M.O.A. (Maitrise en Orthophonie et Audiologie). The prerequisites are a B.A. or B.Sc. in Audiology and Speech Pathology and a knowledge of the French language.

About the same time, the University of Toronto (Toronto, Ontario) established its course in the Department of Rehabilitation Medicine. There is at present a 2-year postgraduate program leading to a Diploma in Speech

Pathology and Audiology; however, an M.A. program has been approved by the faculty, and it is reported that, by the Fall of 1975, the diploma will be phased out.

The University of Western Ontario (London, Ontario) established a program in Communicative Disorders in the early 1970s. It is a 4-year course of study which can only be entered after the completion of 1 year of a general program. At the completion of the course students receive a B.Sc. in Communicative Disorders. The university is also beginning an M.A. program, and students will be encouraged to continue in graduate school. The aim is to provide students with an education in sciences and social sciences and simultaneously prepare them for careers in audiology and speech pathology.

The University of Dalhousie (Halifax, Nova Scotia) is also preparing to establish an M.A. program in Speech Pathology and Audiology by September 1976. This course is intended to serve all the Atlantic provinces.

It must be noted that the programs are generally small. Approximately 15 students are graduated by each university except for the University of Montreal (25–30). Although initially three programs were offered—a master's degree, one a diploma, and two an undergraduate degree—there is a current move toward locating all training at the graduate level.

There has been no attempt to standardize the programs at a national level. Provincial interests override federal involvement for two reasons. The first concerns the provincial role with respect to funding and the second is the unique development of provincial health services with differing types of health care and delivery services. Graduates from the University of British Columbia, for example, may function as both speech pathologists and audiologists, whereas students in other programs must specialize in either speech pathology or audiology.

Although differing philosophies with resultant emphasis in certain subject areas are reflected in the courses offered by each of the universities, there is a commonality of competencies displayed by graduates in the work field, and all programs have a strong internship or practica component. The diversity and yet similarities of the programs are reflected in the following academic curricula:

1. McGill University—Basic Science of Human Communication, Audiology and Aural Rehabilitation, Physiology of Speech and Hearing, Speech and Language Pathology, Advanced Audiology, Advanced Speech Pathology, Rehabilitation of the Aurally Handicapped, Practicum, Research Methods, Seminar in Human Communication Disorders, Lectures, and Research on Selected Advanced Topics, Independent Project.

2. University of British Columbia—Acoustic Phonetics, Instrumental Phonetics, Mechanisms of the Auditory System, Perceptual Acoustics, Developmental Phonology, Acquisition of Language, Speech Perception, Neurological Aspects of Language, Seminar in Problems of Audiology and Speech Sciences, Directed Reading and Conferences, one course in both Psychiatry and Neuroanatomy, Internship, and Thesis.

It is interesting to note that only two provinces, Manitoba, 1961, and Quebec, 1964, have legislative acts regarding the licensing of speech pathologists and audiologists. Bill 250 of Quebec province (which is the professional code) includes both speech pathologists and audiologists in its regulations; basically it states that no one may practice in either field without first obtaining a license from the Professional Corporation of Speech Therapists and Audiologists.

At present, although the other provinces have no legislation concerning certification, the provincial branches of the Canadian Speech and Hearing Society are striving to maintain high standards, and members of professions are expected to join the society. Many of the provincial branches, e.g., British Columbia, Manitoba, Ontario, and Nova Scotia, are currently pressing for legislation which will require that speech pathologists and audiologists be licensed.

As in the related field of education of the deaf, there are many Canadians and immigrants who have undertaken training in the United States, England, and Australia. These persons have brought a diverse array of experiences to university programs and health services which is perhaps unparalleled in any other country.

The first Canadian professional journal, *Human Communication*, was published by Glenrose Hospital, Edmonton, Alberta in the winter of 1973 for the Canadian Speech and Hearing Society.

Hearing Aid Dealers

In 1973 federal regulations were drafted that require persons selling hearing aids in Canada to provide every purchaser (i.e., distributor) with a copy of performance characteristics of the type or model sold and they require that this information would be available to consumers upon request. Furthermore, it was an offense to sell a hearing aid that does not meet the performance characteristics claimed.

At the provincial level there are only three provinces, Quebec, Manitoba, and British Columbia, which have statutory regulations requiring provincial licensing of hearing aid dealers.

The Statutes of Quebec 1973, Bill 270, abolished the Association of Hearing Aid Acousticians of the Province of Quebec incorporated in July

1966 and, among other things, set out the legal and illegal practices of the profession and set up a bureau of nine persons to license hearing aid dealers and a board of examiners to set qualifying examinations. The corporation empowered to issue the permit was established by Bill 250 (1973), and hearing aid dealers found their professional corporation rubbing shoulders in the same bill with the many corporations for advocates, notaries, physicians, dentists, pharmacists, opticians, accountants, nurses, dieticians, social workers, psychologists, speech therapists, and audiologists and others.

In British Columbia there are the Hearing Aid Regulation Act (1971), Bill 31 (1972) and Bill 137 (1973) and, in Manitoba, the Hearing Aid Act (1971) which has very similar wording. The main features of these acts were to set up boards (compositions varied slightly between provinces) appointed by the Lieutenant Governor in Council. The board was empowered to regulate the education of hearing aid dealers and consultants, to appoint an examining committee, to make regulations to provide for licensing, to authorize types of services, and to inquire into, hear, and determine, by its own motion or upon complaint, any misconduct or incompetence. The board has the power to reprimand and suspend a dealer or cancel his license and registration.

Some other provinces have loose knit voluntary groups of hearing aid dealers who have tried to establish standards and provide some form of certification to members who meet standards in regard to training experience, character, and ethics (e.g., The National Hearing Aid Society, Nova Scotia). The Ontario Hearing Aid Association has gone further and set up a disciplinary board made up of three consumer protection bureaus to handle complaints from dissatisfied individuals. In a few instances it is interesting to observe that qualified audiologists have entered the commercial field.

The British North America Act hinders federal and national regulations concerning hearing aid dealers, and provincial governments appear to have been reluctant to enter into this field of legislation. Perhaps the relatively new legislation in British Columbia and Manitoba or the umbrella professional corporations legislation of Quebec will act as a model to the legislatures in other provinces. With pressure group activities by organizations of the hearing impaired (see section entitled "Organizations and Associations Serving the Hearing Impaired"), there may well be further legislation in the near future.

Audiometrists and Hearing Aid Technicians

Some community colleges have begun courses, and others are examining the feasibility of training technicians at a lower level than undergraduate and graduate studies at universities. In this way simpler routine tests and repairs may be carried out in a more economical fashion. In order to alleviate the shortage of personnel in these areas, the universities are encouraging these developments.

Other Support Personnel

Some community colleges are now running full-time and part-time programs in manual communication and offering courses for rehabilitation workers, child care counselors, and teacher aides in residential schools. Nowhere, however, is there a program which will certify interpreters nor is there an organization similar to the National Registry of Interpreters which exists in the U.S.A. This crucial need must be resolved.

RESEARCH RELATING TO HEARING IMPAIRMENT

In his report on services available to the deaf and hard of hearing across Canada, Wallace (1973, p. 65) commented that there was "a complete lack of definitive ongoing studies of the size, characteristics and location of the deaf population." He went on to comment on the lack of information about counseling, job placement, mental health, vocational skills training, and other services for the deaf, and on areas such as employer attitudes toward the hearing impaired.

Wallace's condemnation of Canadian research relates particularly to information about services for deaf adults and seems to have been based primarily, and perhaps somewhat optimistically, on his survey of provincial departments of Health, Education, Welfare, and Labour which requested details of current research related to deafness being carried out in each province. Certainly the response to this inquiry was scanty; the 40 provincial departments polled listed nine studies, one of which (the report of the committee set up by the governments of the four Atlantic provinces to make recommendations about educational services for severely handicapped children—see section entitled "The Background of Current Educational Programs for the Hearing Impaired") was in no sense intended as a research report. Of the other eight studies, one was concerned with play patterns of hearing-impaired children, one with the status of the deaf in Ontario in relation to their educational experiences, three with audiometric studies (effects of noise on farmers; base line hearing levels in Northern Saskatchewan; reliability of evoked response audiometry), while the remaining three consisted of a study of the interest and competency in manual communication by speech and hearing professionals, a study of the psychiatric correlates of deafness in children, and a report on the development of a multidisciplinary health care delivery system. From two provinces there were no reports. Wallace concluded "if this is all that is being carried out, it shows a very limited uncoordinated research effort in no way appropriate to the magnitude of the problem. If (it) is incomplete, it demonstrates a further need for a national directory of current research being undertaken into deafness" (p. 66).

However, it is surprising that Wallace's dismissive review does not mention other published studies in the small, fragmented, but growing body of Canadian research. Some of these have admittedly been carried out and reported by isolated individuals, but some—notably the work from the School of Human Communication Disorders at McGill and from the University of British Columbia—already form a more systematic, directed corpus, concerned with several aspects of hearing impairment. In this brief review, it is impossible to list in any comprehensive fashion, let alone discuss, the research work of individuals and groups, scattered as it is through so many diverse publications and related to so many different disciplines and professions. What we have tried to do is to present some examples of recent Canadian work, under five main headings.

Clinical and Epidemiological Studies Apart from isolated reports of clinical programs in large Canadian cities (e.g., McHugh, 1961, 1962), there has been one extended attempt, by Robinson and his co-workers from the Department of Paediatrics, University of British Columbia, to carry out a clinical and epidemiological study of children with hearing impairment (Kendall, 1963, 1964; Robinson et al., 1963a, 1963b, 1964, 1965, 1967, 1973; Budden et al., 1974). In the most recent report from this group (Budden et al., 1974), it was shown that there had been no major changes in the etiologies of deafness among children referred for assessment in British Columbia during the past 18 years, with the genetic, rubella, and meningitic groups, in that order, making the greatest contribution to cases with known etiology, and 48.4% of cases (N=500) characterized as of unknown etiology. Robinson et al. (1963a) further showed that about 38% of all young deaf children in their survey suffered from other disabilities. Budden et al. (1974) speculated that the relatively large number of cases of unknown etiology probably reflected their rather stringent criteria governing the assignment of cases to a genetic category. They concluded that preventive and other measures will begin to reduce the incidence of congenital causes of hearing loss, specifically through the greater availability and use of rubella vaccine, the preventive use of RH immune globulin, and the therapeutic use of phototherapy.

Psychiatric and Social Casework Studies Two Canadian studies (Hefferman, 1955; Varwig, 1960) suggest that families with a deaf child have a greater than average risk of stress and marital breakdown. A recent and more extensive study reported by Freeman (1973) was concerned with the psychiatric correlates of deafness in 121 severely and profoundly deaf children with age of onset under 2 years; a control group matched for age, sex, and neighborhood was included for some parts of the analysis. Freeman's population was drawn from that collected by Robinson et al., and was almost completely representative of the lower mainland area of British Columbia. His preliminary findings were that, compared with the controls, his deaf subjects: (1) were hospitalized more in early life; (2) their families moved more; (3) they changed schools more often; (4) had fewer friends or friends their own age; (5) had mothers who were more likely to work; (6) had fathers who more often had to turn down opportunities for advancement in their work because of services required by the children; (7) had parents who permitted them to engage in fewer independent activities. The delay between suspicion and confirmation of deafness was excessive, ranging from 8–25 months. There were significantly more reports of behavior problems in the deaf population, particularly in the areas of stealing, over-particular behavior, and destruction of belongings. Half of the parents had been frustrated in communicating with their deaf child, and the educational controversies about methods of communication were continuing to affect many families and children in complex ways.

Audiological Studies A small number of audiometric studies have been reported. In addition to the three recent studies referred to by Wallace (1973), the descriptions of audiometric findings in the British Columbia series (Kendall, 1963; Robinson et al., 1963a, 1963b); and some specific reports from McGill (e.g., Dayal and Swisher, 1967; Swisher and Gannon, 1968; Baxter and Ling, 1972) and the University of British Columbia (Clarke and Conry, 1974), a series of studies on early (neonatal) audiometric screening of infants has been reported by Ling and his colleagues from the McGill School of Human Communication Disorders (Ling, Ling, and Doehring, 1970; Ling, Heaney, and Doehring, 1971; Sommer and Ling, 1970; Ling, 1972a, 1972b). This work, which clearly demonstrated the limitations of behavioral audiometry with newborns, was reviewed above in the section entitled "Diagnostic Procedures and Interprofessional Relationships." Ling and his colleagues have also been interested in several aspects of coded speech with the deaf, including the transposition of high frequency sounds in the delivery of speech signals to deaf children (Ling and Druz, 1967; Ling and Mechan, 1967; Ling, 1968; Ling, 1969; Ling and Doehring, 1969; Ling, 1971; Ling and Maretic, 1971; Ling, 1972c). This work has shown that deaf children can learn to discriminate coded speech as effectively as conventionally amplified sound but, as other workers have found, appear to derive no specific benefits in auditory discrimination from frequency transposition.

Psychological and Educational Studies Apart from attempts to standardize an intelligence scale for deaf children at the Ontario School for the Deaf, early Canadian work in these fields was restricted to occasional, isolated individual projects. However, in the past 10 years the quantity and quality of Canadian research in this area have increased markedly. Doehring and his colleagues at the McGill School of Human Communication Disorders have shown a consistent interest in the auditory perceptual and language abilities of normal and hearing-impaired children and adults and in training and educational procedures related to these (Doehring, 1965; Doehring et al., 1967; Doehring, 1968a; Doehring, 1969; Doehring and Rabinovitch, 1969; Doehring and Rosenstein, 1969; Bartholomeus and Doehring, 1971a, 1971b; Doehring, 1971; Doehring and Ling, 1971). Clarke and his students at the University of British Columbia have been interested in both the visual perceptual and linguistic correlates of deafness (Clarke and Leslie, 1971; Bunch, 1972; Leslie, 1972; Bunch, 1975; Ling and Clarke, 1975). Wallace (1972) and McDougall (1973) have also reported work on short-term memory and coding strategies in deaf children. Finally, there is growing evidence of research covering a wide range of topics reported from schools for the deaf (Darbyshire, 1973; Roberts, 1973; Forde, 1973).

Vocational, Employment, and Social Studies These were deservedly singled out by Wallace as neglected areas. Two studies, one of which was referred to in his report, should, however, be mentioned. In 1963–1964, Boese carried out a survey of the hearing handicapped in the Greater Vancouver area sponsored by the Western Institute for the deaf (Boese, 1966). The survey attempted to reach by questionnaire a representative sample of the deaf and hard-of-hearing population aged between 15–65, living in a defined geographical area. Several methods of identifying potential respondents were used—newspaper and radio announcements; clubs, organizations, and associations of the deaf and hard of hearing; otologists; schools for the deaf; welfare organizations. A total of 1,013 questionnaires were filled out; of these, 600 fitted the criteria, and 465 (287 deaf and 178 hard of hearing) provided reasonably detailed information. The survey clearly reached a larger and more representative population of deaf than of hard-of-hearing persons. The results showed: (1) that a relatively high percentage (27.2%) of the deaf working force was unemployed, and (2) that 18.6% of those employed had part-time or seasonal jobs, with the majority earning well below the national average income for employment, (3) 20% of the hard-of-hearing respondents were employed in professional, technical, and managerial positions, compared with 4% of the deaf, (4) individual interviews with deaf respondents showed a significant number of employment problems, mostly centering around communication difficulties, (5) 79% of those in the working force stated that their chances of promotion were poor, (6) less than 3% of the deaf had attained college education, as compared with 12% in the hearing community. However, the greatest needs revealed by the survey appeared to be in the area of personal and social counseling, where existing community facilities were found to be unsatisfactory by more than two-thirds of the respondents. The survey further showed that very few (13%) of the deaf respondents had learned a trade at school, but that more than two-thirds of them now had a trade they wished to learn.

The Boese survey was neither conceived nor carried out as a sophisticated piece of sociological research. It was intended mainly to provide information on the basis of which agencies concerned with services for the hearing impaired could make the best use of their limited resources by making their services more sensitive to identified as opposed to perceived needs. In this respect it seems to have succeeded admirably (see section entitled "Organizations and Associations Serving the Hearing Impaired").

Reich and Reich (1973) have more recently reported on their follow-up study of graduates of Ontario Schools for the Deaf. They found that only about 20% of these former students were working at jobs for which they had been trained. Their findings also showed that the academic levels of the former students were low, i.e., an average grade level of grade 4–5 in reading, with writing skills that were similarly retarded. They comment that, for deaf adults, communication by signs is especially important, particularly in situations which demand precise expression and reception of information. These conditions were not easy to meet in many job situations.

In summary, there is at present no provincial or national body concerned with the coordination of research efforts in the field of hearing impairment nor with the systematic collection and dissemination of information about completed research or about ongoing studies, funded or nonfunded. Some projects related to hearing impaired have been federally funded by National Health Grants (these are the ones likely to be known to provincial departments of health), the National Research Council and by Canada Council; information about these is not, however, readily available, although it has recently been announced that information about Canada Council grants will be published regularly, beginning late in 1975. There is, thus, no readily identified group, committee, or organization of mandarins which might serve at a national level as a policy-making body, overseeing and determining the priorities for federal support to research relating to the hearing impaired; the usual practice has been for individual applications to be submitted to panels of referees whose work is largely anonymous. However, there are now at least two university centers from which a more coordinated, directed, systematic series of publications has begun to emerge, and, as we have noted, a growing body of research from the schools for the deaf.

ORGANIZATIONS AND ASSOCIATIONS SERVING THE HEARING IMPAIRED

Historically the churches (and, in particular, the Lutheran Church) provided the first services for the deaf; recreational activities and social clubs grew out of lengthy sidewalk conversations following church meetings. Members of the clergy, perforce, had to take on the roles of interpreter, social worker, marriage and vocational counselor. From these modest beginnings, a multiplicity of organizations for the deaf and of the deaf grew up across Canada—first at the local scene, then provincially, regionally, and nationally. In the following overview, however, the order of development is reversed so that we may first examine the function and structure of the more broadly based organizations.

National Organizations

The largest and oldest is the Canadian Association of the Deaf (CAD) which is a coordinating and consulting body founded in 1940 and federally incorporated in 1948. The Board of Directors is composed of 25 deaf persons. Five are representatives of regional affiliates, and the remaining 20 are directors-at-large from different geographical areas across Canada. The regional affiliates are the Western Canada Association of the Deaf, the Ontario Association of the Deaf, the Quebec Federated Associations of the Deaf, the Eastern Canada Association of the Deaf, and the Canada Club of Washington, D.C. A sixth affiliate, the Canadian Deaf Information Centre, prefers to remain neutral on controversial issues and does not have a director on the board. Through its affiliates, the membership is over 2,000. The association depends upon donations from the deaf and investment income to cover its expenses, and none of the officers or directors receive remuneration for their services.

The CAD does not provide services to individuals but strives to maintain and improve the well being of the deaf population as a whole. It acts as a spokesman for Canadian deaf and as a watchdog on legislation and other such matters to ensure that the interests of the deaf are protected. It deals with federal officials on behalf of its affiliates and assists them at the provincial and local level on matters which are of national interest. For example, the CAD for years has proposed a program to recruit, train, and register interpreters but has been unable to secure the necessary financial support. Paradoxically this is one of, if not the most, serious shortcoming on the Canadian scene.

In May 1974, the CAD voted in favor of joining the World Federation of the Deaf.

Another national organization is the Federation of Silent Sports of Canada. This is a nonprofit sporting organization which obtained a federal charter in 1963. Its special function is to encourage and coordinate special sports programs of the deaf and to select, train, and sponsor deaf Canadians for the Winter and Summer World Games of the Deaf. It is affiliated with Le Comité International des Sports Silencieux and of the Canadian Amateur Sports Federation. It is financed by public contribution and assistance from the Federal Fitness and Amateur Sport Directorate.

A further national organization, The Canadian Coordinating Council on Deafness (CCCD), is emerging. The idea and plans for this organization stem from the National Consultation on Hearing Impairment in Toronto, March 1971, which was sponsored by the Welfare Grants Division, Department of National Health and Welfare, Ottawa, and organized by the Canadian Rehabilitation Council for the Disabled. One of the principal recommendations of this conference was that a national advisory committee for the hearing impaired (including the hard of hearing) be established. Later in the same year delegates from the Canadian Hearing Society, Toronto, and the Western Institute for the Deaf, Vancouver (both of which hold federal charters) approached the federal government in Ottawa for financial support for a national organization. These joint discussions resulted in a grant in July 1972 to support a research study to determine the need for and the design of a national organization. Dr. Graeme Wallace was appointed project director of this study and his report (Wallace, 1973) was published in the following year. Although the report came in for some heavy criticism (Kitcher, 1973; Wick, 1973; Carbin, 1974; Wallace, 1974), the CCCD held further meetings and, in September 1974, through an enlarged consortium of 24 provincial representatives, met to draw up a constitution and by-laws so that the new organization could be incorporated by the federal government. The basic membership is to consist of provincial councils each of which is entitled to two representatives on the governing board except for Ontario and Quebec which are entitled to four delegates because of bilingualism in Quebec and the size of their populations. In each case, half of the delegates are to be deaf.

In March 1975 the CCCD held their inaugural convention in Ottawa, together with nonvoting representatives from other concerned agencies and government. The constitution and by-laws were approved, and the following aims were formulated:

1. To provide a forum for discussion for voluntary and professional groups serving the hearing impaired on a national level.
2. To coordinate facilities for the hearing impaired across Canada.
3. To act as an advisory body to the federal and provincial governments and to agencies on matters relating to hearing impairment.

Regional Organizations

At the interprovincial level there are several organizations (see Canadian Association for the Deaf earlier), but one example will suffice to illustrate their function. The four western provinces set up the Western Canadian Association of the Deaf as early as 1923, and its various activities have included campaigning for a school for the deaf in Saskatoon (1931); successfully fighting the ban on deaf drivers in British Columbia in 1929 following an incident when a deaf driver was in an unwise collision with the Vancouver police chief's car; successfully pressing for radical changes in facilities and staffing at the then British Columbia School for the Deaf and Blind (1932); fighting tirelessly to keep the Manitoba School for the Deaf open during the depression and finally a continuous campaign from 1945–1965 to have the Manitoba school resited in its original building.

Provincial Organizations

It is not practical to describe in detail all the associations at provincial and local levels which operate across this country. Several publications list many of these organizations (The Canadian Hearing Society, 1972; Wallace, 1973; Plummer, 1974; Ling, D., 1975), but mere listing does not illustrate the diversity of programs which in fact exists. In order to highlight the variety of structures and functions, the following recent developments were selected at random and described in some detail.

In 1950 the Community Chest, Vancouver, invited Mrs. Lena Clarke, a charter member of the local Quota Club, to chair a committee to see what could be done to assist people with hearing problems. As a result of her work, the Society for Advancement of the Deaf and Hard of Hearing was founded in 1956, bringing under one board of directors the Vancouver Association of the Deaf (VAD) and the Vancouver League of the Hard of Hearing (VLHH). The newly revived Parent Teacher Association of Jericho Hill School for the Deaf and the Metropolitan Health Services sent delegates to the new society. Upon recommendations by the Community Chest, the society became the Western Institute for the Deaf (WID), a less unwieldy nomenclature and more consonant with the future plans of the society. From this period on, services later spelled out in the Survey of Hearing Handicapped (Boese, 1966) were developed and expanded.

Today the WID has its own quarters, a board of directors, a paid executive director, and a service team. More than 20 separate local organizations in British Columbia are affiliated with the institute and these can be grouped as follows:

1. Associations of the deaf and hard of hearing. These separate groups include the VAD, the VLHH, the FSSC, the Western Canadian Association of the Deaf (Vancouver Chapter), and the Jericho Hill School Alumni. Each group has its own constitution, but the WID building is made available for business, social, recreational, sporting, and cultural activities. Requests for group or individual assistance are forwarded through the executive director either to the board or to the service team.
2. Parents' groups. Throughout the province, parents have organized societies to initiate and/or maintain contact with educational programs. Some of these who have elected to affiliate with WID include Jericho Hill, the Vancouver Oral Center, Vancouver Island, Alberni-Clayoquot, Fraser Valey, Quesnel, Prince George, and the Okanagan.
3. Religious organizations. Church group affiliates include the Trinity Lutheran Church of the Deaf which this year celebrated its 40th anniversary, the Vancouver Catholic Deaf Association, and the Vancouver Church for the Deaf.
4. Professional groups. These include the British Columbia Speech and Hearing Association, the University of British Columbia Program in Education of Teachers of the Deaf, the Children's Hospital Diagnostic Centre, and the ENT Section British Columbia Medical Association. Although they have mainly a consultant role, individuals from these groups have given extensive service to the board. All accredited local organizations have one representative on the Council of Organizations Serving the Hearing Impaired of British Columbia. This council, which meets several times a year at various places in the province, provides a forum for the identification, discussion, and presentation of the needs of the hearing impaired which in turn are brought to the attention of the WID by the four members of the council who are elected to the board.

WID's income is obtained from the provincial government, United Community Services (formerly Community Chest), the city of Vancouver, and other municipal councils, donations, and bequests, local campaigns and membership fees. (The nominal fee of $3.00 allows all who are interested in the work of the institute to attend and vote at all general meetings and also receive the monthly WID Newsletter.)

Services provided by the 11 full-time staff members include interpreting, social work, audiological consultations, speechreading instruction, leisure time programs, sign language classes, and public education and information. Counseling is available concerning employment, family matters, financial problems, health, housing, and rehabilitation.

WID also produces a weekly half-hour television show for the deaf entitled "Show of Hands," and has been active since 1969 in the provision of a teletypewriter (TTY) network which enables the deaf to enjoy telephone communciations via obsolete 5 Code telecommunication equipment and an acoustic coupler. This network has spread to Edmonton, Calgary, Winnipeg, Toronto, and Montreal.

The institute has a close association with the King's Daughter Manor, a residence for elderly deaf. The visual alarm system is designed specifically for them, and a special vibrator unit gives warnings at night. Future plans include providing a closed circuit television system between the main entrance and each of the apartment units to identify visitors.

Other multipurpose homes for elderly deaf exist in Winnipeg and Montreal at the School of St. Denis. The Ontario Mission also has extensive plans for a community center and housing for the deaf in Toronto.

The Manitoba Coordinating Council for the Hearing Impaired was established in 1970 and is composed of representatives of all agencies and personnel serving the deaf. Through the activities of various committees, the general public is made more aware of the handicap of deafness; and hearing-impaired persons and professional personnel work cooperatively to improve educational, social, economic, cultural, and spiritual opportunities for the deaf. The council now speaks with a united voice on behalf of the hearing impaired; fosters cooperation between parents, teacher organizations, and educational authorities; evaluates services and facilities; encourages early detection, diagnosis, and treatment; and coordinates and strengthens the services of its member organizations. A current project concerns a new Community Centre for the Deaf in Winnipeg which provides a residence for deaf senior citizens, accommodation for deaf persons taking vocational training, and facilities for recreational and social gatherings.

Other similar coordinating provincial bodies have recently been established in Alberta (The Alberta Council for the Hearing Handicapped), Nova Scotia (Maritime Council of the Deaf), and Saskatchewan (Saskatchewan Coordinating Council on Deafness).

The Canadian Hearing Society (CHS) consists of an executive committee of five members and a board of 50 (including some deaf people). The board does most of its work through committees–e.g., aims, objectives, information services, medical and audiological, parent-child guidance, management, media, projects, public relations, membership, campaign, and finance. Apart from the head office in Toronto, there are branch offices in London, Hamilton, and Ottawa.

The CHS is financed by the Ontario government through Social and Family Services, by individual and corporate donations, trust funds, and some fees. Although its major aim is to encourage the coordination of public and private agencies involved with the hearing handicapped, it operates various services at the grassroots level:

1. Through its news letter, "Vibrations," information is provided concerning community resources and educational materials. The CHS also sponsors speech and hearing month (May) in Ontario and makes an all out drive on public education at this time.
2. Trained audiologists perform hearing evaluations and aid fittings. The CHS makes aids available direct from the manufacturers. Sales cannot be made to the general public, but government agencies and nonprofit organizations underwrite the cost for a hearing-impaired person who is under CHS sponsorships.
3. A telephone answering service is available for all the local agencies in the province, and overnight accommodation is made available for out-of-town parents whose hearing-impaired child may be hospitalized for on-going assessment.
4. For graduates and postschool students of the various schools, placement offices offer vocational services which include assessment, guidance, counseling, training and retraining, and job placement. Although the high employment rate among the deaf in Ontario is well publicized, little information is available about the type of employment.

The Ontario Mission for the Deaf has established throughout Ontario, interdenominational independent churches which are owned and operated by and for the deaf. Services, meetings, and social activities are conducted in total communication.

The mission also runs the Ontario Summer Camp of the Deaf, for deaf and hard-of-hearing children and hearing children of deaf parents, aged 8 years and older. The supervised program includes worship, sports and crafts, and there is also a special program for multiply handicapped deaf children. Facilities are available for unstructured family camping.

In addition, the mission runs the Ontario Farm for Deaf Children. This is a treatment and training center which houses eight or so homeless and disturbed deaf boys and girls of school age. Younger children will be accepted if the need should arise. The children attend the nearby Provincial School at Milton.

Recently the Ontario Mission for the Deaf purchased six acres of land to build a community center in Toronto. The center is to provide court, legal and medical interpreting services, social work and counseling services, English instruction for deaf new Canadians, instruction in manual communication, cooperation with other community organizations and services, recreational and social facilities, apartment units for deaf senior citizens, a worship center, and residential training facilities.

In May 1975, three inventors from the University of Toronto (Van Douglass, Doyle, and Lancee) patented a new device, not much larger than a cigarette package, which will allow the deaf to communicate by telephone. The key parts of the system which take advantage of the existing telephone network are a touch tone telephone and a container which can be instantly affixed to the telephone ear piece. It contains small panels on which illuminated letters rapidly spell out words in much the same way as news is printed out on television sets by cable TV. The device will be manufactured at a cost of approximately $100 in the nonprofit workshop established by the Mission and operated by the deaf.

Programs by the Deaf for the Deaf

In recent years the deaf themselves have organized two very promising ventures. The first is a nonprofit organization–The Canadian Cultural Society of the Deaf (CCSD)–set up in 1971 with national headquarters in Winnipeg, Manitoba but with provincial and local centers in other provinces. The aims of the CCSD are:

1. To preserve, guide, stimulate, encourage, and motivate deaf Canadians to strive for excellence and reach higher levels of "culturama."
2. To promote the development of cultural programs so that the deaf may achieve a state of well being in which they will function most effectively at home, at work, and at play.
3. To challenge the deaf and to recognize and honor outstanding achievements through a series of national awards.
4. To arrange for cultural contests on the local and provincial level and to present national awards.

The national award for the winners will consist of the Golden Defty Trophy (Defty being derived from the pronunciation of deaf and the word deft) in four fields–physical, literary performance, recreation, and home arts.

The periodical, *Cultural Horizons*, of the deaf in Canada was first published in June 1973.

The second was the arrival in September-October 1972 of a bimonthly magazine, *The Deaf Canadian,* a belated relative of the *Deaf American.* In the first issue it states the following purposes:

1. As a first duty, to educate the general public to an awareness of deafness and its causes.
2. To publicize problems of the deaf concerning education, discrimination, vocations, and injustices.
3. To report any mishappenings to the deaf and hard of hearing.
4. To publicize any difficulties that hearing people, especially bureaucrats, are creating for deaf people who want the chance to show their ability in employment, vocations, education, and other situations; and to suggest solutions to these problems.
5. To inform the deaf of news of their fellow deaf countrymen.
6. To urge the deaf to speak up about anything that others (including professionals) should know so that something might be done.

This acceptance of responsibility by the deaf was for a time in the U.S.A. referred to as "deaf power." In Canada, the preferred term is "deaf pride."

CONCLUDING THOUGHTS

It will have become abundantly clear from our review of Canadian developments in aural rehabilitation that the overall picture is blurred, uneven, and difficult to discern. To some extent, this lack of clarity reflects the biases of our own background and interests; as artists we may indeed have been maladroit with our brushes and colors in our attempt to depict the Canadian scene. But there are other reasons for this confusion: the relegation of responsibility in critical fields of health, education, and welfare from the federal level to the 10 provincial administrations; the dearth in any province of legislation protecting the interests of the hearing impaired; the imbalance in funding between services for children and those for adults; the marriage of convenience between the public sector and the voluntary organizations; problems within the voluntary bodies; the struggle between those organized by the hearing for the hearing impaired and those organized by the hearing impaired themselves.

Yet, in the last analysis, we should have to record our conviction that the story is one of considerable achievement. For hearing-impaired children, at least, the physical plant, amenities, equipment, and staffing in classes, schools, clinics, and training programs are at least equal to, if not superior to, those found in any other country. And as we have tried to stress, throughout the whole field there is an increasing ferment of activity, a growing recognition of the unmet needs of both children and adults, and a readiness to discuss contentious issues rather than sweeping them under the rug.

ACKNOWLEDGMENTS

To our many respondents, who are too numerous to name individually, we offer sincere thanks for the oral, manual, and written information we received. On recognizing their contributions, they will appreciate that it was their efforts which enabled this chapter to be completed.

The opinions expressed, however, belong to the authors; full responsibility is accepted for any bias shown in our selection of illustrative examples and apologies are made for unwitting inaccuracies. Special thanks are given to our research assistant, Judy Cherniak, and our secretary, Grace Holmes, for their encouragement and untiring assistance.

LITERATURE CITED

Anthony, D. A., and Associates. 1971. Seeing Essential English. University Northern Colorado, Greeley.

Bartholomeus, B., and D. G. Doehring. 1971a. Development of naming responses to meaningful non-verbal sounds. Percept. Motor Skills 32: 195–204.

Bartholomeus, B., and D. G. Doehring. 1971b. Effect of verbal content and stimulus order on visual-auditory association. Percept. Motor Skills 33:891–897.

Baxter, J. D., and D. Ling. 1972. Ear Disease and Hearing Loss Among the Eskimo Population of Pangnirtung. McGill University Baffin Zone Project. Canad. J. Otolaryngol. 1: 337–343.

Boese, J. R. 1966. Survey of the Hearing Handicapped, Greater Vancouver Area. The Western Institute for the Deaf, Vancouver, Brit. Col. 122 p.

Budden, S., G. Robinson, C. Dunnella MacLean, and K. G. Cambon, 1974. Deafness in Infants and Preschool Children: An Analysis of Etiology and Association Handicaps. Am. Ann. Deaf 119(4): 387–395.

Buell, E. M. 1968. Outline of Language for Deaf Children. Books I and II. The Volta Bureau, Washington, D. C. 107 p. and 121 p.

Buller, G. 1973. Special Classes for the Multi-Handicapped Hearing Impaired Child. *In* G. O. Bunch (ed.), Proceedings of the First National Conference of Canadian Teachers of the Deaf, pp. 56–65. Ontario School for the Deaf, Belleville, Ont.

Bunch, G. O. 1972a. Concept development studies and the classroom

reading performance of deaf children. Canad. Teacher Deaf 1(3):14–23.
Bunch, G. O. 1972b. The retarded deaf child in residential schools for the deaf in Canada. Presented at the American Association on Mental Deficiency, Region 1 Conference, October, Vancouver, Brit. Col.
Bunch, G. O. 1973. Canadian services for multiply-handicapped deaf children. Canad. Teacher Deaf 2(4):27–31.
Bunch, G. O. 1975. An Evaluation of Natural and Formal Language Programs with Deaf Children. Unpublished Ed.D. dissertation, University of British Columbia, Vancouver, Brit. Col.
Canadian Hearing Society. 1972. Why Go it Alone. Canadian Manpower Local Initiatives Program, Toronto, Ont.
Caniglia, J., N. J. Cole, W. Howard, E. Krohn, and M. Rice. 1972. Apple Tree. Centre for In-Service Education, Colorado. 205 p.
Carbin, C. F. 1974. Editorial. Deaf Canadian 3(5):6–7.
Clarke, B. R. 1972. Total communication. Canad. Teacher Deaf 2(1): 22–29.
Clarke, B. R. 1974. Overall impressions of the Canadian scene: A study of Canadian programs in education of the deaf. ACEHI J. 1(1):3–21.
Clarke, B. R., and R. Conry. 1974. Hearing impairment in children of low birth weight. *In* H. Dunn (ed.), Neurological and Ophthalmic Disorders in Children of Low Birth Weight. In press.
Clarke, B. R., and P. Leslie. 1971. Visual-motor skills and reading ability of deaf children. Percept. Motor Skills 33:263–268.
Clarke, B. R., and D. Ling. 1975. Cued speech: A follow-up study. Volta Rev. In press.
Clarke School for the Deaf. 1972. Language. Massachusetts. 163 p.
Commission on Emotional and Learning Disorders in Children. 1970. One million children. Leonard Crainford. Toronto. 521 p.
Cornett, O. R. 1972. Cued speech. *In* G. Fant (ed.), International Symposium on Speech Communication Ability and Profound Deafness, Stockholm, 1970, pp. 213–223. Alexander Graham Bell Association for the Deaf, Washington, D.C.
Cory, W. 1959. Education of the Deaf in Canada. Unpublished Master's thesis, University of British Columbia.
Darbyshire, J. O. 1973. Recent research into the play patterns of young hearing impaired children. *In* G. O. Bunch (ed.), Proceedings of the First National Conference of Canadian Teachers of the Deaf, pp. 132–137. Ontario School for the Deaf, Belleville, Ont.
Doehering, D. G. 1965. The validity of intelligence tests for evaluating deaf children. J. Speech Hear. Disord. 50:299–300.
Doehering, D. G. 1968. Picture-sound association in deaf children. J. Speech Hear. Res. 11:49–62.
Doehering, D. G. 1969. Temporal sequence effects in auditory oddity discrimination. Percept. Psychophysics 6:65–68.
Doehering, D. G. 1971. Serial order effects in auditory discrimination by oddity and matching to sample. Percept. Psychophysics 10:137–141.
Doehring, D. G., J. G. Dudley, and L. Coderre. 1967. Programmed instruction in picture-sound association for the aphasic. Folia Phoniat. 19: 414–426.

Doehring, D. G., and D. Ling. 1971. Programmed instruction of hearing impaired children in the auditory discrimination of vowels. J. Speech Hear. Res. 14:746–753.

Doehring, D. G., and M. S. Rabinovitch. 1969. Auditory abilities of children with learning problems. J. Learn. Disab. 2:467–474.

Doehring, D. G., and J. Rosenstein. 1969. Speed of visual perception in deaf children. J. Speech Hear. Res. 12:118–125.

Downs, M. P., and G. M. Sterritt. 1964. Identification audiometry for neonates: A preliminary report. J. Aud. Res. 4:69–80.

Downs, M. P., and G. M. Sterritt. 1967. A guide to newborn and infant hearing screening programs. Arch. Otolaryngol. 85:15–22.

Ewing, I. R., and A. W. G. Ewing. 1943. Ascertainment of deafness in infancy and early childhood. J. Laryngol. Otol. 59(9):309–317.

Ewing, Sir A., and E. C. Ewing. 1967. Teaching Deaf Children to Talk. Manchester University Press, Manchester. 255 p.

Fitzgerald, E. 1965. Straight Language for the Deaf. The Volta Bureau, Washington, D. C. 97 p.

Forde, J. 1973. Characteristics of a day-residential school population. *In* G. O. Bunch (ed.), Proceedings of the First National Conference of Canadian Teachers of the Deaf, pp. 121–124. Ontario School for the Deaf, Belleville, Ont.

Freeman, R. 1973. Correlates of Psychiatric Disorder in Deaf Children: Report on Public Health Research Grant No. 609-7-343. Vols. I and II. Mimeographed.

Freeman, R. 1975. Counselling and Home Training Program for Deaf Children. Presented at Symposium Language, Society and the Preschool Deaf Child, March 14, Vancouver, British Columbia.

Groht, M. 1965. Natural Language for Deaf Children. Alexander Graham Bell Association for the Deaf, Inc., Washington, D. C. 185 p.

Gustason, G. 1972. Signing Exact English. Modern Signs Press, Rossmore, Calif.

Harris, G. 1971. Language for the Preschool Deaf Child. Grune & Stratton, Inc., New York. 346 p.

Hefferman, A. 1955. A psychiatric study of fifty preschool children referred to hospital for suspected deafness. *In* G. Caplan (ed.), Emotional Problems of Early Childhood, pp. 269–292. Basic Books, Inc., New York.

Interdepartmental Committee on Consumer Affairs. 1970. Subcommittee on Hearing Aids, Report on Hearing Aids. Ottawa.

Interprovincial School for the Deaf Annual Reports, Amherst, Nova Scotia.

Kendall, D. C. 1963. The assessment of young hearing impaired children in a medical center. *In* P. V. Doctor (ed.), Report of the Proceedings of the International Congress on Education of the Deaf and of the Forty-first Meeting of the Convention of American Instructors of the Deaf, pp. 391–401. United States Government Printing Office, Washington, D.C.

Kendall, D. C. 1964. The audiological examination of young children. Volta Rev. 66(10):735–742.

Kendall, D. C. 1971. Evaluation Report to the Managers of the Interprovincial School for the Deaf, Amherst. Unpublished.

Kennedy, A. 1972. For Readers We Need Writers. Canad. Teacher Deaf 2(1): 5–8.

Kitcher, P. W. 1973. A critique of the Canadian Study of Hard of Hearing and Deaf. *In* G. O. Bunch (ed.), Proceedings of the First National Conference of Canadian Teachers of the Deaf, p. 159. Ontario School for the Deaf, Belleville, Ont.

Kysela, G. M., and S. Masciuch. 1972. A program for multiply-handicapped children. Canad. Teacher Deaf 1(3): 24–34.

Leslie, P. 1972a. Selected Linguistic Skills in Young Deaf Children. Unpublished Ed.D. thesis, University of British Columbia.

Leslie, P. 1972b. Some Considerations of Language Acquisition in Deaf Children. Canad. Teacher Deaf 1(2):16–22.

Ling, D. 1968. Three experiments on frequency transposition. Am. Ann. Deaf 113:283–294.

Ling, D. 1969. Speech discrimination by profoundly deaf children using linear and coded amplifiers. IEFF Trans Audio. Electroacoust. 17: 298–303.

Ling, D. 1971. Deaf Children's Audition of Distinctive Features within Frequency-Shifted Speech. Proceedings of 2nd Louisville Conference on Rate and Frequency Controlled Speech. Louisville University Press, Louisville, Ky.

Ling, D. 1972a. Acoustic stimulus duration in relation to behavioral responses of newborn infants. J. Speech Hear. Res. 15:567–571.

Ling, D. 1972b. Auditory discrimination of speech altered by a sample and hold process. *In* G. Fant (ed.), International Symposium on Speech Communication Ability and Profound Deafness, pp. 323–333. Alexander Graham Bell Association for the Deaf, Inc., Washington, D. C.

Ling, D. 1972c. Response validity in auditory tests of newborn infants. Laryngoscope 82:376–380.

Ling, D. 1975. Conseil Consultatif de Québec Pour la Déficience Auditive. Mimeographed.

Ling, D., and B. R. Clarke. 1975. Cued speech: An evaluative study. Am. Ann. Deaf. In press.

Ling, D., and D. G. Doehring. 1969. Learning limits of deaf children for coded speech. J. Speech Hear. Res. 12:83–94.

Ling, D., and W. S. Druz. 1967. Transposition of high frequency sounds by partial vocoding of the speech spectrum: Its use by deaf children. J. Audit. Res. 7:133–144.

Ling, D., C. Heaney, and D. G. Doehring. 1971. The use of alternated stimuli to reduce response decrement in the auditory testing of newborn infants. J. Speech Hear. Res. 14:531–534.

Ling, D., A. H. Ling, and D. G. Doehring. 1970. Stimulus, response and observer variables in the auditory screening of newborn infants. J. Speech Hear. Res. 13:10–18.

Ling, D., and H. Maretic. 1971. Frequency transposition in the teaching of speech to deaf children. J. Speech Hear. Res. 14:37–46.

Ling, D., and S. R. Mecham. 1967. Frequency transposition of speech for deaf children. Proc. Internat. Congr. Educ. Deaf 1:856–865.

McCarr, J. 1973. Lessons in Syntax. Dormac Publishing Company, Oregon. 164 p.

McDougall, J. 1973. Short term memory and language in the deaf. *In* G. O. Bunch (ed.), Proceedings of the First National Conference of Canadian Teachers of the Deaf, pp. 145–149. Ontario School for the Deaf, Belleville, Ont.

McHugh, H. E. 1961. The Brain Injured Child with Impaired Hearing. Laryngoscope 71:1034–1057.

McHugh, H. E. 1962. Hearing and Language Disorders in Children. Postgrad. Med. 31:54–65.

Neveu, F. Herve. 1974. Letter to the Editor. ACEHI J. 1(3):18.

Nova Scotia Laws. 1960. An Act to Establish an Interprovincial School for the Education of the Deaf. Assented to April 13, 1960. Chapter 7, pp. 48–62.

Peck, G. 1969. Patterned Language for the Deaf. *In* W. J. McClure (ed.), The Report of the Proceedings of the 44th Meeting of the Convention of American Instructors of the Deaf, pp. 195–203. Berkeley, Calif.

Plummer, D. M. (ed.). 1974. Services to the Deaf and Hearing Impaired in the Province of Manitoba. Mimeographed.

Pugh, B. 1965. Steps in Language Development for the Deaf. The Volta Bureau, Washington, D. C. 71 p.

Reich, P. A., and C. M. Reich. 1973. Presentation 1: A follow-up study of the deaf. *In* G. O. Bunch (ed.), Proceedings of the Provincial Conference on Aims and Objectives of the Deaf Individual in Ontario, pp. 4–6. Queen's Park, Toronto, Ont.

Rhodes, M. J. 1972. From a parent's point of view. Deaf Am. September, p. 20.

Roberts, W. 1973. A comparison of rehearsal techniques in visual information processing among deaf adolescents. *In* G. O. Bunch (ed.), Proceedings of the First National Conference of Canadian Teachers of the Deaf, pp. 150–158. Ontario School for the Deaf, Belleville, Ont.

Robinson, G. C., J. R. Brummitt, and J. R. Miller. 1963a. Hearing loss in infants and preschool children. II. Etiological considerations. J. Pediatr. 32:115–124.

Robinson, G. C., and K. G. Cambon. 1964. Hearing loss in infants of tuberculous mothers treated with streptomycin during pregnancy. New Eng. J. Med. 271: 949–951.

Robinson, G. C., and M. M. Johnston. 1967. Pili Torti and sensory neural hearing loss. J. Pediatr. 70:621–623.

Robinson, G. C., D. C. Kendall, and K. G. Cambon. 1963b. Hearing loss in infants and preschool children. The development of a provincial preschool hearing program and some preliminary results. J. Pediatr. 32: 103–114.

Robinson, G. C., J. R. Miller, and L. I. Saepardan. 1965. Waardenburg's syndrome: The risk of recurrence of congenital deafness in a kindred. J. Pediatr. 67:491–494.

Robinson, G. C., L. S. Wildervanck, and T. P. Chiang. 1973. Ectrodactyly, ectodermal dysplasia, and cleft lip-palate syndrome: Its association with conductive hearing loss. J. Pediatr. 82:107–109.

Sommer, F. G., and D. Ling. 1970. Auditory testing of newborns using eyeblink conditioning. J. Audit. Res. 10:292–295.

Statistics Canada. 1974. Canad. Statist. Rev. 50(3):18.
Statutes of British Columbia. 1972. Bill 31. The Act to Amend the Hearing Aid Regulation Act. Assented to March 14, 1972.
Statutes of British Columbia. 1972. The Hearing Aid Regulation Act. Assented to April 2, 1971. Chapter 24, pp. 107–111.
Statutes British Columbia. 1973. Bill 137. The Act to Amend the Hearing Aid Regulation Act. Assented to April 13, 1973.
Statutes of Manitoba. 1971. Bill 26. The Hearing Aid Act. Chapter 22, pp. 67–78.
Statutes of Nova Scotia. 1974. In press.
Statutes of Quebec. 1973. Bill 250. Professional Code. Assented to July 6, 1973. pp. 1–71.
Statutes of Quebec. 1973. Bill 270. Hearing Aid Acousticians Act. Assented to June 29, 1973. pp. 617–621.
Statutes of Saskatchewan. 1973. An Act Respecting the Establishment of a Program to Provide Hearing Aids to Certain Persons with Defective Hearing. Chapter 44, pp. 1–2.
Stokoe, W. C. 1974. Seeing and signing language. Hearing Speech News. September-December 1974, pp. 32–37.
Streng, A. 1972. Syntax, Speech and Hearing. Grune & Stratton, Inc., New York. 290 p.
Swisher, L. P., and R. P. Gannon. 1968. The comparison of auditory and vestibular responses in hearing impaired children. Acta Otolaryngol. 66:89–96.
Tonkin, R. S., 1974. Regionalization Task Force Committee to Study the Needs of the Communicatively Impaired in British Columbia. Province of Brit. Col. Dept. of Health, British Columbia.
Van Uden, A. 1970. A World of Language for Deaf Children. Rotterdam University Press, The Netherlands. 233 p.
Varwig, R. 1960. Family Contributions in the Preschool Treatment of Hearing Handicapped Children. Unpublished Master's of Social Work thesis, University of British Columbia.
Wallace, G. 1972. Short-term Memory and Coding Strategies in the Deaf. Unpublished Ph.D. thesis, McGill University.
Wallace, G. 1973. Canadian Study of Hard of Hearing and Deaf. Canadian Rehabilitation Council for the Disabled, Ottawa. 88 p.
Wallace, G. 1974. Globe and Mail, September 18, 1974. Reprinted in the Deaf Canad. 3(4):5.
Walsh, J., M. Ross, M. Hanson, M. Gilbert, K. MacLaren, and M. M. Moore. 1974. Hearing Aids. Task Force Committee to Study the Needs of the Communicatively Impaired in British Columbia. Province of British Columbia Department of Health, Brit. Col.
Wampler, D. 1971. Linguistics of Visual English. Santa Rosa, Calif.
Washington State School. 1972. An Introduction to Manual English. Vancouver, Washington. 207 p.
Wick, M. 1973. Quoted in Deaf Canad. 2(3):6.

chapter 5

Communication for Hearing-handicapped People in Argentina

Oscar Tosi, Ph.D.

In the history of the healing arts, three different stages or approaches can be distinguished. These stages have always overlapped in one way or other, but, in general, it can be stated that from a chronological point of view the first one corresponds to curative medicine, the second one to preventive medicine, and the last one to habilitative or rehabilitative medicine (Quiros, 1973).

Habilitative and rehabilitative audiology, whether considered a branch of medicine or not, according to each country, should maintain the philosophy of this third stage of the healing arts, i.e., to integrate the patient into "normal" society, since cure or prophylaxis alone will not suffice. As a consequence of this philosophy, the habilitated or rehabilitated patient should be provided with voice communication and not with a specialized type of communication, solely intelligible to the initiated: the oral communication method should be learned by the hearing handicapped in all possible cases. Auditory perception, of course, can be complemented by visual clues, like lipreading, but, in the opinion of the writer, methods of habilitation other than the oral one should be used only in those cases when voice communication is not practical or possible, that is, when central pathways and cognitive areas rather than peripheral structures are impaired.

The habilitated or rehabilitated patient should live a life not too different from that of the normal hearing person if at all possible. Certainly, some capabilities of the latter are absolutely denied to the former, such as enjoying a symphony, but proper substitutes must be searched for to provide the hearing handicapped with the same amount of happiness that any human being is entitled to enjoy.

In summary, a habilitative audiological program should be aimed, at least ideally, at developing, within the hearing handicapped, language and auditory skills that are as close to normal as possible. Such a program should provide also for the necessary psychological adjustments. This is not only the personal opinion of the writer, but also the predominant point of view in Argentina since programs for the deaf started in 1867.

Considering that this chapter is concerned with habilitative and rehabilitative audiology in Argentina, it seems important to give, at this point, a general idea about that nation.

Argentina, a 4,024,45-km^2 (1,553,844 sq. miles) country with approximately 22,000,000 inhabitants, is situated in the southern part of South America, extending from the subtropical areas to the Antarctic regions. A variety of climates are, therefore, included in Argentina, from the temperate in the north to the polar in the south. Most inhabitants are from European extraction, mainly descendents of Italians, Spaniards, and Germans, although other nationalities are also very well represented. The official language is Spanish, but most people speak a dialect of that language that identifies them as Argentinians. In spite of the present economic chaos, Argentina is a well developed and rich country, one of the major world producers of wheat and beef. Average annual income per capita is estimated at approximately $3,000. During past decades Argentinians were considered the best fed people in the world; today this could be still true. Illiteracy is limited to 8% of the population, the lowest figure in all Latin America. Population growth rate is only 1.8% per year.

The political structure of Argentina is similar to that of the U.S.A. Argentina is a federal republic integrated by a federal district (Buenos Aires City) and 23 autonomous provinces. The word "national" is reserved for the federal government and federal institutions, to distinguish them from the "provincial" ones. Municipal governments are also similar to those of the U.S.A., although with one significant difference: schools do not depend on local boards but national or provincial ones. The practical effect of this organization is that all schools offer the same programs irrespective of the social or economic status of the section of a city where they are located.

From the point of view of its economic, social, and political structure, Argentina has been compared to a giant with an enormous head and a rachitic body. Indeed, the out-of-proportion head is Buenos Aires City and nearby towns, where about 9 million persons live; the remaining 13 million are located in four or five other big cities or dispersed in remote places of the vast Argentinian pampas. All communications converge to Buenos Aires City, including railroads, highways, airways, etc. This odd situation came from the colonization times and has molded the idiosyncracies, characteristics, and development of the Argentine institutions. The people of Buenos Aires are called the "porteños," i.e., the people of the "port," since the Spanish rule allowed only one port for importing and exporting merchandise from the vice-royalty of the River Plata (Argentina) during the three centuries it lasted. This port was Buenos Aires, so, consequently, it became the economic, political, and social center of the country. At present this is still true, in spite of some efforts made by the federal government to somehow shift this center of gravity from Buenos Aires City. Some characteristics of habilitative audiology in Argentina may find their reason in these facts. Indeed, most programs of habilitative audiology are offered in Buenos Aires City, a situation essentially different from the one prevalent in Spain or Italy, countries where the different regions had parallel development through the centuries, allowing them, therefore, to offer similar facilities all over the nation. Implications for Argentina are even worse than they are in European countries because of the vast expanse of Argentina and the poor means of communication in the remote areas.

Education in Argentina is free at all levels, including the universities, with exception, of course, of the private schools.

Grade school is obligatory and takes 7 years. These schools are either national (federal), provincial, or private, all with uniform programs regulated by the Federal Board of Education (Consejo Nacional de Educacion) and the respective Provincial Boards of Education. High schools through all the nation offer also very similar 5- or 6-year programs. There are four types of high schools: (1) "colegio nacional," which offers a general humanistic and scientific preparation for the university; this type of high school is very similar to the French "lycee" or the Italian "ginnasio"; (2) "escuela industrial," which prepares technicians in construction, chemistry, etc., similar to the German "real schule"; (3) "escuela commercial," which offer programs to train business clerks, secretaries, and accountants; and (4) "escuela normal," which trains primary school teachers.

In Argentina there are 13 national or provincial universities and 12 private universities. Most of these universities possess a high standard of quality, the National University of Buenos Aires being the most prestigious one, with approximately 80,000 students. Universities are divided into "facultades" (colleges) and usually do not have a campus. Each facultad functions quite independently as a small specialized university in a building, located in an arbitrary place within the respective city, very often far from the other sister facultades. Also, the pedagogical structure of the Argentine university is very similar to the French or Italian one, i.e., in Argentina, there are not graduate and undergraduate programs as there are in the U.S.A.; most facultades offer a straight 6- or 7-year program in engineering, medicine, architecture, pharmacy, or law, leading to a professional degree similar to professional degrees in the U.S.A. Pure scientific programs (physics, chemistry, biology, etc.), which are less common, lead to a doctorate or a "licenciatura." Some facultades offer also a combination of a professional degree and research doctorates. Some facultades also offer a shorter and lower level, a 3-year program to train paraprofessionals. For instance, the facultades of engineering offer 3-year programs to train surveyors; law facultades train notaries; facultades of medicine train optometrists, nurses, phonoaudiologists, etc., within this "paraprofessional" concept. Some facultades offer also programs of specialization for professionals, although it is not common practice.

The prospective university student must make up his/her mind concerning the desired field of studies before applying to the proper facultad for admission. The system is very rigid; in general, there are no optional equivalent courses once the student has chosen a profession. Usually every facultad has rather stringent entrance examinations that often require a year of preparation beyond high school.

It is generally admitted that the content of the first 2 years of undergraduate studies in the U.S.A. is covered in the Argentine high school programs, which are similar to those in Europe. The reader must consider these facts when comparing audiological programs among the different countries.

In Argentina there exists also a third level of education that does not belong to the university. This third level corresponds to pedagogical schools which depend upon the ministry of education. These schools train high school teachers and teachers of the deaf. Programs are 3- or 4-year extensions according to the specialty.

Traditionally, primary and secondary schools in Argentina are separated according to sex.

Although the percentage of illiteracy in Argentina is very low, only 20–25% of the youngsters who complete primary school attend high school. About 40% of the high school graduates continue on to university studies. Statistics show that less than 50% of the students enrolled in universities manage to graduate (Esmay, 1971).

HISTORICAL OVERVIEW OF HABILITATIVE AUDIOLOGY IN ARGENTINA

Domingo F. Sarmiento (1811–1888), an outstanding Argentine teacher, who eventually became president of Argentina in 1868, was instrumental in the creation of the first school for the deaf in South America in 1843. At that time Sarmiento was a political exile in Chile. Sarmiento's school for the deaf was founded there, sponsored by the Chilean government. After the political enemy of Sarmiento, the dictator Juan M. Rosas, was overthrown, Sarmiento returned to Argentina, becoming first senator and later president. In that position, he tended to favor the programs for deaf children as part of his effort toward education in general. Indeed, Sarmiento was quoted as saying: "I can be a senator, a general or even the president of the nation, but above all I am a teacher" (Barlaro, 1927). In 1868 Sarmiento received a "Doctor Honoris Causa" degree from the University of Michigan.

The first school for the deaf actually established in Argentina was founded in 1857 in Buenos Aires City by Karl Keil, a German who was a former student of S. Heinicke (Itarburu and Vailanti, 1966). Heinicke had championed the oral method of habilitation, as opposed to the sign language taught in France by L'Epee. Keil emphasized the oral aspect of habilitation in his school, but he also used the L'Epee method to some extent. In addition to the habilitative teaching, Keil provided his students with instruction on the Bible, on reading and writing, and on drawing. Keil's school for the deaf had two sponsors, the private philanthropic society "Regeneracion" and the government of the province of Buenos Aires. Indeed, by a decree of 24 October 1857, signed by governor Valentin Alsina, funds to support the school were granted to Keil. Mr. Keil kept the school working until approximately 1870, 1 year before he died from yellow fever that erupted in Buenos Aires City (carried in by an oriental ship). Fortunately, by that time, Mr. Jose Facio, who fathered a deaf child, felt the urge to do something for his child, as well for other deaf children. Wih this purpose he traveled to Italy to receive training as a teacher of the deaf. After returning to Argentina, he opened a private school for the deaf in Buenos Aires City in 1870. Facio's school received financial support from the government in 1873. In 1875, it became an official institute, with Facio appointed as a director. This school utilized also the oral method of habilitation. In addition, it offered primary instruction and training in practical trades to the pupils.

In 1882, a pedagogical international congress was held in Buenos Aires City, promoted by the National Board of Education. One of the participants, Dr. Jose Terry, presented a paper entitled "The Argentine Deaf-Mute Child; his Habilitation and Instruction." This paper attracted the attention of the authorities. Wishing to have more information on the subject, they appointed an ad hoc committee to report on the methods and results obtained by Facio in his school. This committee was formed by Drs. Emilio Coni, Guillermo Rawson, Lucio Menendez, and Jose Terry. After the task of this committee was completed, a report was presented to the

Argentine authorities, recommending: (1) creation of a new institute that should use exclusively the oral method of rehabilitation with programs similar to the Italian ones; (2) to import Italian teachers for the deaf to staff this institute; (3) to train Argentine teachers who eventually could take over the habilitative process and train other Argentine teachers. Following these recommendations, the Argentine government contracted Friar Serafin Ballestra, a professor at the University of Como, Italy, to develop these courses. Friar Ballestra arrived at Buenos Aires in May 1885, assuming his position as Director of the National Institute for the Deaf in April 1886. Four months later, he was fired because of proved immoral events that took place in the institute. Good Mr. Facio was immediately called to replace Ballestra.

In 1890, a special commission, headed by Dr. Emilio Coni, was appointed to reorganize the institute. This task was satisfactorily accomplished. Dr. Coni contracted a new Italian teacher for the deaf, Luiggi Molfino, from Milano the same year. Molfino assumed the direction of the institute and continued with excellent success for 4 years. Molfino created a special school to train teachers of the deaf, as a separate department within the institute. One of the first Argentine teachers graduated from this school was Bartolome Airolo, who, in 1894, became director of the institute. Since that year the habilitation of the deaf children has been completely the responsibility of Argentine personnel.

In 1897, Airolo funded a department for deaf girls, adjunct to the Institute for the Deaf that admitted only deaf boys. Until that year, habilitation of deaf girls was in charge of the Beneficial Association of Buenos Aires City (Associacion de Beneficencia de la Capital Federal). In 1899, this department became an Institute for Deaf Girls.

A second school to train teachers of the deaf was created in 1900, following programs and suggestions provided by Airolo. The first director of this school was Mrs. Maria Ana Mac Cotter-Madrazzo, a pioneer in this field in Argentina.

These early Argentine schools for the deaf were official, or became official, shortly after their foundation. The first permanent private Argentine Institute for Deaf was the General Belgrano Institute, established in 1886 in a section of Buenos Aires City. The oral method of habilitation was also used exclusively in that institute. The most important provincial institute for the deaf functioning at that time was the one created in 1890 by the government of the province of Buenos Aires. Another provincial institute for the deaf functioned from 1899 until 1903 in the province of Santa Fe. It was discontinued because of lack of funds. Most of the present schools for the deaf in Argentina were established between 1900 and 1950.

Studies on the science of hearing were initiated in Argentina at the turn of the century by otorhynolaryngologists of the National Institute for the Deaf and acquired more relevance after 1930. Argentine audiometry received great attention and developed during the decade 1940–1950 because of the efforts of Drs. Juan Manuel Tato, Aldo Remorino, and Renato Segre. After 1960, Dr. Julio Bernaldo de Quiros became the leading audiologist in Argentina and throughout Latin America.

PROGRAMS AND PROCEDURES OF AURAL HABILITATION AND REHABILITATION IN ARGENTINA

Programs for the hearing handicapped in Argentina can be classified into four general groups: (1) diagnostic; (2) otological treatment; (3) habilitative and rehabilitative training; and (4) schooling. No institute or center in Argentina offers all four types of services. Diagnosis and otological treatment are usually offered by hospitals and special medical centers. Habilitation of deaf children is normally entrusted to schools for the deaf or to audiological centers that may function within a private hospital. Rehabilitation of deaf adults usually is provided by phonoaudiologists acting as paramedical professionals within a medical setting. Schooling for the deaf children is accomplished within the "normal" schools when possible or as soon as it becomes possible. In other cases, educational work is done in differential schools or in differential grades within a normal school. An exception to this rule is the National Institute for the Deaf (both the male and female branches), where diagnosis, habilitation, and schooling altogether are offered to the pupils. It should be especially noted that only primary schools specialized for the deaf are available in Argentina. There are no specialized high schools for the deaf. This is a direct consequence of the general tendency in Argentina to use the oral method of habilitation; that is, to provide the patients with voice communication and to send the individual as soon as possible to cope with the normal environment. This is done immediately after the child has acquired a minimum of communication skills compatible with a learning situation within a normal school. In addition, the deaf child may continue with his habilitation program outside the school. Those deaf youngsters who want to pursue secondary, special, or even university studies have to cope the best they can with their handicaps. Usually they receive extracurricular help from a teacher of the deaf. Few deaf undertake secondary studies and even fewer attend a university. Nonetheless, this situation does not differ drastically from the normal population trend concerning studies in Argentina, as it was discussed in the Introduction.

Concerning the habilitative aspects, children may receive specialized therapy in accordance with the diagnostic evaluations made in special centers, like the Medical Center of Audiological and Phoniatric Investigations (directed by Dr. Julio Bernaldo de Quiros), or within a private hospital, like the Israelite Hospital of Buenos Aires, or in schools for the deaf, like the Instituto Oral Modelo. All these centers utilize the oral method, using sign language only when diagnosis indicates a low probability of being successful with the oral method. Normally people who are peripherally deaf respond very well to oralization. Subjects with auditory central pathways syndrome are difficult subjects to provide with voice communication. The situation is further complicated when mixed syndromes are present.

As a general rule, if a phonoaudiologist is in charge of the habilitative program, he will follow the indications of the physician in charge of the case, usually an otorhynolaryngologist and seldom a specialized phoniatric or audiological physician. Such a physician may consider the opinion of other physicians involved in the diagnosis, i.e., pediatricians, psychiatrists, neurologists, and sometimes also he would request the opinion of phonoaudiologists to outline the treatment. On the other hand, when a teacher of the deaf is devoted to the habilitative program, he has more latitude to exercise personal criteria, since the teacher of the deaf in Argentina is responsible only to pedagogical authorities rather than to physicians. But whoever is in charge of the habilitative program, frequent checkings are normally performed to follow up on the results of the program. Most of these programs are quite standard. Essentially, they consist of stimulating the patient with exercises designed to teach the deaf to differentiate between sound and silence; teach him to make gross discriminations among different types of sounds; teach him to discriminate among the different phonemes of the Spanish language; help him to improve the intelligibility of his utterances; assist him in localizing the source of sound; and assist him to adjust socially (Quiros, 1974).

Deaf children may receive this habilitative training groups of four or five. Group therapy is considered in Argentina to be more functional than individual therapy since it provides the social contact and sense of competence that are essential factors encountered in real life situations where the deaf are expected to be integrated.

Most settings for habilitative programs in medical centers consist of a special room with mirrored walls to provide visual feedback to the patients. Amplification may be used alternatively within the same therapy session, depending upon the particular case. Children are stimulated with standard techniques, using toys, musical instruments, and visual aids. They are rewarded according to their therapeutic needs and their mental age. Therapeutic sessions of this type are usually administered by phonoaudiologists. Proper screens facilitate observation by other therapists. Usually vegetative functions of children are observed and considered for the evolutive process.

Concomitantly with a habilitative program, a child may attend a school, either a normal or differential school, according to his particular situation. Centers that offer specialized habilitative programs usually are located only within the five or six largest cities of Argentina. If a deaf child lives very far from these centers, the trend is to secure the services of a teacher for the deaf at his home, even an itinerant one, to keep the child within a familiar environment while receiving help. He is taken to the center for the initial diagnosis and habilitation and, afterwards, periodically for routine checks. Parents are often counseled and advised on how to provide their child with proper auditory stimuli and exercises that they may be able to handle.

In Argentina there are approximately 40 differential schools which provide special programs for deaf children, in addition to programs for other types of handicapped. From south to north, provinces and cities which possess these differential schools are: Santa Cruz Province–Cipolletti and C. Rivadavia cities; La Pampa Province–Santa Rosa and Gral. Lamadrid cities; Buenos Aires Province–Bahia Blanca, Tandil, Azul, Moron, Lanus, Bolivar, San Isidro, San Nicolas, Pergamino, and Lujan cities; Cordoba Province–Rio Cuarto, San Francisco, Cordoba cities; Santa Fe Province–Venado Tuerto, Rafaela, Santa Fe cities; Entre Rios Province–Gualeguaychu, Parana, Santa Fe cities; Corrientes Province–Goya and Corrientes cities; Chaco Province–Resistencia City; Santiago del Estero Province–Santiago City; Catamarca Province–Catamarca City; San Juan Province–San Juan City. Provinces of Chubut, La Rioja, Formosa, Misiones, and Tierra del Fuego do not have differential schools, but in La Rioja, Formosa, and Misiones there are available teachers for the deaf.

Some educators believe that these differential schools, where different types of handicapped children interact, provide a good learning experience for all which is beneficial to their social adjustment.

In addition to these differential schools, in Argentina there are 18 schools exclusively devoted to the deaf. The list of these schools is as follows: Buenos Aires City (Federal District)–six schools; La Plata city (Province of Buenos Aires)–two schools; Mar del Plata (Province of

Buenos Aires)–one school; Rosario (Province of Sante Fe)–one school; Sante Fe (Province of Sante Fe)–one school; Cordoba (Province of Cordoba)–one school; Mendoza (Province of Mendoza)–one school; Tucuman (Province of Tucuman)–one school.

Three other schools for the deaf, as yet not providing full services (1975), are located in: Olavarria (Province of Buenos Aires); Corrientes (Province of Corrientes); and Salta (Province of Salta).

The total number of deaf children in Argentina, excluding the mild hypoacusics, but including deep peripheral deaf, aphasics, and children with other types of syndromes related to deafness and mutism, is estimated to be approximately 80,000, i.e., 8.5% of the population under 14 years of age. Only 27,000 out of these 80,000 deaf children are registered in habilitation courses. The reason for this "absenteeism" is difficult to determine. Indeed, clinical services and schools are free in Argentina. So, economic reasons are really not a cause. There is also a superabundance of teachers of the deaf. Actually, Argentina exports teachers of the deaf, especially to Latin America. Classrooms have an average of one teacher for every 10 deaf children.

Therefore, one of the reasons for lack of attendance may be found in the fact that most teachers and services for the deaf are concentrated in the big cities. The long distances a deaf child from the country must travel to these centers discourage the family; as a result the child remains with no habilitation. To solve such a problem is a very difficult task that would require a complete demographic restructuring of Argentina. It is a kind of specific evil of large countries with relative small populations. Another reason could be ignorance or lack of concern of the parents. Education and advertisement of the available service for the deaf may correct this situation, although it would require considerable time and effort to disseminate this information.

There are approximately 3,000 professionals concerned with habilitation and rehabilitation programs for the deaf in Argentina. This number includes teachers of the deaf, phonoaudiologists, psychologists, phoniatric physicians, etc.

The total number of otorhinolaryngologists in Argentina is approximately 1,250. From this number, some 45 are devoted to audiology and phoniatry on a part-time basis and only 15 on full-time basis. The total number of physicians in Argentina is approximately 27,000, i.e., 1 physician per 900 inhabitants, although the distribution is uneven, since in the Greater Buenos Aires area there is 1 physician per 400 inhabitants.

In addition to the national and provincial schools for the deaf, there are also some private schools for the deaf in Argentina, for example, the Instituto Oral Modelo and the Colegio Provolo, both in Buenos Aires City.

Among the federal centers for the deaf, two very important ones are: the National Institute for Deaf Boys and the National Institute for Deaf Girls, also in Buenos Aires City. These institutes offer well equipped facilities for diagnostic, habilitative programs and regular primary schooling.

Buenos Aires City has 28 hospitals that offer habilitative and rehabilitative training for the deaf. Within the national institutes for the deaf also should be mentioned a school managed by the Secretary of Public Health.

DIAGNOSTIC PROCEDURES

Diagnosis of auditory deficit in Argentina follows international standards, as used in the U.S.A., Germany, etc.

Batteries of audiological tests for diagnosis are used in all clinics, hospitals, and centers specialized in this particular field. In addition to pure tone audiometry (air and bone conduction), speech audiometry, recruitment, Fowler, Reger, Jerger, and Harford tests are widely used for auditory threshold detection. Adaptation and auditory fatigue are tested through the methods of Hood, Carhart's (or Fournier's) "tone decay" technique, etc. Automatic (Bekesy) audiometry is also available in most institutions. The Sensorineural Acuity Level (SAL) test to determine neurosensorial losses, and the Short Increment Sensitivity Index (SISI) test utilized for differential diagnosis of cochlear pathology, are currently used in Argentina, although impedance audiometry, vestibulometry, Electroencephalography (EEG), Evoked Response Audiometry (ERA), are techniques used only in some centers of large cities, like Buenos Aires, Rosario, and Cordoba. This means that in those difficult cases where a clear-cut diagnosis cannot be established, children must be transported from their home towns to these few places where such sophisticated differential diagnosis can be performed. More and more, the ERA is used in Argentina to establish whether or not a hearing-impaired child is actually peripherally deaf or suffers from aphasia.

Naturally, the correct diagnosis is imperative for indicating the appropriate habilitative procedures that should be used with each particular child. The tendency is to send the child back to his home after the diagnosis is established. School authorities, physicians, etc., then try to provide the child with the services of a local teacher for the deaf that can help in the process of habilitation. Usually, the family also interacts with the program, after receiving proper counseling within the center in which the diagnosis was made.

Children are submitted to audiological tests according to their mental and chronological ages. Common tests used, according to age, include: 0–24 months–survey of hearing, exploration of the Moro, palpebral, and cochlear reflexes, exploration of asymmetries, etc.; 2–3 years—sound toys, free field pure tone audiometry, peep-show, Suzuki test, etc.; 3–6 years—conditioned audiometry through play and games, subjective and objective pure tone audiometry, visual aids; 6 years and up—pure tone audiometry to determine thresholds. Speech audiometry, mainly administered to adults, is based on several special lists of Spanish words.

The lists prepared by Tato and associates (1949) are widely used. A list of phonetically balanced monosyllables (in Spanish there are not too many monosyllabic words) prepared by Lopez Estrada (1958) is used together with a similarly phonetically balanced list of bisyllabic acute and grave words by the same author.

Another list of words used in speech audiometry was prepared by Cruz (1967). She managed to collect a list of words that are commonly used in approximately 10 different dialects of the American-Spanish language. It is to be noted that although Spanish is the official language of most South American countries and Mexico, local dialects vary widely and all of them differ from the Castillian language and other dialects spoken in Spain.

Quiros and Morgante (1961) produced other lists of words expecially adapted to clinical needs. Ferrer (1960) experimented with nonsense monosyllables to establish a good discrimination test since the usage of the few monosyllabic words existing in Spanish limited the validity of such type of a speech audiometric test.

Tosi, Cruz, and Black in 1969 presented a report on the two multiple choice intelligibility tests they constructed in Spanish following the same criteria used by Black (1957) in the development of his well known multiple choice tests in English.

In all Argentine audiological centers, musical instruments are used for auditory exploration with children up to 5 years of age. Normally, these instruments include: a gong, a small drum, a bell, a whistle, a wood xylophone, etc. Knowing the frequency and dynamic range of these instruments makes them useful in determining the approximate limits of auditory acuity of patients if the examiner manages to obtain responses to the stimuli provided by the instruments.

A proper anamnesis is a vital part of the diagnostic procedures. Leading physician-audiologists in Argentina, like Dr. Julio Bernaldo de Quiros have expressed their opinion (Quiros and D'Elia, 1974) that a good anamnesis serves as a tool to establish a differential diagnosis, sometimes better than relying solely on audiometry. Quiros, in his Medical Center for Phoniatric and Audiological Investigation in Buenos Aires City, routinely produces a comprehensive anamnesis from his patients, divided into six parts: (1) identification of the patient and the informer; (2) hereditary and familiar antecedents; (3) personal antecedents; (4) history of the process of maturity of the patient; (5) diagnostic antecedents and referrals; and (6) social factors involved.

The rationale for each of these items is as follows: identification of the informer or the informers is crucial since data on the child released by different informers could be contradictory or biased. Heredity and familiar factors can explain very often the etiology of the child's impairment, i.e., similar ailment in grandparents or brothers, tensions within home, parents in the process of divorcing or speaking different languages because of different nationalities may explain some psychodeafness, etc. Personal antecedents disclose details of the gestation period; they could reveal whether or not the mother took drugs or antibiotics that may have produced the child's hearing loss. The knowledge of the Rh factors in the father's and mother's blood may also help to clarify the diagnosis. Mother's nutrition may be responsible for the child's impairment according to experiences obtained during World War II. Type of delivery also may effect the child's condition. The history of the process of maturity of the child is most relevant to the differential diagnosis. Questions on this item refer to the development of the motor skills of the child that allows the clinician to detect deviations from normal. Normal development of motor skills is: at 3 months of age, a child can hold his head up straight; at 6 months of age a child can sit up alone voluntarily; at 9 months of age, a child can stand voluntarily; and at 12 months of age, he starts walking. The language process bears a most direct relationship to the diagnosis. There are clues that may help to establish whether or not the child is really deaf. For instance, both deaf and hearing 10-month-old children may say "mama." The difference observed in the anamnesis is that the deaf child may say "mama" only as a reflex act whereas the hearing child will use the word to actually call his mother. Illness sustained by the child will complete this part of the case history. A professional can extract important conclusions from these data for diagnosis, treatment, and habilitation. Items of the Quiros' anamnesis concerning "diagnostic antecedents" refer to the behavior, communication, and conditioning of the child. In general, if case history data from a particular patient reveal normal behavior, apart from an apparent auditory deficit, a peripheral deafness is to be strongly suspected. Other clues may be found in the case history to rule out or to suspect mental retardation or other neurological or physical problems, very often labeled "aphasia." This part of the case history may indicate the need to continue the diagnosis with a special test, like the Vineland scale of maturity, adapted to Spanish by Quiros and Glotter (1964).

Conditioning aspects of the child should be disclosed also in this part of the case history. Very often the response of a child to some event consists of a simple conditioning rather than to an auditory perception. A skillful clinician can discriminate adequately during this part of the examination. Quiros believes that questions like: does the child listen better to the father or to the mother, or is he able to listen to a motorcycle or to a doorbell, are more relevant, in some cases, than formal pediatric audiometry.

There are approximately 340 audiological clinics, hospitals, and public and private institutions which have centers for diagnosis and treatment of the hearing impaired in Argentina. The level of sophistication and the availability of these facilities vary. In general, the farther a place is from Buenos Aires City, the less well equipped is the facility. The distribution of these audiological centers is as follows:

Buenos Aires City:
audiological clinics–37; hospitals (public and private) with audiological centers–28; universities with audiological centers–3.

Province of Buenos Aires:
audiological clinics–31; hospitals (public and private) with audiological centers–27; universities with audiological centers–3.

Province of Cordoba:
audiological clinics–25; hospitals (public and private) with audiological centers–18; universities with audiological centers–2.

Province of Sante Fe:
audiological clinics–16; hospitals (public and private) with audiological centers–14; universities with audiological centers–1.

Province of Entre Rios:
audiological clinics–9; hospitals (public and private) with audiological centers–8.

Province of Corrientes:
audiological clinics–6; hospitals (public and private) with audiological centers–6; universities with audiological centers–1.

Province of Misiones:
audiological clinics–1; hospitals (public and private) with audiological centers–2.

Province of Chaco:
audiological clinics–3; hospitals (public and private) with audiological centers–3.

Province of Formosa:
audiological clinics–2; hospitals (public and private) with audiological centers–4.

Province of Jujuy:
audiological clinics–6; hospitals (public and private) with audiological centers–4.
Province of Salts:
audiological clinics–6; hospitals (public and private) with audiological centers–4.
Province of Tucuman:
audiological clinics–7; hospitals (public and private) with audiological centers–5; universities with audiological centers–1.
Province of Santiago del Estero:
audiological clinics–1; hospitals with audiological centers–2.
Province of Catamarca:
audiological clinics–1; hospitals (public and private) with audiological centers–2.
Province of LaRioja:
audiological clinics–1; hospitals (public and private) with audiological centers–2.
Province of San Luis:
audiological clinics–1; hospitals (public and private) with audiological centers–2.
Province of San Juan:
audiological clinics–3; hospitals (public and private) with audiological centers–2; universities with audiological centers–1.
Province of Mendoza:
audiological clinics–9; hospitals (public and private) with audiological centers–5.
Province of La Pampa:
audiological clinics–4; hospitals (public and private) with audiological centers–4; universities with audiological centers–2.
Province of Neuquen:
audiological clinics–3; hospitals (public and private) with audiological centers–2.
Province of Rio Negro:
audiological clinics–3; hospitals (public and private) with audiological centers–3.
Provinces of Chubut, Santa Cruz, Tierra del Fuego, and Malvinas:
audiological clinics–2; hospitals (public) with audiological centers–3.

TRAINING OF PROFESSIONALS FOR THE FIELD OF AUDIOLOGY IN ARGENTINA

There are approximately 3,000 professionals in Argentina concerned in one way or another with habilitative and rehabilitative audiology. This number includes phonoaudiologists, teachers of the deaf, psychologists, phoniatric physicians, etc.

Training of phonoaudiologists during the last two decades showed a trend toward the U.S.A. model rather than the traditional European one still predominant in all other Latin American countries. Concretely, in Argentina, phonoaudiology has shown some tendency to become a profession independent of medicine, although related to this art by a close interprofessional interaction. However, as yet, the phonoaudiologist is considered for all practical purposes a paramedical person in Argentina; he is not allowed by law to engage in diagnostic procedures or even to prescribe hearing aids. Training of phonoaudiologists is usually offered by the schools of medicine. After 3 years of study, some schools grant a degree of technician in phonoaudiology; other schools grant a degree of phonoaudiologist. Only a private university in Buenos Aries City presently offers more advanced studies in phonoaudiology: a 5-year course leading to a degree of "licenciado" and also a doctorate of phonoaudiology or perturbations of human communication that requires 6 years of study plus a thesis. The number of graduates from these advanced studies is very small and, as yet, has not had a significant effect upon the audiological profession in Argentina. Phonoaudiologists are assistants to attending physicians, usually otorhinolaryngologists or otologists. Phonoaudiologists perform audiometry, vestibulometry, impedance testing, and speech therapy to patients but always under the supervision of a physician. A phonoaudiologist is allowed a private practice but with patients under medical prescription.

There are a few physicians in Argentina who have received formal training in phoniatry and audiology. The University of Buenos Aires offers a course on Pathology and Human Communication only for physicians and psychologists. Two private universities, San Salvador and Museo Social Argentino, offer postgraduate courses in this subject for physicians who want to specialize in Pathology of Human Communication.

On the other hand, there are several institutes that train teachers of the deaf. These institutes usually do not belong to universities. They offer a standard 3-year program to high school graduates who desire to become teachers of the deaf.

The first course ever offered in phonoaudiology was given at the School of Medicine, University of Rosario (Province of Sante Fe) in 1943 (Segre, 1972). It was an accelerated course of 6 months. Several persons graduated with the degree "Technician in Phonoaudiology." The course was eventually discontinued. In the year 1950, Dr. Juan Manuel Tato reinstituted it permanently at the School of Medicine, National University of Buenos Aires. Later on, several other universities organized similar programs on a permanent basis.

There is still some confusion in Argentina between the role of the teacher of the deaf and the phonoaudiologist. It seems that the prevailing concept is that the teacher of the deaf, rather than the phonoaudiologist, should be the one concerned with the habilitation of deaf children. Rehabilitative and medical assistant's tasks are considered proper for a phonoaudiologist. Since the phonoaudiologist is considered a paramedical person in Argentina, she works directly under the supervision of a physician within the hospital or clinical setting. The teacher for the deaf has no business within a hospital. These distinctions are also emphasized by the fact that the teacher of the deaf registers his degree within the Ministry of Education as an educator and the phonoaudiologist registers his degree within the Ministry of Public Health as an auxiliary to medicine.

In 1972, there was a round table discussion in the Argentine Association of Logopedics, Phoniatrics and Audiology discussing the role of the teacher of the deaf and the phonoaudiologist (Tato, 1972). The opinion expressed at that meeting seems to coincide with the general trend in this matter as expressed above.

In summary, although phonoaudiologists and teachers of the deaf are different professionals with different goals, there is not a clear-cut distinction between the two. This is because of the lack of precise definitions and differentiation between their respective training programs and reflects the fact that audiology and speech pathology always were concerned with both medical and pedagogical aspects. The phonoaudiologist is biased toward the medical aspects, and the teacher of the deaf toward the pedagogical aspects of the field, but obviously they overlap in many areas. Only the official bodies can regulate the sphere of activity of each profession in Argentina. Authorities have not been too anxious to create such regulations.

A sample of programs to train phonoaudiologists and teachers of the deaf follows (Arcella, 1972).

The course in phonoaudiology at the University of Buenos Aires in the first year includes: Phonetics, Physics (Acoustics), Phoniatric Semiology, Psychopathology I, Anatomy and Physiology of the Hearing and Speech Mechanisms, Psychometry, Practicum, and Monography. In the second year it includes: Clinical Audiology, Clinical Phoniatry, Psychopathology II, Audiometry, Phoniatric and Kinesiological Therapeutics, Evolutive Psychology, Social Serivices, Practicum, and Monography. In the third year, it includes: Clinical Practicum in Audiometry and Phoniatry, Psychology and Psychopathology of Language, and Monography Based on Treatment of a Patient. An entrance examination and a high school diploma are required in order to pursue these studies. Graduates must register their title within the Ministry of Public Health to practice, although there are no Board Examinations of Clinical Competence, which, incidentally, do not exist in Argentina for any healing profession or any profession.

At the School of Phonoaudiology at the University of Museo Social Argentino (Buenos Aires City), studies in the first year include: Anatomy and Physiology, Neurophysiology, General and Evolutive Psychology, Communicology, Evolutive Deontology, and Practicum. In the second year, they include: Physics (Acoustics), Phonetics, Audiometry, Structural Linguistics, Orthophony, Cerebral Palsy, and Practicum. In the third year, they include: Psychology Applied to Speech Pathology, Endocrinophoniatry, Phoniatric Therapeutics, Audiology, Didactic Methods of Habilitation and Rehabilitation for Voice Communication Handicapped, and Practicum. After successful completion of these 3-year courses, a title of "phonoaudiologist" is granted. Entrance examination, a high school diploma, and passing a Psychophysical Aptitude Test are required for candidates to this program. Upon successful completion of another 2-year course, a title of "Licenciado" in Phonoaudiology is granted. Entrance examination and a diploma of Phonoaudiologist are required to register as student in the fourth year of studies. In the fourth year, the program covers: Advanced Phonoaudiology, Psychopedagogy, Psychoacoustics, Mental Retardation, Biology and Genetics, and Practicum. In the fifth year, it includes: Kinesiology and Kinosiotherapy, Laberintology and Postural Systems, Pediatric Psychology, Specialized Pedagogical Therapeutics, Seminar I, Practicum, and Monography.

Upon successful completion of 1 more year of studies and a thesis, a title of Doctor of Phonoaudiology (Human Perturbations of Communication) is granted. The title must be registered within the Ministry of Public Health to practice. The content of this sixth year of studies follows: Statistics and Scientific Methodology, Basic Sciences, Psychiatry, Neuropathology, and Seminar II.

According to the catalog description, the Doctor of Phonoaudiology is expected to become interested in research, to teach at the university level, or to interact on clinical practice at equal level with other university professionals. However, according to the law, he cannot produce medical diagnosis but rather "phonoaudiological" diagnosis in order to guide the process of habilitation or rehabilitation of patients.

In Argentina the teacher of the deaf is considered to be a specialized teacher rather than a clinician. Therefore, he is free to follow any habilitative or rehabilitative program as educational officers consider fit, independent of physician's prescriptions. However, in most cases, a good interaction and relationship exist between teachers of the deaf and phoniatric physicians or otologists.

Teachers for the deaf register their title within the Ministry of Education rather than within the Ministry of Public Health, as is the case with the paramedical phonoaudiologists.

TRAINING PROGRAMS FOR TEACHERS OF THE DEAF

In the first year at the Teacher's School Osvaldo Magnasco (Ministry of Education and Culture), classes include: Normal Pedagogy, Psychology, Anatomy and Physiology, Physics (Acoustics), Pure Tone and Speech Audiometry, Introduction to Phoniatry, Structural Linguistics I, and Practicum. In the second year, they include: Special Pedagogy for the Deaf and Hypoacusic, Evolutive Psychology, Psychometry, Semiological Phonoaudiology, Clinical Audiology and Speech Pathology, Structural Linguistics II, and Practicum. And, in the third year, they include: Special Pedagogy for the Handicapped (Speech, Reading, and Writing), Psychopathology, Phonoaudiological Clinic, Tests Used in Audiology, Habilitation and Rehabilitation Techniques, and Practicum.

Upon successful completion of the 3-year course, a title of Teacher of the Deaf ("Professor Especializado on Deficientes del Oido, la Voz y la Palabra") is granted. Entrance requirements are that he be able to pass a Psychophysical Aptitude Test and have a degree of teacher (a 6-year special high school program). The maximum age to enter is 30 years.

Other programs to train teachers of the deaf, such as the one offered by the Teachers School of the Province of Cordoba, are very similar to the one offered by the "Osvaldo Magnasco" School.

PROGRAMS FOR SPECIALIZATION OF PHYSICIANS IN PATHOLOGY OF HUMAN COMMUNICATION

These programs are presently offered only by two private universities: San Salvador and Museo Social Argentino Universities. Both are similar and were organized by Dr. Quiros (1975). They include the following courses: Communicology and Learning, Psychophoniatry, Orthophony, Evolutive Neurophysiology, Biology and Genetics, Audiology and Audiometry (I and II), Cerebral Palsy, Neuropathology, Laberyntology, Electrostygmography, General and Evolutive Psychopathology, Phoniatric Pathology and Recuperative Methodology, Scientific and Statistical Methodology, and seminars in related matters.

There are very few physicians who have pursued these studies.

INTERPROFESSIONAL RELATIONSHIPS

The different persons involved in habilitative and rehabilitative audiology in Argentina work as extensions of an attending physician, who makes the diagnosis, makes recommendations for treatment, and corrects it according to periodic checks of the patient. The teacher of the deaf works relatively independent of the attending physician since his tasks are mainly pedagogical ones; however, the teacher of the deaf usually will consider the medical diagnosis and prognosis in order to select the proper educational approach in each case when possible.

Several medical specialists may work as a team in the audiological centers of big cities in making diagnosis, i.e., a pediatrician, a neurologist, and a psychiatrist could be involved in the diagnosis, but they will report to the attending physician, usually an otorhinolaryngologist, who will make the final decisions and give instructions to his subordinates, the phonoaudiologists. On some occasions, the otorhinolaryngologist in charge may have formal training or practical experience in audiology, but, in other cases, this may not be true.

The social worker is almost nonexistent in Argentina. Normally, parents of deaf children may be advised by the physician in charge or by some phonoaudiologist. Rarely is a psychologist involved in counseling of parents.

There is a tendency of phoniatric physicians, phonoaudiologists, and teachers of the deaf to form separate associations, in spite of the fact that the Argentine Association of Logopedics, Phoniatrics and Audiology is composed of physicians and phonoaudiologists. Within this association, interprofessional relations are cordial. Usually phonoaudiologists will accept without resentment the authority of physicians.

ORGANIZATIONS AND ASSOCIATIONS RESPONSIBLE FOR THE HEARING HANDICAPPED

The Federal Government in Argentina, through the National Office of Differential Schools, takes care of habilitation programs for deaf children. The National Service of Rehabilitation and the National Committee to Fight Deafness also serve similar purposes. Private, professional institutions concerned in one way or another with habilitative and rehabilitative programs for the hearing handicapped are: The Association of Teachers for the Deaf, The Argentine Association of Logopedics, Phoniatrics and Audiology, and The Foundation to Help Deaf Children. The newly formed Association of Professional Phonoaudiologists is also partially concerned with the same goals. Another related association, still in the initial stages of formation, is the Argentine Association of Human Communication Medicine. This association was founded in 1973 by 15 physicians devoted to phoniatry and audiology.

These physicians are the most prominent professionals in Argentina in the field of audiology and phoniatry. A list of their names follows: J. Bernaldo de Quiros, L. E. Bustamante, A. Etchegaray, J. N. Gonzalez, F. Z. Gueler, E. Jager, A. Lombi, C. Longo, J. L. Montonati, D. G. Postan, J. M. Salvatori, O. L. Schrager, R. Segre, J. Seoane, J. Somaschini, E. E. Tormakh, and J. C. Tripputi.

There are also some lay associations in Argentina related to the hearing handicapped. These associations include deaf adults and parents of deaf children; their goals are to help the hearing handicapped both socially and also economically. One of the oldest associations of this type is the I.A.D.A.L. (Argentine Institute of the Audition and Language). Another is the F.A.N.S. (Argentine Federation for Deaf Children). Five of these lay associations are in Buenos Aires City, two in the Province of Buenos Aires, two in the Province of Santa Fe, two in the Province of Cordoba, two in the Province of Mendoza, and one in each of the other provinces of Argentina.

The oldest of the professional associations in the field of Audiology and Phoniatry is the Argentine Association of Logopedics, Phoniatrics, and Audiology; it was founded in 1948. This association publishes a journal, *Fonoaudiologica*, which has a wide circulation in Latin America and also in Spain. In 1970, the Spanish Association of Logopedics, Phoniatrics and Audiology signed an agreement with the sister Argentine association to use *Fonoaudiologica* as the official organ of the Spanish association.

FAMILY INVOLVEMENTS

Counseling the parents of deaf children and families of deaf adults in order to better cope with the social, economic, and therapeutic aspects is practiced in Argentina, but not in a regular and standard fashion. It would be most desirable to have a formal program to train parents in order that they could provide habilitation effectively to their deaf children, especially for those who live in places distant from the big cities where professional programs are available.

In this respect Argentina has a similar situation to that of India where good centers for diagnosis and treatment exist only in the big cities. Those children from remote places can be helped directly only by their parents. Recently, a proposal to train parents and to test their ability to provide habilitation to their children was proposed by Dr. Pal Kapur from the Department of Audiology and Speech Sciences, Michigan State University. Experience obtained from such programs could easily be applied to Argentina. This would eventually save effort, time, and money; it also might provide a good example of international cooperation in this field, bringing into reality one of the goals of the editor of this book.

RESEARCH

Research in audiology and habilitation procedures is not too significant in Argentina. To the best knowledge of the writer, the most important institution that could be cited in this aspect is the Laboratory of Sensorial Research, directed by Dr. Miguelina Guirao, a graduate from Harvard University and a former student of Professor S. S. Stevens. This laboratory publishes an annual report.

There are several physicians in Argentina very well known for their publications in audiology. One of the most prominent Argentine authors in this field is Julio Bernaldo de Quiros, who has produced a formidable output in audiology and related matters. He has been very well known internationally, since the early 1960's. Competing among prominent U.S.A. audiologists, Quiros won the Beltone Prize (Quiros, 1964), awarded by a committee that included von Bekesy and Carhart.

Another Argentine author of international prestige in audiology, but devoted mainly to surgery, is Juan Manuel Tato, professor at the University of Buenos Aires and Chief Otologist at the Italian Hospital of Buenos Aires.

Although Argentine audiologists do not perform significant experimental research, they are busy testing and adapting international methods and procedures. The difficulty in carrying out experimental research in Argentina is lack of financial support. Also, importing laboratory devices and supplies proves to be an extraordinary hardship on researchers. Argentine industry does not produce most of these special instruments.

In general, Argentine scientists and professionals are research conscious and have excellent theoretical backgrounds. Many of those who emigrated to the U.S.A. and Europe during the last part of the 1950's and early 1960's have succeeded in these countries.

ACKNOWLEDGMENTS

This chapter could not have been written without the generous help of Dr. Julio Bernaldo de Quiros. He kindly supplied complete and authoritative data, although he declined to be a co-author. Also, thanks are extended to

M. Morrone, A. Zielinsky, D. Itarburu, and R. Vallati, all of them "licenciadas" in phonoaudiology, who contributed data included in this chapter.

LITERATURE CITED

Arcella, A. I. 1972. Planes de estudio 1971 de las Carreras Oficiales y Privadas reconocidas por el Estado en la Capital Federal y la Provincia. Fonoaudiol. 18:249–257.

Barlaro, R. 1927. Sarmiento, maestro. Monitor Educ. Comun. LXI(3): 85–89.

Black, J. W. 1957. Multiple choice intelligibility tests. J. Speech & Hearing Disorders 22:213–235.

Cruz, C. A. 1967. Logoaudiometria en español. Otorinolaringo. 8(3): 258–263.

Esmay, M. 1971. Institutionalization of the Facultad of Agronomia at Balcarce, Argentina, Research Report #8, Institute of International Agriculture, Michigan State University, p. 28.

Ferrer, O. 1960. Speech audiometry: A discrimination test for the Spanish language. Laryngoscope 70(11):154–155.

Itarburu, D., and Vailanti, R. 1966. La enseñanza del sordo en la Argentina en el siglo XIX. *In* J. Quiros and F. Gueler (eds.), La Communicacion Humana y su Patologia. Vol. 1, pp. 250–262. CEDIFA, Buenos Aires.

Lopez, E. J. 1958. Listas de monosilabos y bisilabos balanceados foneticamente. *In* Poch Vinals, R. (ed.), La Exploracion Funcional Auditiva, pp. 238–247. Paz Montalvo, Madrid.

Quiros, J. B. 1964. Accelerated speech audiometry. Trans. Beltone Instit. Hearing Res. June 17.

Quiros, J. B. 1973. El Centro Medico de Investigaciones Foniatricas y Audiologicas. Paper presented at the I Seminar of the CEDIFA, November 24–30, Buenos Aires.

Quiros, J. B. 1975. Personal communication.

Quiros, J. B., and D'Elia, N. 1974a. La Audiometria del Adulto y del Niño, p. 413. Paidos, Buenos Aires.

Quiros, J. B., and D'Elia, N. 1974b. La Audiometria del Adulto y del Niño, pp. 309–336. Paidos, Buenos Aires.

Quiros, J. B., and Glotter, R. 1964. Vineland test. El lenguaje en el niño, CEDIFA, Buenos Aires.

Quiros, J. B., and Morgante, D. N. 1961. Seleccion de una lista para uso logoaudiometrico en Latino America, CEDIFA. 023A, Buenos Aires.

Segre, R. 1972. Mesa Redonda: El campo de accion del profesor de sordos y del fonoaudiologo. Fonoaudiolo. 18:260–261.

Tato, J. M., and Alfaro, A. 1949. Audiometria del lenguaje hablado. Otorinolaringol. 1(2):207–213.

Tato, J. M. 1972. Mesa Redonda: El campo de accion del professor de sordos y del fonoaudiologico. Fonoaudiolo. 18: 248–261.

Tosi, O. 1969. Estudio Experimental sobre la Inteligibilidad de un test de multiple eleccion en idoma espanol. Fonoaudiolog. 15(1):28–35.

chapter 6

Communication for Hearing-handicapped People in the United Kingdom and the Republic of Ireland

Kevin P. Murphy, Ph.D.

Without full discussions with all the contributors of this book, it is impossible to assume that each of us means the same thing when we talk of impairment, handicap, and rehabilitation. In this chapter, the terms are used as follows:

1. Impairment: any modification of human performance arising from sensory, neural, neuromotor, intellectual, or psychological deficits or malfunction.
2. Handicap: the aggravation of disability associated with the intellectual, psychological, social-emotional, or physical consequences of impairment. It is also emphasized that the consequences of impairment cannot be limited to the impaired individual alone. As a member of a community, the individual discharges a complementary function, and limitations upon such function cannot but affect the community or group within which the impaired individual finds himself. In this sense, the individual with a hearing impairment can expect such social reactions as rejection, withdrawal, aggression, distrust, embarrassment, to name but a few of the ways in which society reacts to underfunctioning. We see, then, the hearing-impaired individual as a potential social contaminant within the very community from which he would normally expect support and help.
3. Rehabilitation (as defined by The British Council of Rehabilitation of the Disabled, 1974): "The whole range of services from the time of onset of the individual's disability to the point at which he is restored to normal activity or the nearest possible approach to it." In using this definition, one has deliberately avoided discussion of the difference between "habilitation" and "rehabilitation" because teachers of the deaf and

therapists in the United Kingdom (England, Scotland, Wales, and Northern Ireland) do not normally use the term "habilitation." The main reason for separating impairment from handicap arises from the fact that, in the majority of severely deafened individuals, there is little or nothing that can be done to cure the impairment, and, hence, remediation concentrates on the prevention of handicap or its amelioration in those cases where the condition has already begun to occur. Most workers in the field of hearing impairment will have met individuals with extensive impairments who, nevertheless, are less severely handicapped than are other individuals affected by relatively minor disabilities. In other words, we recognise that the extent and nature of handicap are only partly related to the impairment. The work of Ling (1959) provided a useful example when he showed that minor hearing losses led to major modification of auditory attention. The writer, therefore, differentiates between hearing and listening. Relatively minor decrements of hearing lead to severe listening failure and, after surgery to restore normalcy of thresholds, postoperative auditory training may be required to re-focus attention on environmental noise and particularly on the discrimination of speech.

During the last few years there have been major legislative and social changes designed to improve the lot of persons suffering from various disabilities. Hearing-impaired individuals stand to gain to a considerable extent from the effects of these as time goes on. However, in spite of heroic endeavours on the part of a number of people working alone or in organizations, it would be false to pretend that the present situation is at all satisfactory. There is, however, a danger that frustration will lead to loss of objectivity and the good which undoubtedly is happening will be lost sight of. It is essential, therefore, to strike a balance between objectivity and a natural desire to pretend that all is well. All is by no means well (Toomin, 1974). On the other hand, all is by no means ill. Even in the face of acute financial stringency, there are encouraging signs of progress, and these will be referred to in the following pages.

Two major strands are woven into the pattern of provision in the United Kingdom, and to a certain extent in the Republic of Ireland. These are the effects of educational facilities embodied in law and the structures of the Nationalised Health Services. Because these enactments were so important, there is a tendency to assume that the whole of such provision began then. Such an assumption is, of course, wrong. One does not need to be a historian or a politician to recognise that most social enactments develop from, and are based on, earlier patterns of provision and tend, in democracies, to represent the slow growth of social or educational awareness and their interaction with experience of the efficacy of those previous provisions. Hence, the 1944 Education Act (see below for more full discussion), regarded at the time as a historic act of parliamentary wisdom, never pretended to be the innovator of all education under governmental direction. Similarly, the 1946 Health Enactments, although establishing a National Health Service (NHS), did not spring, as it were, from nowhere. They were based on the fact that earlier legislation had begun limited forms of medical services for certain categories of people. For the sake of brevity, however, this account will not deal with the medical, educational, and social factors relating to hearing impairment before 1944.

SIZE OF THE PROBLEM

The United Kingdom and the Republic of Ireland share a total population of some 58½ million people. Of these, 55½ million reside in the United Kingdom in an area of 93,000 sq. miles and 3 million in an area of 26,600 sq. miles in the Republic of Ireland. The balance between these two sets of figures needs to be kept in mind when considering comparable provision. The annual budget of the Inner London Education Authority exceeds by a considerable amount the whole of the annual budget for education in the Republic of Ireland. Such facilities as are provided in Ireland face all the problems associated with scattered populations, low and sporadic incidence of disability, and relative restrictions on the numbers of professional workers required, which to a certain extent inhibit the process of recruitment and training. This phenomenon is typified by the fact that until the Dominican Sisters established their training programme for teachers of the deaf in Dublin some 20 years ago, teachers of the deaf either left the country for training or followed correspondence and "in service" courses. In encouraging the development of the Dublin College, the government of the day were no doubt aware of the value to a country of a specialist teacher training programme which is integral with and based upon its own educational and cultural heritage.

SCOPE AND COMPLEXITY OF THE PROBLEM

Some of the problems of rehabilitation in these countries stem from its traditional basis in medicine. This is not to say that rehabilitation ought necessarily to be based otherwise but that a clinical basis has negative as well as positive features. We can recognise that all work in the field of impairment or disability begins with the process which brings the patient to diagnosis. The processes of detection depend to a considerable extent on an amalgam of community pressures, the energy and enthusiasm of individual clinicians and the support they receive from their colleagues. It is a disagreeable fact of life that chronicity and preventative medicine generate less excitement both socially and clinically than does the acute condition. Hence, the medically trained clinician interested in audiology tended in the recent past, with some honourable exceptions, to be either a nonsurgical specialist or more interested in audiology as a support system for surgery than as a discipline in its own right (Rawson, 1973). This cannot but affect the attitude to audiological diagnosis within both the clinical and the general community. To a certain extent, the same phenomena have affected preventative medicine. Although clinicians have been aware of the danger of noise for nearly half a century, other aspects of ecological stress tended, until recently, to receive greater publicity, partly because of their novelty and partly because their effects appear more suddenly and dramatically. Fortunately, there are signs of considerable change in this respect. A review of Parliamentary Questions reveals that the topic was raised 45 times in the House of Commons during 1974 and was the subject of three debates. As a result, the sense of urgency so basic to research and to community involvement tends to depend upon such factors as parental pressures, the appeal of the child with an impairment, or a certain sentimentalising of the predicament in which the hearing-impaired individual finds himself. The danger of overprotection and paternalism, particularly in the case of children, is often stressed in the literature (Robinson, 1958; Gorman, 1960). If workers who know deaf individuals so well are prone to regard them as helpless or incompetent, we can hardly blame the general community for falling into the same error. As a result of these attitudes, work with hearing-impaired individuals has, in the past, smacked more than a little of unction in certain groups. Particularly in the area of social work, the notion of charity and vocation appealed more effectively in this part of the world than did the kind of professionalism that one met in such countries as the United States or Australia. However, an increased professionalism, even in voluntary work, has emerged in the last decade, and one has noted the development of a new pattern of administration with increased objectivity and a diminution of those aspects mentioned above.

Changing public attitudes have led to changes in laws, regulations, structures, and organizations.

Another aspect of rehabilitative work with hearing-impaired people, as mentioned earlier, is the need to emphasize amelioration rather than cure. In the case of children, this has led to the development of various kinds of pressure groups, usually established by parents or teachers, which aim to alert the public to the phenomenon of hearing loss. Although primarily aimed at helping children who have already been diagnosed, they do tend to publicise the fact of hearing loss and, as a result, put pressure upon community services for improved detection and diagnostic facilities and for further remedial measures. Public Health Authorities in the United Kingdom now provide systems aimed at recognising the possibility of hearing loss and encouraging referral to diagnosis and therapy. The results of the pioneer work in the field of risk registration (Sheridan, 1962) have spread rapidly, and improved detection procedures have led to a slow reduction in the age at which a child is brought to diagnosis and treatment.

In nearly all cases of infantile hearing impairment, the early stages of diagnosis and therapy are inextricably related. The term "diagnostic therapy" represents the complex process involved in identifying hearing impairment, experimenting with various forms of amplification, and attempting to guide parents and community in the first steps of rehabilitation. It is stressed that, although the notion of remediation might be thought to exclude the notion of preventative medicine, such a conclusion would be unwarranted in the case of deafness. The vulnerability of a person affected by sensorineural conditions to a further impairment arising from undetected or untreated conductive overlays demands preventative medicine, and is an integral part of rehabilitation. This is dependent upon detection and diagnosis and demands a close cooperation between the community services and the specialist clinical workers. The need for such cooperation has led to a recent reorganisation of the National Health Service, designed to integrate community health and hospital serivces within Area Health Authorities. These, in turn, are grouped into Regions under the central control of the Department of Health and Social Security through which funding is channelled.

DEFINITION OF AURAL REHABILITATION

Aural rehabilitation may be narrowly defined as the restoration of normality of auditory function. The temptation to luxuriate in such a definition will be eschewed, and this account will deliberately widen the field to all attempts to maximise the complete and harmonious development of all the hearing-impaired individual's potential.

So many factors are necessary to initiate, maintain, and coordinate the rehabilitative process that it is impossible to exclude the work of the clinician at the one hand or the support and guidance services on the other. Hence, one sees a role for otologist, audiologist, paediatrician, and psychologist with relative precision in the initiation of services; one sees a role for psychologist, social worker, and teacher at the continuation of services. To separate them in this way would certainly make for simplicity of exposition, but would, in fact, cause loss of precision when we look beyond the period of initiation of services to the joint supportive role of diagnostic therapy and of the involvement of so many disciplines, separately and together, in the process of guidance. There is a marked difference between the initiation of services and their refinement. Deciding on the best hearing aid for a young infant demands certain patterns of information both about the child and the choice of amplification systems. A decision about the aid which the child requires in a domestic situation may involve additional factors or, more commonly, may be designed to meet the needs and developing sophistication of the parent in matters audiological. Entry to school poses more problems; evaluation of school progress, differential diagnosis, educational audiology, still more; the list lengthens. All are relevant to aural rehabilitation. Each specialty has its part to play which is different in emphasis, extent, or urgency at different times. In my own experience, the notion of teamwork, although relevant, has a certain constrictive quality; working with a deaf individual demands a blending and shifting of roles which seem more akin to the function of an orchestra, where the quality of the music demands a discipline of coordination, skill, and dedication which is of a higher order than simple teamwork. Emphasis on the integrity of the individual requiring rehabilitation creates one level of involvement in the support services. Recognition that the individual, even as an infant, is part of a social community creates another emphasis. The eventual independence of the individual within the community and the extent to which the support services create this independence are the yardstick by which they will be judged. In justice to the individual and also to the legitimate demands of any community, the potential of the person with disability must be realised. When we see the slow shift from a dependent to a communally supportive role in our client, we can begin to sit back. The aim of rehabilitation is to maximise potential and to assist the individual, as far as possible, into an attitude to himself and to the community in which the significance of the impairment is subordinate to the reality of his own achievements. Perhaps the time may come when we can concentrate on people first and impairments afterward. When we do, it will be because we have recognised that the person with the hearing impairment is also a member of the orchestra and that, without him, the performance will be sadly incomplete.

DEVELOPMENT OF SERVICES

In this country, the pressure to develop speech and language as the major avenue of communication for deaf children was central to the early work of the Ewings (1958). In the face of current methodological controversies, it is well to remember that, even when the writer first began a research career in this field at the end of World War II, the oral-manual controversy was still rumbling in England and was even fiercer in Ireland.

Education

Personal research on the part of the present writer into aspects of deaf education began some 25 years ago. Even after this period of time, one finds it impossible to separate aural rehabilitation from general rehabilitation. In particular, it is impossible to separate the various strands of the educational process (which in the majority of prelingually deafened children in these countries begins before the age of 2 years with the exception of the Republic of Ireland, where 75% of children with severe hearing impairments attending special schools in 1972 did not begin school until the age of 6 years or more) into the relevant emphases of parent support and counselling, auditory training, language development, communication readiness, or the host of other elements subsumed within the expression "deaf education." One can say, however, that deaf education has the same aims as general education and that the teacher of the hearing-impaired child is deeply concerned to optimise the potential of the child in every possible dimension conducive to his own well being and that of the community. In this sense, certain patterns of the educational structure for hearing-impaired children merit discussion.

Because education for hearing-impaired children was subject to a radical change in 1944, this date has been selected for a historical starting point. Clause 33 of the 1944 Education Act stated that the Minister of Education would identify the categories of children requiring special education "and make provisions as to the special methods appropriate to each category." The Secretary of State for Scotland and the Minister of Education of Northern Ireland received similar powers. Two sets of regulations came into being subsequently; these were published in 1945 and 1953 (HMSO) respectively, and the latter defined (inter alia) two categories of children with hearing impairments who required special educational treatment. These were described as "deaf pupils and partially deaf pupils." The former were defined as "pupils who have no hearing or whose hearing is so defective that they require education by methods used for deaf pupils without naturally acquired speech and language." Although apparently circular, such a definition neatly avoided responsibility for attempting to define in law those educational methods which are required for deaf children. In this sense, there was a grey area of hearing impairment which lay between that defined as relevant to children who have no hearing and those who, regardless of the extent of their impaired auditory acuity, had no language and "required education by methods used for children without hearing." Partially deaf pupils were defined as those who had "some naturally acquired speech and language but whose hearing is so defective that they require for their education special arrangements or facilities, though not necessarily all the educational methods used for deaf children." With hindsight, one can discern in this clause (Clause 14) a faint hint that the partially deafened child did not need as much in the way of special methods as did his profoundly deaf colleagues. In terms of aural rehabilitation, a strong case can be made for the provision of different rather than fewer facilities, and it is interesting to note that the development of such additional methods is still taking place.

A further distinction in the educational methodology for these two groups occurred as a consequence of the statement that a blind or deaf pupil required education in a special school "unless the Minister otherwise approves," but that a wider choice existed for partially deaf children since these were permitted to attend special schools or ordinary schools "as may be appropriate" (Clause 15). Care was taken in the following clause (16) to ensure that, for every handicapped pupil attending an ordinary school, special educational treatment should be provided "appropriate to his disability." Increased flexibility resulted from the 1959 regulations which, besides demanding that methods "shall be efficient" (that is, open to government inspection and supervision), also stated that they should be "suited to age, ability and aptitude of the pupils, with particular regard to their disability of mind or body." A later clause (21) forbade admission to, or retention in, a school "unless it is suitable for him having regard to his age and sex and to the nature of his handicap." In some cases, anomalies arose because auditory training produces excellent results for some children. If language comprehension and usage were to be the major criteria, then there was evident need for change in the regulations. These were published in 1962 and redefined categories of pupils with hearing handicaps as follows: deaf pupils were those with impaired hearing, "who require education by methods suitable for pupils with little or no naturally acquired speech or language." Partial deafness was dropped as a category and the term "partially hearing pupils" was substituted. These latter were "pupils with impaired hearing whose development of speech and language, even if retarded, is following a normal pattern, and who require for their education, special arrangements or facilities, though not necessarily all the educational methods used for deaf pupils." Once more we see an emphasis on methodology which is concerned with amount rather than type of educational measures. As our information in psycholinguistics increases, it may well soon prove possible to look more closely at the term "normal" in reference to language development. Even so, in terms of the then status of information, the new amending regulations were a welcome improvement on early ones especially in the light of the accompanying circular (October 1962). In the circular, one saw a more forceful emphasis on the virtue of early diagnosis as a basis for the improved use of residual hearing. Although rightly pointing out the complexity of factors thought to affect prognosis and, therefore, to be taken into account when placement was to be decided, they were predominantly articles of faith and were not supported by research, current or planned. Even today, although no one in these countries would deny their validity, research is still patchy, relatively superficial, and short of funds in such areas as the analysis of linguistic development, lipreading ability, auditory discrimination, and personality factors. The stress placed on consultation, team diagnosis, regular review, and the significance of complex or multiple disability was a more positive factor which set in train a more widespread use of a multidisciplinary approach than had existed hitherto.

Having made provision in law for early diagnosis and therapy, followed by "provisions as to the special methods appropriate for the education of pupils in each category," the various parts of the United Kingdom were faced with an almost total shortage of separate special facilities for children designated as "partially deaf" (and subsequently "partially hearing"). In Scotland there had been some facilities since 1908 but, except for a short-lived attempt to provide separate facilities in the schools administered by the then London County Council during the period of World War I, there were no separate facilities in England, Wales, Northern Ireland, or the Republic of Ireland. The advisability of separate educational facilities was explained in a 1946 Ministry of Education document (pamphlet no. 5) which also gave notice of intent to the establishment of separate boarding schools for the two categories. Separate boarding facilities began to emerge at the same time. The Bodies responsible for the Liverpool School for the Deaf achieved separation in 1948 by opening the Liverpool School for the Partially Deaf in Birkdale, Lancashire. Brighton School for the Deaf changed function and name to specialise in the education of partially deaf pupils in 1949. The profoundly deaf children in the Brighton School were transferred with few exceptions to the School for the Deaf in Margate. Subsequently, Tewin Water School was opened in Hertfordshire (1953) and Needwood School in 1954. Provision in these new schools took advantage of a new climate of opinion in educational architecture and, besides providing the most advanced electronic group hearing aids then available, the buildings themselves were lighter, more cheerful, and less forbidding than many of the earlier Victorian buildings which were positively penitential in character. At the same time, there was an interesting growth in the provision of partially hearing units. These units began again in the London County Council, taking the form of one or two classes with special equipment and staffed by teachers of the deaf. Attached to county primary schools, they began slowly, with considerable reservations on the part of a large proportion of members of the National College of Teachers of the Deaf. Any grouping of children with hearing impairments which is derived from small populations faces additional problems stemming from such factors as the possible need to travel long distances to and from school, dependence on one teacher, who is faced with a wide span of age or intellectual skills, the attitude of the rest of the pupils and staffs of the schools to which they are attached. These and other factors plague the partially hearing unit system. As a result, some parents who preferred day placement moved to other more favoured areas or sought alternative placement in other day schools (in some cases, schools for normally hearing children maintained by voluntary bodies). In such schools, there were small classes and sympathetic staff who, in spite of lack of formal training in deaf education, were prepared to learn. Where Local Authorities did not have special classes for hearing-impaired children, or in those cases where the parents had been able to persuade them that their educational facilities did not meet the special educational needs of their child, interpretation of the law was sufficiently generous for the child to be admitted to a school for children with normal hearing (sometimes an independent boarding school) and all the fees, travel, and a proportion of uniform costs were defrayed.

Social Services

The writer has relied upon two excellent unpublished sources in preparing this section. Lyssons (1965) and Gorman (1960) have approached their topics from different points of view and, consequently, each complements the other. The wealth of information they present merits careful study but is obviously too much for the present section and a deliberate limit has, therefore, been set. Partly because the passage of the Act was important in itself and also because the date in which it was passed fits the time scale of the visit of the present review, the National Assistance Act 1948 has been selected as a logical starting point.

As Lyssons says, "The statutory authority for the welfare of Deaf Persons in the United Kingdom is to be found in section 29 of the National Assistance Act of 1948 which empowers County and County Borough Councils to make arrangements for promoting the welfare of persons who are blind, deaf or dumb and other persons who are substantially and permanently handicapped by illness, injury and congenital deformity." Because these powers were permissive, their usage tended to be restricted to those authorities in which there were sufficient finance and public interest to facilitate some involvement. At this time, the majority of voluntary organizations were well established and providing a modicum of supportive services which reflected the intentions of their original founders. That is, they were, in the main, philanthropic bodies, usually stemming from religious organizations and designed to provide supportive and interpretive services combined with an active evangelical role [Booklet 485 National Institute for the Deaf (1950) places the church before any other facilities in its recommended minimum accommodation as a welfare centre for the deaf]. Many of the organizations had come into being in the latter half of the 19th century. They were, in fact, highly uncoordinated, variable in quality, paternalistic in outlook, excruciatingly short of funds, and hampered by public indifference and official ignorance at best or, indeed, official hostility in certain cases. To understand the situation they faced, it is necessary to remember the virtues and vices of the Victorian era from which they had recently emerged; the upsurge of wealth and philanthropy on the one hand and the appalling poverty, cruelty, intolerance, and bigotry on the other. That particular period of British history was probably one of its most vigorous phases of radical social concern. The emergence of powerful and wealthy philanthropists who had access to the ear of government, aided by the developing power of the press and the effects of a national education policy, eventually brought about a slow growth of official concern of which the passage of such laws as the Disabled Persons (Employment) Acts 1944 and 1958 are useful examples. Before the latter enactments, other signs of governmental concern can be seen from the various Committees of Enquiry established by various government ministers. In particular, the "Younghusband report" 1959 (HMSO) made the following recommendations. The provisions of Section I are summarised as follows: (1) assistance to overcome the effects of their disabilities and to obtain treatment; (2) an advisory service on personal and other problems; (3) encouragement to take part in social activities; (4) visitation by voluntary workers.

In addition, the following services were given permissive approval: (5) practical assistance in the home; (6) wireless, library, and other recreational facilities; (7) provision in social centres or by way of visits or outings of lectures, games, and other recreational facilities; (8) special religious services; (9) travelling facilities to enable hearing-impaired people to take advantage of the services provided; (10) holidays at holiday centres; and (11) provision of social centres and holiday homes.

They also suggested the following: (a) Local Authorities should take a more direct interest in the welfare of the deaf; (b) a proportion of Local Authority welfare officers should learn to make adequate contact with deaf people; (c) the use of voluntary organizations or specially trained and experienced staff was advocated for interpretive purposes; (d) the provision of a "high standard of service without establishing a separate service" was recommended; (e) while ensuring the availability of "spiritual ministration" Local Authorities should not take such functions over themselves; and (f) A casework service for deaf people should be provided even if this meant the initial involvement of an interpreter.

Even so, 12 years elapsed before the clauses relating to deaf people contained in the 1948 Act were made mandatory in a Ministry of Health circular (1960). During this period, both voluntary organizations and Local Authorities now depended heavily on the guidance of another Ministry of Health circular (1951). This circular contained a "model scheme," which was intended to be applicable to deaf and hard-of-hearing people. Because the model was designed to guide agencies seeking approval and financial assistance for their services, there was more than a little force in its "Suggestions." Because funds were limited, the draft consisted of two parts. The first detailed services without which the Minister "would be reluctant to approve schemes." The second dealt with the progressive build-up of services, as the availability of resources permitted.

In the following section, it will be seen that, although a slow build-up of Local Authority services is to be expected, the intentions of the Younghusband report had not by any means led to the absorption of the voluntary bodies. Although widely forecast at that time, the development of a generic social work system throughout the Local Authorities still has a long way to go. The attitude of successive governments may be judged from the fact that the Chronically Sick and Disabled Persons Act (1970) was A Private Members Bill which, although supported by Parliament to the extent that it reached the statute books, did not have the same force or provide the financial support that could have been expected if it had been a government bill.

Development of National Groups

From 1890 on, the following national groups came into being: The British Deaf and Dumb Association (BDDA) (1890); The Council of Church Missioners to the Deaf and Dumb (1904); The National Institute for the Deaf (NID), later The Royal National Institute for the Deaf (1911); The Church of England Council for the Deaf (1922); The Deaf Welfare Examination Board (1929); The National Deaf Children's Society (NDCS) (1945); The National Council of Missioners and Welfare Officers to the Deaf (1962); The British Association of the Hard of Hearing (founded in 1947; now affiliates more than 300 clubs throughout the United Kingdom); and the British Deaf Amateur Sports Association (1930).

PROVISION OF SERVICES

Education

In attempting to cover the total field of hearing impairment, there is a danger of ignoring the very real problem of prelingually profoundly deaf children. Although there has been some slightly increased usage of traditional signing and fingerspelling and a more recent introduction of the Paget Gorman, Mouth-Hand and Cued-Speech systems in the schools in the last 5 years, the recommendations for controlled research published in 1968 (Lewis report) have been barely implemented (for a well reasoned and objective account of the present position with regard to manual education see Denmark (1973) and The Dublin Report (1972)). There is apparently no government plan in the United Kingdom to permit formal training in manual systems as part of the education of Teachers of the Deaf (Thatcher, 1972).

In a survey of children born in 1947 (HMSO, 1964) who were in schools for the deaf during the years 1962 and 1963, no more than 22.3% had intelligible speech (and 23% had not). These children were regarded as profoundly deaf (77% had losses in excess of 70 decibels across the speech range) and were educated in schools for the deaf. When children who were not prelingually deaf or who had losses below 70 decibels were excluded, the figure for intelligibility now shrinks to 11.6%. Because of national circumstances from 1947 forward, it would be invalid to extrapolate from these figures to a reasoned judgement about present prognosis for speech intelligibility. Even so, there is obviously no basis for complacency either at parent or at teacher level.

Further Education

These countries have not reached the levels achieved by the United States in the provision of further education facilities especially designed for adults with hearing impairments. The two major reasons for this are that there is a shortage of candidates of adequate education and that resources have been concentrated on the provision of support centres or on providing special tutors for students attending higher education centers or universities designed for, and attended by, students with normal hearing. The development of the Open University (1969), based on an admixture of radio and television services, correspondence courses, and occasional residential seminars, has provided opportunities for hearing-impaired adults to follow courses of a modular nature leading to eventual conferment of a first level degree. Support services are provided by The City Literary Institute in London and the Whitebrook Centre in Manchester. Since March 1974, the Inner London Education Authority has planned a considerable increase in the role of the City Literary Institute in cooperation with the Education Departments of the other London boroughs and the home counties. To be redesignated as a "Regional Centre for the Deaf," it will provide a wide range of courses as well as a vocational guidance centre within its own campus for all hearing-impaired adults in that catchment area. In addition, it will provide peripatetic teachers for hearing-impaired adults attending full- or part-time vocational courses in further and higher education colleges. Staff from the centre would act as interpreters at the beginnings of courses to enable hearing-impaired students to adjust and also to provide tuition in technical or other specialised terminology which the students might find difficulty in understanding at first. They would also seek to develop the interest of lecturers and staff in their hearing-impaired pupils and also to ensure that satisfactory electronic aids were available if needed. Even today, over 500 students attend the department, mainly in the evening, and the wide range of classes includes a total of 20 lipreading classes per week. There are also classes for teachers of lipreading (the only ones in Britain) and courses in manual communication.

In addition to the above, there are eight other centres which provide similar services, although on a less ambitious scale. Academic needs for high school children are met partly by five secondary schools for deaf children, including the Mary Hare Grammar School in Newbury, Berkshire and Burwood Park School in Surrey; the latter combines a Sixth Form College and also a Secondary Technical College for deaf pupils. Many of the other all-age schools also contain effective secondary departments which either meet all the secondary or technical educational needs of their pupils themselves or are in cooperation with local colleges of further education, in which the deaf pupils participate on a full- or part-time basis. There are approximately 100 lipreading classes spread throughout these countries (see Table 11). The numerous social clubs run by, or for, hearing-impaired adults might well be included under the category of educational establishments but, although many of them do in fact provide lipreading training facilities, they serve as a welfare or social service in the main.

A separate category of special provision merits discussion; this ranges from a custom-built special school for hearing-impaired children with emotional disturbances to schools for partially sighted and hearing-impaired children at Condover Hall in Shrewsbury. In Dublin, a courageous experiment has begun in both major schools for the deaf to provide special manual education for children who are deaf and have specific learning or communication problems. Similarly, a small group of children who are visually and auditorily affected are placed in Jordanstown Schools in Belfast, Northern Ireland. Some 300 more hearing-impaired children affected by mental subnormality are educated in an additional six special centres. There are two more special centres for deaf adults with psychiatric or behavioural problems. At present these are in Preston and Devon, and an extension of facilities for such people is under consideration in the Manchester area.

Children in schools for the deaf are allowed to take public examinations later than normal (up to 19 years of age for Advanced Certificate of Education). Hence, such children may begin the long haul to advanced education before the age of 2 years, be supported in the home by their parents and a peripatetic teacher until entering nursery school, transfer from there to primary school between the ages of 5 and 7 years, move to secondary school by the age of 11 years, and remain there until they are over 19 years when they begin higher academic, technical, or professional training.

It should be remembered that higher education is uncommon for profoundly deaf students. The majority of them face a severe restriction on potential life style. Choice of occupation may well be limited to no more than a dozen openings and possibly even fewer for women. Pay scales are similarly depressed (Dublin Survey, 1973). Many are dependent on a social worker to help them choose and find an occupation and may well rely on his services to explain their problems to the employer and to explain the job specification to themselves. In the case of the hearing-impaired person, much depends on the extent of the hearing loss, age of onset, parental support, educational facilities, and a host of other factors, particularly of intellect and personality. Even the partially hearing person is prone to educational hazard, stress, disappointment, modification of self-image (Goffman, 1968), and, as age advances, a heightened sense of isolation, loneliness, and confusion.

Changing Patterns

Partial Hearing Units As is seen in Table 1, special educational provisions for children with impaired hearing in England and Wales have not only increased numerically but also have changed dramatically since the days (1957) when there were no partially hearing units to the more recent figures (1972) in which the provision has risen by 67% and the balance between provision for partially hearing pupils and deaf pupils has swung from roughly 33% to 132%.

A total of 8,780 hearing aid wearers are educated in special schools and a further 8,230 are educated in nonspecialist schools supported, where feasible, by a total of over 148 peripatetic teachers of the deaf (Table 2). Provision of special schools in these countries is illustrated by Tables 3 and 4 which list the location of separate special educational facilities for deaf and partially hearing children.

Health Services

Figures on the incidence of deafness are imprecise in the countries under review. In the case of young children, it is traditional to assume that approximately three per 1,000 live births will be complicated by significant hearing impairment (Davie, 1972). In a follow-up study of 16,000 children born in March, 1958 (National Child Development Study, (Cohort) (1958)), Davie reports, "The results from the analysis of the audiograms indicate that with one exception all the children with a moderate, 'serious' or 'severe' hearing loss could have been detected by

Table 1. Changing pattern of educational provision for hearing-impaired children in England and Wales

Impairment	1957	1962	1965	1969	1971
Deaf	3,692	3,247	3,110	3,333	3,799
Partially hearing	1,337	1,557	1,617	2,216	2,422
Partially hearing units	–	672	1,254	1,709	2,559
Totals	5,029	5,476	5,981	7,258	8,780

Table 2. Teachers of the deaf employed in England and Wales (1973)

Location	Number
In schools for the deaf or partially hearing	941[a]
In partially hearing units	173
In peripatetic services	148
In hospitals and clinics	15

[a]Of the 941 teachers in special schools for deaf or partially hearing children, 269 (31%) are not qualified to teach deaf children. Of the 672 qualified teachers, 216 have received in-service training leading to the diploma of the National College of Teachers of the Deaf.

audiometric screening on three frequencies only (250, 1000 and 4000 Hz)."

Of children tested, 5.7% had losses in excess of 35 dB on at least two frequencies. Of these, 4.2% of the total sample had a loss in one ear only. Of children with bilateral losses, 1.3% had losses in the range of 35 dB, 0.2% had losses in the range of 55–70 dB, and 0.1% had losses of 75 dB.

Assessment of the incidence of mild conductive conditions varies between 5 and 20% at any one time according to age. With regard to adults, a number of factors make for difficulty in identifying incidence, but the majority of writers agree that such numbers as are known do not represent the total and, moreover, that detection and diagnosis are the major aspects of rehabilitation. Provision of NHS hearing aids is illustrated by the Tables 5 and 6.

Approximately one in nine of all new patient visits to ENT departments led in 1973 to the first-time issuance of a hearing aid. If we add the numbers who purchase commercial hearing aids, we may assert that between 2.5 and 3% of the population of these islands wears a hearing aid. It would appear that, in these countries, between 6 and 7% of the population suffer from some degree of impaired hearing at any one time. (If on the other hand we accept the higher figures of incidence, then the proportion rises to almost 15%.)

The reader will find useful descriptions of therapeutic services in Dale (1967), Whetnall (1964), Ewing (1967), and a series of valuable publications by HMSO and the Dublin Stationery Office. Increasing provision of paediatric audiology services has led to the employment within hospitals of a complex of disciplines including otology, paediatrics, medical

Table 3. Units for partially hearing children attached to schools for children with normal hearing in England, Scotland, Wales, Northern Ireland and the Republic of Ireland (1973)

Country	Numbers of units
England	
Bedfordshire	6
Berkshire	14
Buckinghamshire	9
Cambridgeshire	5
Cheshire	8
Cornwall	3
Derbyshire	3
Devonshire	6
Dorset	1
Durham	12
Essex	12
Gloucestershire	14
Hampshire	8
Herefordshire	9
Hertfordshire	1
Huntingdon and Peterborough	3
Kent	6
Lancashire	11
Leicestershire	4
Lincolnshire	1
London (ILEA)	13
London (Greater London)	13
Norfolk	6
Northamptonshire	3
Northumberland	6
Nottinghamshire	2
Oxfordshire	4
Shropshire	3
Somerset	4
Staffordshire	7
Suffolk	5
Surrey	3
Sussex	4
Warwickshire	8
Yorkshire	10
Scotland	
Clackmannanshire	1
Dunbartonshire	1
Stirlingshire	1

Continued

Table 3—*Continued*

Country	Number of units
Wales	
Caernarvonshire	1
Carmarthenshire	2
Denbighshire	1
Flintshire	2
Glamorgan	23
Monmouthshire	4
Northern Ireland	
Co. Antrim	9
Co. Armagh	1
Belfast	1
Co. Londonderry	3
Co. Tyrone	1
Isle of Wight	1
Isle of Man	1
Channel Isles	1
Republic of Ireland[a]	
Dublin	3
Cork	3[b]

[a]Two hundred and seventy-two severely hard-of-hearing children in three schools and six classes.

[b]One special area of provision in Cork consists of a two-class nursery unit in which 16 hard-of-hearing children aged 3–6 years attend. Forty-five other children in this category were not in receipt of special education.

otology, audiology, psychology, nursing, technology, and education. In one or two unique centres medical social workers are involved, but no centre for early paediatric diagnostic therapy has been discovered in which a social worker with special skills in assisting hearing-impaired people is employed as an integral member of the team. Beginning with Ewings and Whetnall, early diagnosis attempted to compare patterns of auditory responsivity to a variety of crude stimuli likely to prove interesting to the child. In recent years, Taylor and Sheridan have produced rattles which, properly used, have minimal low or high frequency components. Other workers have used monitored live voice, pure and complex tones (Martin, 1971; Fisch, 1964) and have studied the effects of visual reinforcement, tactile reinforcement, maturation of intersensory function (Murphy, 1972), the effect of acoustic conditions, illumination and domiciliary versus hospital testing. These are well summarised in a Scottish Education Department report (1967) and will not be dealt with in detail.

Table 4. Special schools for deaf and partially hearing children in England, Wales, Scotland, Northern Ireland, and the Republic of Ireland (1973)

Country	Number of special schools
England	
Berkshire	1 VR[a]
Buckinghamshire	2 1 R and 1 VR
Cheshire	1 VR
Derbyshire	1 VR
Devonshire	2 1 VR and 1 day
Gloucestershire	1 Day
Hampshire	1 R
Hertfordshire	1 R
Kent	1 VR
Lancashire	7 2 VR, 2 R, 3 day
Leicestershire	1 Day
London (ILEA)	10 5 VR, 1 R, 4 day
Greater London	5 1 VR
Norfolk	1 R
Northumberland	1 VR
Nottinghamshire	1 Day
Staffordshire	2 1 R, 1 day
Surrey	3 1 VR, 2 R
Sussex	3 VR
Warwickshire	3 2 day, 1 VR
Worcestershire	2 VR
Yorkshire	8 2 VR, 3 R, 3 day
Wales	
Glamorgan	1 R
Radnorshire	1 R
Scotland	
Edinburgh	2 1 VR, 1 day
Glasgow	2 Day
N. Ireland	
Belfast	2 1 VR, 1 day
Republic of Ireland	
Dublin[b]	3 2 VR, 1 day

[a]VR, voluntary residential; R, residential.

[b]Total of 390 pupils: 312 residential and 78 day students, 26 from N. Ireland and 364 from the Republic of Ireland.

Table 5. Department of Health and Social Security national summary of ear, nose, and throat patients for all England in the year ended 31/12/73

Services	Number of all patients	Number of new patients
Total	1,986,613	616,799
Audiometry	362,298	187,505
Hearing aid departments	869,083	89,540
Aids issued	277,799	71,438

The writer was privileged to work with an otologist and two paediatricians wherein close daily collaboration at the clinical level led to a pattern of identification of middle ear pathologies and their effects which formed the basis for an attempt at early differential diagnosis.

Throughout these countries, it became increasingly apparent to all workers in the field that a reappraisal of diagnostic and therapeutic services was needed, particularly when otologists were allowed to prescribe a wider range of amplifying equipment than was originally provided by means of the Medresco hearing aids. Extended research into objective audiometry began and, following closely upon the work of Davis in the U.S.A., preliminary work in ERA began at the Burden Neurological Institute in Bristol. Grey Walter, a neurophysiologist of international repute, pioneered work on evoked potentials before the advent of averaging computors, and other centres in London, Oxford, and Manchester followed suit in more recent years. Because of the problems of differential diagnosis and particularly because of the need to describe the prognosis for the development of speech and language, such programmes did not spread

Table 6. Full-time equivalent staffs in hospitals in England, Wales, and Scotland (ENT) during 1973

Position	England	Wales	Scotland	Total
Consultants	321	17	48	392
Senior registrars	64	5	42[a]	249[a]
Registrars	130	8		
Other	211	10	7	228
Total	732	40	97	869
Physical measurement technicians (audiology)	264	71	41	376

[a]Figure includes both senior registrars and registrars.

widely. For similar reasons the use of psychogalvanometry and vasculometry was limited to one or two research centres. Stapes impedance audiometry and tympanometry developed more rapidly and became routine clinical tools in major diagnostic centres (Swannie, 1965; Brooks, 1971, 1973; Bennett, 1973). In older patients, standard audiometric techniques were generally in the hands of nongraduate technicians, and the quality of development of techniques tended to be patchy and dependent on the information available in American and Scandinavian reports. The use of techniques such as vestibulometry for evaluating labyrinthine function was also restricted and tended to depend on the interest of individual otologists, neurosurgeons, or medical physicists. In this context, it should be remembered that audiology forms no part of the present education of otologists in these countries. This is not to say that individual otologists have not developed skills and interests in audiology as part of their ongoing clinical experience during training. Many of them have attended short courses at Manchester, Grays Inn Road, London, or Southampton. Others have spent periods with the Portmans in Bordeaux but, until the advanced techniques of audiology become a more integral part of otological training, it is unlikely that a routine nationwide use of audiological techniques will develop to the level that may be found in Denmark or the U.S.A. New departments of Medical Physics in some of the British teaching hospitals are likely to lead to the development of valuable clinical tools (Douek, 1974), and the research into hearing aids developed at the Royal National Institute for the Deaf, London (Martin, 1975), has led to encouraging progress in the provision of a wide variety of hearing aids for children by the National Health Service. A series of research proposals are at present before the Medical Research Council which, subject to the availability of funds, might eventually lead to the development of national hearing aid evaluation services which do not yet exist in these countries.

Parallel with, and often preliminary to, the involvement of hospital services, the Local Authorities play a tremendous part in early diagnosis, screening, parent guidance, auditory training, and subjective evaluation of hearing aids. In England, Northern Ireland, Scotland, and Wales, screening programmes are carried out by public health nurses under the supervision of a doctor, assisted in some cases by a teacher of the deaf. Although by no means 100% accurate, the Local Authority procedures not only find a large proportion of profoundly deaf children in the first year of life, but also keep the problem of hearing impairment before the public, remind family doctors of the need for vigilance, maintain a flow of information to public health and hospitals, and serve as a primary source of help for parents who suspect hearing impairment in ther children in the early months of life when they bring their infants to postnatal evaluation clinics. A report published in 1969 showed that, of 157 Local Health Authorities who responded to a questionnaire, 138 (87%) had a scheme for routine screening of infant hearing during the age range 6–12 months. Of these 138, only 45 (less than 35% of the total) managed a virtually complete survey. A similar proportion did not try to give a complete screening service but concentrated on vulnerable groups (Risk Registers).

The approach to hearing impairment in school-age children shows similarly wide discrepancies. Some Local Authorities employ audiology technicians, others employ teachers of the deaf, others employ school nurses or other school health staff with varying degrees of training and skill to visit schools and test all children in their first year of school life. This results in the routine screening of approximately 60% of all school entrants during their first year and a further 26% during the second year. For 7.8% of all school entrants, there is no routine audiometry, although there may well be audiometry on referral by a teacher or parent, and 4.5% do not have their hearing tested routinely until they have been at school for more than 2 years. Twenty percent tested children at age 6 years, 6.5% children at age 7 years, and 3.5% children at age 8 years.

A more detailed survey may be found in a report published in 1974. Although these figures appear good on the surface, a series of caveats has been produced up and down these countries in Local Authority Medical Officers' Annual Reports. They may be summarised as follows:

Testing Conditions These vary from bad to tolerable. Ambient noise levels are high, some tests are done in the presence of groups of children, and other distractions are variably controlled.

Test Materials These vary from pure tone audiometry with portable audiometers, in various stages of age or recency of calibration, to simple gramophone speech tests in free field or even "forced whisper" tests.

Examination of Ears This is rarely carried out by anyone but the medical officer when impairment is suspected or by the otologist on referral.

Frequency of School Visits Because of the pressures on staffs, children may have to wait long periods for testing within the school situations if a teacher suspects hearing impairment unless the parents take the child to the family physician (HMSO, 1972).

The use of audiometry by family physicians depends very much on the interest of the doctor who is usually a general practitioner and not necessarily specifically interested in child health. Recent developments of group practices within the Area Health Authorities have led to an increase in specialization, and, in those areas where the interest of the family physician is supported by a similar degree of interest in hospital otologists, a more widespread use of audiometry is slowly developing (Williams, 1968).

In the Republic of Ireland, responsibility for child audiometry has been vested in the Hearing Aid and Educational Guidance Service. Two teams based on Dublin, consisting of a doctor, a nurse, and a teacher of the deaf, travel throughout the republic to 26 centres and, in cooperation with local otologists, provide a diagnostic service. Although a praiseworthy attempt to initiate a service, the minister's own Committee of Enquiry (1973) has expressed extreme disquiet over the results.

Social Work Services

Recent legislation and restructuring of Local Authorities (1970, 1973, 1974), have created temporary stress in all areas of disability. However, a wide range of hearing impairments (deafness without speech, deafness with speech, and hardness of hearing) are now included in the category of severe disability meriting inclusion (should the individual so desire) on the Register of Disabled Individuals held by each Local Authority, and placement on which provides access to all relevant existing welfare services. Persons failing to register are in danger of exclusion from services in the present state of the social work agencies. By refusing registration, the independent person may place an additional burden on the family or immediate community. Once a hearing-impaired individual is registered with the Disablement Resettlement Officer, he may be helped to find employment in either open or sheltered conditions. The latter are provided in rare cases where other personal factors lead to a high degree of social incompetence. Registration with the Disablement Resettlement Officer has the added advantage that all but the smallest firms with less than 20 employees are compelled to employ a percentage of registered disabled people who cannot be dismissed without good cause (Wilmot, 1971). The parent of the hearing-impaired child may turn for advice to her local teachers of the deaf, the youth employment officer, the local welfare officer, the disablement resettlement officer, the generic social worker, the designated welfare officer to the deaf, or to the advisory services of the various voluntary agencies listed on p. 213). Should the hearing impairment be complicated by other features which make undue demands on domestic care or preclude employment, special grants are provided in law for parents or for the individual concerned.

The situation in the Republic of Ireland is less structured. Although industrial placement officers have an overall responsibility for helping any applicant to find suitable employment and it is natural that a significant proportion of their clientele should be suffering from a variety of disabilities, there is no specific responsibility for such advisory work, and training does not yet exist for these officers in skills which would be relevant to the person affected by hearing problems. A series of recent reports has drawn attention to the need for specialist social workers (National Association for the Deaf, 1973) and other measures which would draw the attention of various agencies, employers, the information media (press, radio, and television), and the general public to the effects of hearing impairment (National Association for the Deaf, 1973).

Burton (1972) examines the distribution of services to hearing-impaired individuals and finds that there has been an inequitable distribution in favor of the profoundly prelingually deafened community. He describes six different types of classification into which hearing-impaired people can be incorporated and describes the extent and quality of the pattern of services provided for them. The groups are: (1) deaf children and their families; (2) deaf and dumb adults who use manual communication; (3) prelingually deafened adults who reject manual communication; (4) hard-of-hearing persons; (5) traumatically deafened adults; (6) blind persons with a significant hearing loss.

For group 2, he feels there is a place for the generic social worker. He also suggests consideration of the employment of interpreters who would not necessarily be social workers.

In considering group 4, his suggestions are similar to those made by the two Irish surveys previously mentioned, although he goes further in outlining the needs of older deaf people, particularly those with degenerating manual dexterity or various problems of senility.

Although small in number, the traumatically deafened population which falls into group 5 needs special facilities, and he describes the experimental training scheme established by Link at Eastbourne for deafened individuals and their spouses. The main problem he discerns in regard to group 6 results from failures in communication between the major social work specialists involved with deaf-blind people (Table 7).

Table 7. Employment of social workers for deaf or hearing-impaired people in 1973

Where employed	Deaf	Hearing impaired
Voluntary agencies	242	10
Local authorities	99	53
Total[a]	341	63

[a]Of these, 103 were unqualified.

In June 1974, The British Deaf Association (BDA) produced an *Interim Report* which surveys the developments in welfare services available to deaf people. The report confines itself to a consideration of the services "for those people who consider themselves to be deaf; who may seek their social satisfaction among others of the same conviction using, as their means of communication, a mixture of speech, lipreading, writing, finger-spelling and signs." The working party gave special consideration to the following: "Communication, community life, spiritual needs, continued education throughout life, employment, personal help and participation." Their report is preceded by a statement which merits full quotation. To conserve space, however, it is summarised as follows:

1. Deaf people have the same needs as other people, plus exceptional difficulties arising from the consequences of their impairment.
2. There is an acute need for those in authority to recognise the special needs of deaf people.
3. Deaf people feel they are not sufficiently consulted or involved in matters pertinent to themselves or to the field of deafness in general.

Among a series of recommendations the following relate most directly to the present chapter:

1. That the BDA press the Department of Education and Science to make better provision for deaf people in further and higher education.
2. That efforts be made to improve consultation among all concerned with the assessment and placing of deaf people in employment.
3. That the services of specially trained social workers be made available to deaf people in every locality.
4. That the responsible authorities be advised of the importance of a close and continuous involvement by the social worker for the deaf in and with local deaf groups. (For a more detailed summary, see pages 17–18 of the above report.)

As part of the above review, a questionnaire was sent to all directors of Local Authority Social Services Departments. This achieved an 88.8% return and is summarized as follows:

1. It was disturbing to discover the low numbers registered at present as deaf or hard of hearing (22,325 deaf; 18,524 hard of hearing, i.e., less than 0.2% of the known population of hearing aid wearers).
2. Clubs and their members. The survey revealed that there are facilities for meetings of deaf people (see Table 8).
3. Responsibility for club activities was divided roughly as is shown in Table 9.

Table 8. Facilities for meetings of deaf people during 1973

Description of facilities	Number of facilities
Centres provided by voluntary societies exclusively for deaf people	125
Centres provided by local authorities exclusively for deaf people	9
In a centre used simultaneously by other disabled people	23
In one private room or section within a centre used simultaneously by other disabled people	17
In a community centre	11
In a room or building owned or hired by deaf people	21
In other facilities	40
Total	246

4. Populations and needs provided for in centers (Table 10). The extent to which Local Authorities have merged facilities for deaf, partially hearing, hard of hearing, or other disabled people is unclear.

5. A satisfying picture emerges of the availability of the social workers. Almost 80% were regarded as being "available at all times" to their deaf clients, and I have little doubt that that statement may be taken as substantially correct. A sign displayed prominently in the home of one welfare worker states simply, "The worse the hour, the greater the need."

6. Other sidelights on the role of the social worker are contained in the above report on interpretation in courts of law, interpretation on educational or cultural occasions, work with persons seeking employment and in the course of employment. These are obviously regarded as an important part of the role of the social worker and give some point to the suggestions concerning interpretation made by Burton.

Table 9. Responsibility for club activities during 1973

Responsible person(s)	Number
Committees of deaf people	80
Deaf people and social worker together	108
Social worker and chaplain for deaf	34
Paid community worker	8

Table 10. Populations and needs provided for within the centres

Populations	Number of centres
Elderly deaf	146
Deaf-blind	126
Hard of hearing	135
Deaf youths	124
Deaf children	94
Parents and families of deaf children	115
Physically handicapped deaf	98
Deaf and in psychiatric or mental subnormality hospitals	92
Additional facilities for hobbies, interests, sports group	216

DIAGNOSTIC AND THERAPEUTIC FACILITIES

The psychological, linguistic, educational, and sociological consequences of hearing impairment are now generally recognized throughout the world. Different communities have dealt with them in different ways. The character and extent of provision in these countries have been profoundly affected, as has already been stated, by the fact that education and health are national services. There is insufficient space to enter into discussion of the merits or demerits of a national service, and this chapter will concentrate on a description of the services as they exist. Because the field of hearing impairment is so complex, the number of specialties involved directly or indirectly is equally complex. For the sake of brevity, they can be summarised under three main categories. These are detection, diagnosis, and dealing with (Murphy, 1972a). In the case of children, processes of detection have been helped by the fact that parents have a right in law to seek expert help if they suspect hearing loss in their children and the health services are constrained by law to provide the medical services upon which educational placement is based. In the case of adults, detection procedures depend upon the individual in the majority of cases, except for those circumstances where the patient is already in the care of, or under the supervision of, other health services (e.g., hospitals for mentally subnormal or psychiatrically disturbed patients). The difference in the pattern of detection leads to significant differences in their effectiveness. The adult is free to accept or reject diagnostic and remedial services, and this particular phenomenon is reflected in the relative scarcity of support services for adults affected by hearing impairment (Burton, 1972; Rawson, 1973; Groves, 1974; Rimmer, 1974). Services for adult prelingually profoundly deaf individuals are better organized than are those for adults who fall into the category commonly described as hard of hearing. Some indication of the extent to which deafness is regarded as a "crippling disease" may be gained from the fact that in a recent 87-page report (NFERD, 1973) on the workings of the Chronically Sick and Disabled Persons Act (1970), a mere 10 lines were devoted to hearing impairment. The report states, "By contrast with the blind, services to the deaf have been largely provided by voluntary organizations and there has so far been little change since the Seebohm reorganization. However, some Directors (of social services) expressed dissatisfaction with these services and intend to take over the provision. At least half the Authorities have officers to deal with the deaf. Problems were expressed in recruiting these specialists nowadays and in encouraging social workers to attend training courses for work with the deaf." Although accurate as far as it went, the above report was more remarkable for the points it did not make than for the points it did.

Paradoxically, detection and diagnostic procedures are, to a greater or lesser extent, modified by the quality of the subsequent remedial and rehabilitation services. The primary purpose of any diagnostic approach is to effect a cure; where a cure is not possible, to prevent deterioration; to achieve amelioration by the use of a prosthesis, where feasible, and ultimately to develop sufficient information about causation to facilitate preventative measures for those cases in danger of the condition under investigation. In addition, there are numerous subsidiary aims from which, among many, administrative, sociological, and educational categories may be selected. For instance, although the epidemiology of hearing impairment in association with mental subnormality has not been fully researched in these countries, sufficient research has been done (Simon, 1974; Ives, 1975) to suggest a possible incidence of between 6,000 and 10,000 children within the above category. However, until formal surveys have been completed there is little or no likelihood of the provision of training in specialised diagnosis and education for such children. Without specialist diagnosticians and teachers, the provision of special education support services is even more unlikely. (To date there is special provision for the education of approximately 300 such children in six different centres throughout the countries under review in this contribution.) Other groups needing specialised help are blind, spastic, or language-disordered children with hearing problems. Even when they are detected, we may ask ourselves, how accurate is the diagnosis of the true state of the language acquisition processes and to what extent are decisions about education dependent on sociological rather than educational criteria? Until diagnostic procedures are satisfactory, educational emphases must stem from subjective judgement. Diagnosis is seen as a continuing function throughout the rehabilitation programme centre. Within any special remedial centre for dual handicap there must be sufficient flexibility, based on regular assessment of the child, to allow radical shifts in educational emphasis should they be required. The above statement is made to emphasise that, insofar as rehabilitation of children is concerned, the diagnostic emphases must shift from the factors which lead to detection (hearing impairment and failure to speak) and concentrate more closely on educational and sociological criteria. It is in this particular area that these countries can claim to have given an international lead. The provision of day facilities, the attempt to integrate programmes for partially hearing children within schools for children with normal hearing, the new emphasis on weekly boarding, while to a certain extent dictated by administrative or fiscal criteria, stem, in the main, from sociological thinking and are a logical outcome of the philosophies underlying the early arguments in support of oral education. Discussing educational placement, Reed (1974) states, "The decision should be based on a complete assessment of the child and his environment by a team of trained personnel. Such a team should consist of an audiologist, an otologist, a psychologist, a social worker, a teacher of the deaf, and an audiology technician with the frequent services of a neurologist, a paediatrician and a psychiatrist, as so many hearing impaired children have additional handicaps, or the diagnosis may be clouded by the presenting behaviour pattern." He sees such a team located in a "specially provided and equipped centre, suitably acoustically treated, in association with a paediatric development assessment centre." Such centres are now being developed by the Inner London Area and are a combination of educational, medical, and social services. The emphasis on the early involvement of the social services represents a welcome step forward in current thinking in these countries, and it will be of great interest to observe the extent to which social workers and their educational colleagues can develop a joint approach to parent counselling. A good case can be made for the development of an emphasis in counselling practice in which the relevant skills could be held by one person who would be acceptable by teacher and social worker alike. Having described the ideal situation, in the interest of accuracy, the following description of the current situation is included (Rawson, 1973):

> The group of doctors most closely concerned with deafness, the consultant otolaryngologists, have concentrated on the surgical treatment of conductive deafness. The non-surgical management of adult patients has received little attention, although, since the pioneer work

> of Sir Alexander and Lady Ewing in Manchester (Ewing, 1946; Ewing and Ewing, 1947) and Dr. Edith Whetnall (Whetnall, 1952; Whetnall and Fry, 1964) in London in the 1940s, consultant otolaryngologists have been increasingly aware of the importance of the early diagnosis of deafness in children, together with the provision of hearing aids, the correct use of hearing aids, auditory training, and early parental guidance and teaching. Dr. Mary Sheridan developed simple clinical tests of hearing for very young children, as part of developmental assessment (Sheridan, 1960). Some consultant otolaryngologists concern themselves predominantly with children, and a few concentrate on the assessment and management of children entirely and no longer undertake surgical work. There are conflicts between those doctors with a surgical training and those without, whether undertaking paedo-audiological or adult work.
>
> Child psychiatrists, linguists and clinical psychologists are insufficiently involved in either service or research today; yet it would appear that the skills of child psychiatrists and the research skills of departments of psycholinguistics are urgently needed to explain some of the problems of language development in profoundly deaf children.
>
> The support and management of adults with hearing impairment are not normally the concern of consultant otolaryngologists once a diagnosis has been made and a hearing aid prescribed, and not all understand the technicalities and limitations of hearing aids, or the problems or complexities of lipreading.
>
> The few medical otologists work in the specialist centres mainly in the fields of diagnosis, diagnostic techniques, and the clinical application of the work of many basic sciences.
>
> A re-ablement role would be appropriate if a group of doctors had the training for it, or the interest in it, but neither appears to be the case at present. As a result there is no concerted effort to provide support and management of hard-of-hearing and defened adults.

In the course of the comments quoted above, Reed talks of a "complete assessment" of the child. While agreeing wholeheartedly with the need for this, we are compelled to the reluctant conclusion that, in our present state of knowledge, the notion of "completeness" can be only relative. The tests available to psychologists which are specifically designed for deaf children are unfortunately all too few. Until much more is known about the cognitive structures of hearing-impaired children, and the extent to which linguistic factors confuse rather than inform them, it is difficult to be sure that the present armamentum of adapted test materials is satisfactory. Many psychologists working in the field of hearing impairment have expressed concern over their lack of knowledge of the amount of language saturation in performance tests. As a result, when in-depth testing has been carried out (Ives, 1974; Boscak, 1970), the disquieting results which emerge may well represent test artifacts rather than specific deficits in the population under test. A similar problem arises in the results of early audiometric testing. The emphasis on measurement of acuity of peripheral hearing has tended to divert attention in these countries from the problems of auditory function. Prognostic statements about the value of amplification, the possible relevance of lipreading, signing, fingerspelling, mime, and the interplay of visual and tactile inputs are virtually impossible in the present state of knowledge about young children. The significance of aetiological factors, although part of the folklore of deaf education, has not yet been the subject of rigorous research in reference to educational prognosis. More information is needed on the educational effects of rubella embryopathies, meningitis, hyperbilirubinaemia, and encephalitis, to name but a few. With improved diagnostic facilities, we should be in a better position to correlate pathologies and problems of learning, particularly in the language areas. Such facilities as now exist are adequate to detect gross malfunction, to diagnose peripheral auditory disacuities, to make preliminary provision of amplification on a trial basis. Hence forward, in the case of both child and adult, much more follow-up of the effects of amplification, the significance of acoustic environments, the value or otherwise of one aid, two aids, or of all the various refinements of signal transmission, need the close and continuous investigation of a complex team approach.

Discovery of Children with Hearing Impairment

Responsibility for the discovery and management by Local Education Authorities of children with hearing impairments is defined in the Education Act (1944) as beginning at the age of 2 years. Parents were also granted the right to request an examination for their children if they suspected the presence of an impairment. Beginning at the age of 2 is late for starting auditory training and encouraging language development. Fortunately, most medical officers in the school health service either work in child health clinics themselves or are closely in touch with those who do, so that most babies and young children with a hearing loss severe enough to delay normal language development should be recognised early and known to the principal school medical officer. Local Authorities were permitted to begin special educational provision in nursery schools or classes for children aged 2 years. This led to the extension of early specialised diagnostic facilities into their Child Health and Welfare Services. By 1961, the Ministry of Health was able to issue a circular (23/61) which re-emphasized the importance of early diagnosis and suggested ways in which case finding methods could be improved. In particular, the establishment of Paedoaudiology Units and the value of early auditory training received powerful encouragement.

Screening for Hearing

Taking the information from Form 8M(iv) 1971 as a starting point, Local Education Authorities can be divided by the audiometric services they provide under the School Health Service into six groups as follows (The Health of the School Child 1971–1972 (1974), pp. 32–34): (1) those who have no facility for audiometry; (2) those who arrange audiometry for school children only when it is individually requested, i.e., only when children are referred; (3) those who arrange routine audiometry on all entrants during their first year at school, which, for the purpose of this report, is taken to be at the statutory age of 5 years; (4) those who arrange the first routine audiometry during a child's second year at school, i.e., at the age of 6 years; (5) those who arrange the first routine audiometry during a child's third year at school, i.e., at the age of 7 years; (6) those who arrange the first routine audiometry during a child's fourth year at school, i.e., at the age of 8 years.

Returns for 1971 were made by 145 Local Education Authorities, one making no return. (It should be stated that the Inner London Education Authority made a single return on behalf of the 13 inner London boroughs which have, therefore, been counted as a single authority for this purpose.)

Group 1 Five Local Education Authorities, one county, four county boroughs, and nearly half of another county, fall into the first group, although two of the county boroughs do not use pure tone audiometry but arrange tests, one by forced whisper and the other by spoken word lists.

Group 2 Eight Local Education Authorities arrange audiometry only on referral or for selected groups of school children, such as those known to be handicapped or to be at risk of hearing impairment. Four counties and four county boroughs adopt this practice and at least some of them accept referrals from a wide range of sources, e.g., from parents, teachers, school medical officers, school nurses, and speech therapists.

Groups 3 and 4 One hundred and twenty-seven Local Education Authorities carry out routine screening of all school children during their first or second years at school, i.e., at the ages of 5 or 6, 95 doing it during the first year at school, 32 during the second year.

Group 5 Three Local Education Authorities, all county boroughs, fall into this group.

Group 6 Two Local Education Authorities, one county and one county borough do their first routine test on school children aged 8, i.e., during their fourth year at school.

It is desirable that all school children should have their hearing tested as soon as possible after they enter school, unless it has been done shortly before entry under a system of preschool medical examination. The service provided by Local Education Authorities in groups 1, 2, 5, and 6 most need further examination. Services provided by the Local Health Authorities corresponding to the Local Education Authorities in these groups for preschool and particularly for children under the age of 12 months must be taken into account. In 1969, The Department of Health and Social Security (DHSS) conducted a survey and asked Local Health Authorities the following questions, among others:

1. Have you a scheme for the routine screening of infants between 6 and 12 months? *Yes/No*
2. (a) Is an attempt made to screen ALL infants? *Yes/no*
   (b) If "Yes," are you satisfied that coverage is virtually complete? *Yes/no*
3. If only a proportion of infants is screened, what groups are selected?

Clinic attenders?
At-Risk Register?
Handicap Register?
Other (state________)?

A report on this survey was included in the Annual Report *On the State of Public Health* (1969, pp. 108–109), and can be summarised as follows:

> Replies were received from 157 Local Health Authorities. 138 Local Health Authorities had a scheme for routine screening of infants aged between 6 and 12 months (question 1), 97 such Authorities made an attempt to screen all infants (question 2(a)), but in only 45 of them was coverage virtually complete (question 2(b)). 42 Authorities attempted to screen only selected groups (question 3), some including, as well as the 3 groups on the questionnaire, children referred by, for example, doctors, nurses, teachers or parents and those with speech defects.

Of the 18 Authorities without schemes for routine screening on school entry, 10 do not screen the hearing of all infants, but all but one of them screen one or more selected groups of infants. Five of these 10 Authorities screen the named groups. In some instances, where less than the recommended level of audiometry is provided for school children, there has been fairly substantial coverage of 6- to 12-month-old infants sufficient to detect most of the children with congenital hearing defects. Hearing impairment, particularly that of lesser degree, acquired in later childhood or early school life, would not be detected as early as is desirable, and, of course, the screening methods used in infancy are necessarily less certain than those available at later ages. In terms of coverage of the child population, approximately 60% of school children have their hearing screened routinely during their first year at school and another 26% have it screened during their second year at school. Routine audiometry is not provided for 7.8% of school children (i.e., no audiometry or audiometry on referral only: groups 1 and 2) and a further 4.5% of school children do not have their hearing tested routinely until they have been at school for more than 2 years.

REHABILITATIVE PROCEDURES

Communication Systems

The main systems of communication available to adults are limited to the following: predominantly oral, oral plus gesture, manual plus some speech and lipreading, manual with lipreading but with minimal use of voice. If we consider the total field of hearing impairment, it will be clear that a very large proportion of people with auditory impairments will manage by using amplification and lipreading. Many hard-of-hearing people are effectively profoundly deaf, but few of them resort to formal signing or fingerspelling. There are two reasons for this:

1. The large majority of hearing-impaired people are adventitiously deafened and have had considerable access to, and skill in, the use of normal spoken language.
2. They have a different self-image from the one they attach to profoundly deafened people, and they do not wish to be identified with them.

The situation is different for prelingually deafened individuals or for those who, although deafened later in life, have, nevertheless, been educated in a school for the deaf. Many more of these adults use signing, miming, or fingerspelling than might be expected when we remember that schools for the deaf have not used manual methods to any great extent for the last 30 years. For a large proportion of these manualists, signing or fingerspelling began as a kind of secret system, developed during out-of-class times in residential schools. Because of this, the standards of competency are not high and "manual literacy" is of variable quality. Since the professional users of manual systems have had to modify their own language skills in order to be understood by their clients, the general linguistic quality is not high. Most users of manual systems have learned from each other with the result that the potential language quality had been stultified. Paradoxically, teachers, untrained in manual methods in present schools or departments of deaf education, have to learn the manual system from their pupils or from adults with poor language facility before they can begin to teach through such systems. In the course of the 1974 Congress of the British Deaf Association, teachers explained the approach to different methods of communication in the schools for the deaf in which they worked (Chittenden, 1974; Neate, 1974). The methods described were: the Paget-Gorman systematic signs (PGSS), research project into the use of a one-handed fingerspelling, cued speech, and oralism. With the exception of one-handed fingerspelling, all the other systems were described as complementary to and designed to facilitate a basically oral approach. The research project on one-handed fingerspelling carried out jointly between the University of Newcastle Upon Tyne and the Northern Counties School for the Deaf is supported by a grant from the Department of Education and Science. Generally aimed to discover "more fully the conditions under which finger-spelling may be an appropriate tool in the language development and education of deaf children" (Evans, 1974), it also plans the use of a team of psychologists who will be "concerned with measuring the effects of the use of one-handed finger-spelling on educational progress and language skills and social and personal adjustment." As Evans stresses, although the project is scheduled for a 5-year period "some questions might only be answered in the long term." He also makes the wry comment, "It has taken six years to implement this project as a recommendation of the Lewis Report." In fact, 4 years elapsed between the original invitation by the DES to submit a proposal and the initiation of the first formal use of fingerspelling as part of the project. This was not caused by procrastination on the part of the researchers and illustrates the problems involved in setting up large-scale studies of educational methods for children with hearing impairments. In keeping with the views expressed by other teachers using PGSS, Chittendon (1974) reports, "I find the children are helped in a number of ways." Apparently, they were "more relaxed, understood the teacher more easily, were able to attend for a longer time, during speech they became more interested in words, more oral, less shy or hesitant about speaking and more keen to use correct sentences."

Although the above approaches show that work on alternative communication methods has begun, there is no doubt that there is still a considerable bias against the use of manual methods. Whatever method is tried, preventing contamination by other communication systems will be almost impossible. In the 30 or more years that oralism has been taught in these countries, there can be very few residential schools for profoundly deaf children in which some use of manual systems has not been present.

The greatest barrier to objective research lies in the present lack of knowledge of visual processing systems in profoundly deaf children. Too often manualism has been advanced as *the* automatic alternative for children who fail in oral approaches. No one in these countries has yet been able to indicate: (1) what were the causes of such failures; (2) whether the children who fail would make progress under a different application of the same approach (is the problem in the children, the teachers, or the educational environment?); (3) whether resource to a manual approach would, as the oralists claim, lead to the further isolation of the deaf child from the community of people with normal hearing; (4) what, if any, system would work for children with such conditions as language disorders, mental subnormality, cerebral palsy, or severe visual disability in association with a hearing impairment?

Reading the account of the oral approach (Neate, 1974), it was clear that: (1) great demands are made on technical competence on the part of the staff. Equipment included all those recommended in the preceding section plus the use of video recorders, and teachers needed to be expert in their use; (2) great demands were made on visual acuity, attention, and sequencing; (3) the curriculum was not limited by the emphasis on the development of good spoken language. Although stressing the wide intellectual range of the children, Neate did not analyse results, and we have no way of knowing how the successes and failures were distributed throughout the range of such factors as age, intelligence, hearing loss, double disability, nor do we know what methods were used with the latter group.

Auditory Rehabilitation and Acquisition of Speech and Language

Auditory rehabilitation for infants and young children has been emphasized because considerable evidence has accumulated to show that the normal acquisition of important elements of speech and language is largely contingent upon adequate hearing for speech over the age range of approximately 6 months to 5 years (Renfrew and Murphy, 1964; Rutter and Martin, 1972). Although it has been argued (Katz, 1966; McNeil, 1966; Slobin, 1966; Chomsky, 1968) that a child has an innate or fundamental capacity for language, even the more extreme nativists would accept that much of the shaping of language depends on experiential factors. Although it is clearly recognised that hearing plays an essential role in the development of speech and language, it is extremely difficult, if not impossible, to describe such a role fully, because, although much has recently been written on the acquisition of language in infants and children with normal hearing (Crystal, 1972), we still do not know enough (Friedlander, 1970), and much still remains to be discovered about the way in which speech and language are acquired in those children who suffer from various auditory disorders (Jones and Byers, 1971; Dale, 1972). We also need to know much more than we do at present about the variations which can occur in so-called normally hearing children and the extent, if any, to which they are likely to constitute a threat to language growth in the first few years of life. For instance, it is unlikely that any child could reach the age of 3 without some variation in auditory state. We know next to nothing about such variations and, in particular, we are unable to identify the extent to which they are stable or fluctuating and/or attenuating, and/or distorting. Given such variables, the growth of signal processing (i.e., discrimination, decoding, and encoding) before any expressive function seems to be at risk. Add these phenomena to a sensorineural loss and the problem is further complicated. Nonetheless, enough is already known to compel us to include hearing problems in children within the wider field of what have come to be known as communication problems, in order to achieve effective rehabilitation. This in turn leads on to yet wider issues because: "Children's personality adjustment as well as their development linguistically, socially and intellectually, now clearly have been found to be affected by problems in communication" (Ewing, 1963) and because: "any disturbances of either (the nervous system or the mind) in relation to communication must have the profound social effects, because society is based upon communication" (Brain, 1965).

From the foregoing, it should be clear that we should not fall into the error of regarding problems of rehabilitation as too closely associated with the impairment of the sensory end organ. While recognizing that my topic has its origin in disorders of the ear, the difficulties that ensue are the proper concern of disciplines other than otology, not least because the child is a developing being in many ways which involve complex interactions between a number of variables. Malfunction in *one* particular will have effects on many others, and, in the case of auditory impairment, it is not enough to restore auditory function and then to assume that all will be well. For example, Critchley (1967) has remarked that aspects of hearing involve "brain stem startle reflexes, cortical representation of hearing, development of association areas and feedback mechanism." Lloyd and Frisina (1965) have gone further to remark that hearing is important for "handling auditory symbols mechanically, chemically and electrically, as well as for the subsequent transmission of coded neural impulses to the areas of the brain important for speech and language. Important C.N.S. processes include those such as perception, concept development and ideation." Adopting Hirsch's approach, Bench (1970) has referred to detection, discrimination, recognition, identification, and interpretation of sound, examining the way in which the stimuli which impinge on the ear can be studied and related to past experience. The writer, on the other hand, has dealt with the feedback or self-monitoring processes whereby the child learns to check that his speech sounds conform to his linguistic intentions (Murphy, 1972). Clearly the functions involved in what we refer to as hearing are so multifaceted that even a temporary failure of auditory input has far-reaching effects on other areas, especially for young children whose continuing development will cause higher order derangements to continue to accrue unless appropriate remedial action is taken (Lewis, 1965).

Even in those circumstances where diagnosis is not his primary concern, it is necessary for each person engaged in auditory rehabilitation to have a sound grasp of the strength and limitations of diagnostic methods for assessing hearing impairment. He should also be able to understand the interactions of the findings from his diagnostic and therapeutic colleagues. Paediatrics, psychiatry, clinical psychology, psychometry, education, sociology, and social work all have their place in the balanced assessment of the needs of the young hearing-impaired child. He needs to recognize that no matter how early it begins, the likely success of the training programme is dependent not only on the treatment of the handicap but also on the degree of confidence which can be placed in the estimate of hearing deficit (an especially important point in the case of infants and young children for whom threshold measures are particularly difficult to achieve and which may tend to fluctuate or deteriorate). He needs to be able to judge the extent to which it is possible to help the youngster to begin to understand the nature of his impairment and the effects which the impairment will have on his everyday life. All of these will have to be blended into a coherent whole so that he can begin with confidence to convey to parents, teachers, and the restricted community with whom the child is most likely to come into contact, the behavioural and intellectual concomitants of the hearing difficulties and the importance of each individual's role in the ameliorative programme.

Hearing Aids and Other Equipment

Provision for Children Any hearing aid commercially available may be prescribed free of charge for a child by an otologist should he judge it necessary. Besides the five Medresco aids which have been available for many years, there is now freedom to prescribe any aids to hearing. Depending on the clinical judgement of the otologist, this could include portable speech trainers, tactile reinforcers, or other devices liable to lead to amelioration of individual cases. Group hearing aids are the responsibility of the Local Education Authority (Table 11). Although, in theory, their

Table 11. Centres responsible for the issue and maintenance of Medresco hearing aids and/or holding lipreading classes[a] by county (1973)

Country	Hearing aids	Lipreading classes
England		
Bedfordshire	2	2
Berkshire	2	2
Buckinghamshire	1	1
Cambridgeshire	1	1
Cheshire	3	1
Cornwall	1	–
Cumberland	1	–
Derbyshire	2	2
Devonshire	2	1
Dorset	–	2
Durham	1	4
Essex	6	–
Gloucestershire	1	2
Hampshire	5	6
Herefordshire	1	1
Hertfordshire	3	1
Kent	3	5
Lancashire	14	10
Leicestershire	1	2
Lincolnshire	2	1
London	23	24
Norfolk	1	2
Northamptonshire	2	2
Northumberland	2	3
Nottinghamshire	1	1
Oxfordshire	1	7
Peterborough	1	–
Shropshire	1	1
Somerset	4	2
Staffordshire	2	9
Suffolk	2	1
Surrey	3	4
Sussex	1	16
Teeside	–	1
Warwickshire	3	7
Wiltshire	2	3
Worcestershire	1	2
Yorkshire	9	5

Continued

Table 11—*Continued*

Country	Hearing aids	Lipreading classes
Wales		
Caernarvonshire	1	1
Carmarthenshire	1	–
Denbighshire	1	–
Flintshire	1	–
Glamorgan	6	2
Monmouthshire	2	–
Scotland		
Aberdeenshire	1	1
Angus	1	–
Argyllshire	1	–
Ayrshire	1	1
Edinburgh	1	1
Fife	1	1
Glasgow	5	3
Invernessshire	1	–
Lanarkshire	–	3
Perthshire	1	–
Renfrewshire	2	1
Stirlingshire	1	–
Northern Ireland		
Co. Antrim	2	1
Co. Armagh	1	–
Belfast	3	–
Co. Down	1	–
Newry	1	–
Co. Londonderry	1	–
Co. Tyrone	2	–
Eire	27	6
Isle of Man	1	–
Channel Isles	1	1
Isle of Wight	–	1

[a]Most of the lipreading classes are not held in the centres responsible for hearing aid issue and maintenance.

prescription might well be seen to be the responsibility of the otologist, in fact not many otologists have the necessary information to discharge this function, and Local Authorities tend to rely on the services of teachers of the deaf or educational audiologists or to follow the advice of the larger education authorities.

The system is tending to fall down at present because, although there has been a sudden upsurge of highly sophisticated appliances, the techniques of evaluation and supervision are not consistently utilised (Rawson, 1973). To some extent, this stems from lack of staff and funds and also from lack of information, facilities, and knowledge. Hence, research into reliable evaluation of aids in use still needs to be carried out. Reliable tests of language comprehension, reliable controls of classroom reverberation, reliable techniques for the proper evaluation of induction aerials and for radio microphones may well exist in the laboratory. They are not yet commonly used in these countries. It is difficult to discover why a certain type of hearing aid commends itself to teachers and children. In my experience it has been difficult to know whether a school request for a particular type of aid springs from the general judgment that it is a good aid or that it is particularly good for the particular child for whom it has been requested. Fortunately, the problem of prescription has been recognised, and the Department of Health and Social Security has issued circulars commending trial issue of hearing aids and has agreed to accept financial responsibility for the cost of this and, where necessary, subsequent refurbishment of the aid. The following extracts from Hansard (1973) are relevant: "issue of postaural hearing aids since 1969"—the supplying of ear level hearing aids for children commenced in 1969. Issue in England and Wales, including replacements in each of the last 4 years, is shown in Table 12.

Table 12. Issue of postaural hearing aids since 1969

Year	Number
1969	7,088
1970	6,816
1971	6,376
1972	6,770

Sir Keith Joseph (1973) stated, "I expect the cost of the provision of the hearing aid to rise to a peak of £5 million in 1978–9, and there will be an additional cost of about £1 million per annum when we have recruited sufficient staff."

Provision for Adults Sir Keith Joseph (1973) made a statement in the House of Commons, which included the following:

> We propose, therefore, as part of the National Health Service to provide over the coming years a "behind-the-ear" aid free of charge for all adults for whom it is suitable and for children who already receive this type of aid. This will offer an alternative to Medresco Aid users and help many who do not now use a Medresco aid and cannot afford a commercial "behind-the-ear" aid. These people will for the first time be able to benefit from the hospital-based clinical and allied services in obtaining an aid and using it effectively.
>
> The numbers involved are large, probably a million or more. The cost will be met from the resources available for the expanding Health Service programme, but it will necessarily take time to produce enough suitable aids and to secure suitable staff. We, therefore, aim to begin issuing the new aids in the Autumn of next year, and to complete the operation over five years.
>
> In the first year we plan to give priority to: (1) war pensioners who require aids for accepted disabilities; (2) mothers with young children; (3) children of any age and young people receiving full-time education; (4) young people whose "behind-the-ear" aid has been replaced by a body-worn model on leaving school; (5) people with an additional severe handicap, such as blindness; (6) people with exceptional medical needs not included in these groups.

Sir Keith also promised to consult "the bodies concerned" in deciding priorities for the second and later years of the programme. He also drew attention to the shortage of trained staff and the need for other provisions to help deaf people. To help parents of all handicapped children, the government has set up a £3 million fund to be administered by an independent trust (The Joseph Rowntree Trust, York).

Additional Equipment

Schools The National Deaf Children's Society recommends that every school or unit should have the following basic equipment: group aids in every classroom, individual aids, one or more individual amplifiers (speech trainers), overhead projectors, cine projectors (both 8 mm and 16 mm), cine camera, and film loops. The National College of Teachers of the Deaf recommended the following additions: tape recorder, radiogram, television set, slide projector, and Polaroid camera. The college, however, stressed that circumstances might produce variation of needs and, therefore, suggested a generous allowance with freedom to purchase as needs arose or changed.

Other Equipment in Common Use In a recent parliamentary reply, it was estimated that the General Post Office had 100,000 amplifying telephone headsets rented at a total annual charge of £500,000. There was no present likelihood of this charge being borne by the State Government.

The National College of Teachers of the Deaf and the National Deaf Children's Society strongly recommend to the parents of those children who would benefit from them that they install an induction loop aerial in their houses for use in conjunction with radio, television, and record-playing equipment. These cost approximately £10 per installation if commercially fitted. Some branches of the National Deaf Children's Society run a self-help system which reduces costs of installation considerably. These fittings are not permitted by rental companies who insist on installing them themselves. One or two major companies have fitted them without charge as a philanthropic gesture.

Increased publicity and pressure from interested bodies have led to the slow development of "loop" systems in theatres, conference halls, and churches. There is as yet no consistent policy at the local government level.

Other Miscellaneous Equipment Other equipment includes: Laryngograph, teletype, vibraphone, various pitch and rhythm indicators, various signal presenters, and coders (phonomorse, etc.). At present, the use of most of these can best be described as extremely limited and experimental.

INTERPROFESSIONAL RELATIONSHIPS

There is a temptation in writing this section to concentrate on the negative. It is true, as Rawson (1973) says that cooperation and interdisciplinary contacts are not good enough but, although variable in quality or efficiency, contacts have existed between the disciplines in a tenuous and informal way for many years. For instance, the various joint hospital-local authority schemes have seen the growth of partial hearing unit provision which has demanded considerable integration of services as was outlined in Health of the School Child (1969):

> To be successful, work of this kind calls for close collaboration with special schools and special classes as well as with ordinary schools so that the full range of educational provision in the neighbourhood is well-known and understood by the peripatetic teacher. It is equally necessary that peripatetic teachers should work closely with the doctors (otologists, local authority medical officers and general practitioners) responsible for medical assessment, treatment and supervision and to discuss with them both general policies and the needs of individual children within their families. Close liaison with Youth Employment Officers is also an essential part of the work of peripatetic teachers.

It is interesting that the report should place emphasis on the role of the teacher as the coordinator at an informational level. At the level of decision making, the role of the teacher is acknowledged by all to be important, but the application of this knowledge depends very much on the personal approach of the medical authorities involved. If the doctors see themselves as totally responsible for the child, their ability to draw the teacher into a state of collaborative parity may be limited. If the teacher, on the other hand, sees the role of the medical authorities as almost irrelevant, once preliminary diagnosis is sufficiently developed to lead to the prescription of an aid, cooperation breaks down. If the parents, community, and social workers are not absorbed to a greater or lesser extent, particularly in the case of children with profound or mixed disabilities, there is a danger of stress in ever widening circles of complexity and severity.

When the Manchester Audiology Clinics were beginning in the late 1940's with Irene Ewing, Dorothy Watson, David Kendall, and Aileen Pickles, there was a constant struggle to develop joint services, particularly with otology (Watson, 1969). Over the years, this came into being and the need for the involvement of local authority nurses within the screening services emerged. Fortunately, the nursing service which was selected was already closely linked to social services and, although the quality of screening audiology may be open to criticism, the interdisciplinary results have usually been good. Following the lead of the clinics at Manchester and Gray's Inn Road, London, other centres came into being in which close cooperation between disciplines developed.

A paediatrically oriented programme was established at Guy's Hospital, London, where a fruitful cooperation among paediatrics, otology, and community health developed and from which the recognition of the complexity of multiple pathology associated with hearing impairment began to receive more sustained emphasis. The fact that one of the persons involved in that particular group was also a member of the staff of the then Ministry of Health (now the Department of Health and Social Security) led to a national emphasis on the need for simple tests of auditory acuity, and Dr. Mary Sheridan (1960) not only supplied such tests but also soon became an able protagonist and an international authority in the area of early diagnosis and parent counselling. During the same period, Professor R. H. Hunt Williams established the Audiology Unit at Reading which entered a new building in September 1958, and, as one of its foundation members of staff, the writer had the good fortune to receive the generous advice and support of Edith Whetnall, her colleague, the psychologist Michael Reed, Mary Sheridan, and a succession of brilliant and dedicated teachers of the deaf. In this clinic, as at Manchester and Ealing, there was close cooperation among paediatrics, otology, psychiatry, community health, psychology, teachers of the deaf, and local parents of deaf children. A clinic established at Heston, Middlesex, by Dr. L. Fisch (1964) served as a model for community-based services. During the same period, a less structured situation developed in Dublin where a Dominican Sister, Mother M. Nicholas, having been trained by the Ewings, began the long, slow process of creating a diagnostic, guidance, and education programme which ultimately became an effective national centre upon which the training programme for teachers of hearing-impaired children in Ireland was based. As in England, otologists in Glasgow and Dublin began to develop their own diagnostic centers and the emergence of the Dublin College of Speech Therapists may be traced in part to the cooperation between an otologist, Mr. J. McCauliffe Curtin, F.R.C.S. and a Sister of Charity, Sister M. Supple, a speech therapist with additional skills in audiology. In a different manner, the establishment of the Scottish branch of the Technical Department of the Royal National Institute for the Deaf met the needs of otologists and deaf educators for a reliable audiotechnical support centre which, in company with a group of existing specialties, culminated in the establishment in 1971 of a training programme for teachers of the deaf at Moray House in Edinburgh.

Present problems stem mainly from the following factors:

1. Rigidity of professional and parental attitudes. There is a tendency for the medical profession to establish ownership of the hearing-impaired person because it was responsible for early diagnostic steps; the teachers tend to stress their responsibility, forgetting, in some cases, that no teacher holds more than a delegated responsibility from the parents. In other words, the teacher is a person professionally trained to discharge specific aspects of the parental responsibility. There is a tendency to overprotection and overanxiety on the part of some parents, who behave as though stress-addicted, and complain about lack of services as a substitute for either discovering them or setting them up where necessary.
2. Tendency for workers to be identified with the stereotype associated with their profession; this can make for failure of communication. In any group of people concerned with a hearing-impaired child, there is often a likelihood that, while true leadership stems from one individual's personal dynamism and intelligence, because the hierarchical structure demands it, the leadership may be oblique and perhaps unnecessarily time consuming.
3. Lip service is no substitute for reality. There is acute pressure on hospital and local authorities. Staff in schools are highly mobile; hence, meetings which should be fully attended may not include all the people

who should be there, or even if they do, might find themselves consciously or unconsciously more involved with interdepartmental pressures than with the well being of the child.

PARENT COUNSELLING

Parent counselling in this country has begun informally. Teachers, social workers, and clinicians have learned how to counsel in the course of their normal duties. In spite of the descriptions of counselling programmes, their problems, solutions, and successes, which have emerged in the literature of the last decade (Broomfield, 1967; Ewing, 1967; Broomfield and Campbell, 1969; Society of Teachers of the Deaf, 1970; Darbyshire, 1971; Markides, 1971; and Mohay, 1972), there have been very few major conferences or alternative training schemes, apart from the one-term course held at the University of Manchester, for persons wishing to engage themselves in counselling with hearing-impaired individuals. Social work training does include some instruction in counselling, as does teacher training, but much more is needed. If one were to ask any professional in the field if he felt parent collaboration and communication to be valuable, he would agree heartily. Since the need is recognized, the goodwill apparently there, the question still arises as to why the services are less well organized than they might be. Too many independent bodies, all doing their utmost, are working in isolation from each other. It is possible for patients to be passed through the hands of three or four different professional or clinical agencies and receive guidance from all. More often than not, the advice is consistent, but usually such consistency is quite fortuitous and does not stem from consultation (Tumin, 1971). Where contradictions occur, this is not only bad for the child and the family but also, in the end, bad for the services as well.

Another more subtle problem exists in a nationalised service. Members of the public tend to regard statutory bodies with some scepticism, to expect failures of communication and bureaucracy, and to be pleasantly surprised when they discover signs of humanity and understanding. This does not provide a good climate for the reciprocal function which is essential to good parent counselling. Another contaminant of relationships arises from the fact that the counsellor who has first responsibility usually works in the hospital or clinic in which diagnosis has occurred. This establishes an imbalance in the relationship, tends to place the teacher or counsellor in an authoritarian role (Fraser, B., 1970), and is not a satisfactory basis for the mutual interchange of roles which should be basic to the whole guidance or counselling programme. Unless social factors preclude domiciliary visiting, much of the early work with infants and their parents now takes place in the home (Markides, 1972). As soon as the preliminary diagnosis has been made, Local Authority peripatetic teachers visit the home and, using the child as the ostensible focus, begin the long slow process of creating an informed, confident, and independent family. Some teachers go to the length of involving children, shops, or even bus conductors in the neighbourhood. Neighbourhood children have been encouraged take the hearing-impaired child out in his perambulator from where he begins to relate to the environment and become known as a normal infant in spite of his hearing aid (Wells, 1970). This is sometimes easier to achieve where members of the public can make social contact with the hearing-impaired child in the absence of the parents without fear of embarrassment. Subsequent social contact with the parents is then often facilitated and, properly managed, the social situation is far from hampered by possession of a child wearing a hearing aid.

Parent associations are used by parents, educators, clinicians, and administrators as sources of information and contact (National Deaf Children's Society, 1966). There are now over 60 regional branches of the National Deaf Children's Society, usually completely in the hands of the parents, with the support disciplines available for official or unofficial help. Providing points of contact between parents, a source of advice and help which is not tinged with officialdom, and the freedom to develop personal parity relationships, they are useful adjuncts to the official services. Experimental use of "mother's guides" has been made in some clinics. These are mothers of hearing-impaired children who advise other parents in the light of their own experience. Several parents of deaf children have trained as teachers of the deaf or as audiology technicians. All of these workers can bring practical background experience of the needs of parents to guidance situations. There is a danger that some parent counsellors will regard parents as, in some way, inept or unintelligent because they have a deaf child and may exceed their function as counsellors. Having a parent on the staff is an extremely useful corrective. The provision of training for such workers is difficult. An experimental course started by the National Deaf Children's Society is described by Toomin (1975). Another course under development at present seeks to provide extended training for residential house care staff. Some preliminary courses are provided by the National Deaf Children's Society, but the new course will mark a significant step forward. A useful summary of recent literature has been compiled by Worthington (1974).

TRAINING OF PROFESSIONALS

Twenty-five years ago, workers in the field of audiology arrived there via deaf education, physics, psychology, or medicine. There were, in addition, hospital workers with the title of audiology technicians whose services were so undervalued that they were paid less than hospital cleaners. Except in one or two major centres, their equipment was inadequate, unreliable, poorly calibrated and their role simply designed to assist the prescription and fitting of hearing aids. A few (less than five) centres employed physicists, one or two neurophysiologists pursued personal fields of audiological enquiry, and the bulk of responsibility was divided between those teachers with the scientific or technical skills to involve themselves on the one hand, and the audiology technicians and the otologists on the other. When Ewing edited *Educational Guidance and the Deaf Child* (1957), it gave, albeit inadvertently, a flattering picture of the role of audiology at that time. The book summarised all the major ongoing research of the only university centre for the education of teachers of the deaf in these countries at that time. Five of the 13 topics could be described as educo-audiological (Clarke, 1957; Ewing, 1957; Midgley, 1957; Pickles, 1957; Watson, 1957). For the rest, there were some audiological components in most of the papers, even though there was no formal advanced training leading to qualification in the subject in these countries at that time. Because of its origins, audiology as a science is only slowly reaching a level of academic acceptance here and tends, even now, to be regarded by a number of otologists as almost superfluous to the clinical field or minimally relevant to their own function. The recruitment and training of audiology personnel have tended to remain the Cinderella of hospital science. Faced with a dwindling supply of any audiological staffs and a severe limitation on their technical adequacy, the medical profession has campaigned effectively for the inclusion of audiology technicians within the rest of the disciplines involved in physical measurement. As a result, since 1971, audiology technicians have been designated as "physical measurement technicians (audiology)" and their salaries incorporated into the appropriate pay scales.

As audiometers became more complex and otological horizons widened, the demands for advanced scientific skills became more pressing; more graduates in physics, physiological measurement, and psychology were appointed within hospital and university frameworks. Because of this and the need for educational audiologists, formal training programmes began to develop in the last decade. The University of Manchester now provides undergraduate and postgraduate training programmes which reflect the two emphases of education and medicine. The University of Salford offers postgraduate training in audiology which tends to be technical and scientific in emphasis and includes options in areas of acoustics which the other courses do not. The University of Southampton offers a series of audiological training courses which range from brief introductions to the topic, to specific skill courses, to full postgraduate training and research facilities. Students with audiological interests may also offer theses for partial fulfillment of postgraduate regulations in many universities throughout the country in such departments as Mechanical or Electronic Engineering, Acoustic Physics, Applied Physical Sciences, Ergometrics, Psychometry, Physiology, Neurology, and Medicine, to name but a few. (Historically it may be of interest to note that in order to enable Sir Alexander Ewing to present his doctoral thesis in the University of Manchester, special ordinances had to be passed in the Faculty of Medicine.)

A firmer step toward greater coordination was taken when the British Society of Audiology was founded in 1967. Its aims were: "To promote learning and to advance education in the subject of Audiology, to provide a common platform for discussion among the various disciplines involved in audiological work and to promote the status of Audiology as a discipline."

Training Programmes

As might be expected, programmes for teachers of the deaf predominate and these will be listed below. Persons wishing to qualify as teachers of the deaf may enter upon a 4-year training scheme at the University of Manchester leading to a B.Ed. degree, after they have completed general Certificate of Education (G.C.E.) training at advanced level or, after completing their "A levels," students may train in any university or college of education for either 3 or 4 years (depending on the qualification the applicant wishes to acquire), and then go to either Manchester, London, Dublin, Oxford, Edinburgh, or Newcastle for 1 year of further training in "Deaf Education." The same person could, should he or she wish, take a job after graduation from the university or college of education. While working in a school for the deaf or a school for the partially hearing (although not, at present, in a partially hearing unit), an approximate 2-year in-service training scheme, supervised and examined by the National College of Teachers of the Deaf, may be followed, leading to the "Diploma of Competency to Teach Deaf Children." This diploma is recognized as a valid qualification by the Department of Education and Science and holds parity with all the other qualifications presently available to would-be teachers of children with impaired hearing.

As is seen from the accompanying summary of the "Lady Spencer-Churchill College Syllabus," training is a mixture of theory and practice and all students spend slightly less than a third of the course in supervised classroom observation and teaching. During the courses, students tend to select one specific emphasis for special study. This usually means work under the supervision of a tutor in the area of nursery, infant, primary, or secondary education in all the courses except at Oxford, which provides nursery and primary courses only. Such special emphasis would be recorded in college reports, but does not necessarily limit the freedom of the teacher to accept a job concerned with a different age range of children.

The Lady Spencer-Churchill College of Education
Course for the Certificate
in the Education of Deaf and Partially Hearing Children

Syllabus

The course is based in six main areas of study, all of which include work in both theoretical and practical aspects. Examination of students' competency is based on the following areas and includes assessment and written papers.

I. Child development
  A. Cognitive studies
  B. Social/emotional
  C. Assessment of attainment and abilities
II. Audiology
  A. The physics of sound
  B. Measurement of hearing for pure tones or speech
  C. Types of hearing aids and their usage
  D. Anatomy and physiology of ear, larynx, and central nervous system
  E. Etiology of deafness–types of deafness
III. Language (note: in A, B, and C, there is provision for practical sessions)
  A. English pronunciation and phonetics
  B. Linguistics
    1. Historical outline and development of linguistics
    2. Development of language
    3. Study of English language
    4. Testing of language
    5. Recording of language
  C. Media and methods (including practical sessions)
IV. A. Special curriculum needs at nursery, first, and middle school
  B. A study of progressive primary education
  C. The place of the expressive arts, music, movement, art
V. The history, organization, and administration of facilities for the education of deaf and partially hearing children

VI. Practical work in the education of deaf and partially hearing children, which includes practice in schools, supervised work with individual children in college, and practicum in audiology, etc.

Audiology I. Physiological Measurement Technicians (Audiology)

Entry to training is based on the possession of two or more 0 level qualifications in the General Certificate of Education. With two or more 0 levels, the student enters training as a student technician. After a 2-year period of in-service training which has included a full-time course lasting 3 months, students may be regraded to technical level, subject to the granting of a certificate of competency from the otologist in charge of the department. In large departments, or in those departments attached to teaching hospitals, there will be opportunities for attending a variety of courses of lectures which would not normally be available in smaller departments. The relevant health service circular (PTB283) describes a technician as "one who undertakes the range of techniques routinely employed in a department and assists as required with the less common techniques." Senior technicians are normally in day-to-day charge of the technical work of a department, have at least one other worker or student as subordinate, and are expected to be familiar with the less routine audiological investigations. Eligibility for entry to chief technician grade requires a further 3 years of experience in the senior grading and includes responsibility for the work of three other technicians within the department. Qualification in this field is usually acquired through the Society of Audiology Technicians.

The society conducts periodical examinations for membership, to which are admitted candidates who have taken an approved course.

Syllabus of Membership Course

The membership course is taken in two parts; the first consists of a 3 months' course of lectures and demonstrations, including practical instruction as detailed below, in a recognized hearing aid distribution centre. The second part of the course consists of 9 months' practical work as a trainee technician at a recognized distribution centre.

Part I

Elementary Anatomy and Applied Physiology of the Nose, the Larynx, and the Ear
Mechanisms of Hearing and Speech
Elementary Electricity
Pure and Physiological Acoustics
Audiometry
Electro-Acoustics
Hearing Aids
Medical Aspects of Hearing Loss

Rehabilitation–Disability of Deafness
Deafness in Children
Deafness in Adults
Auditory Training
General–Hospital and Ministry of Health Procedures
Practical work: impressions, simple fault tracing and minor repairs to aids; pure tone and speech audiometry.

Part II

After the first 3 months of the course as outlined above, candidates for membership may take the Part I examination in: (1) Elementary Anatomy and Applied Physiology and (2) Applied Audiology and then acquire further experience of the audiology technician's work by attachment to a recognised distribution centre for a period of 9 months' practical work as a trainee technician.

Candidates who have passed in the written papers, after obtaining the necessary practical experience comprising Part II of the course, may proceed to the practical examination and vivas. The latter consists of tests under working conditions of most aspects of the work of an audiology technician (Royal National Institute for the Deaf Information File, 1974). There are five training centres in these countries at present, though two more are planned.

Advanced Qualifications

University of Manchester

One year "Diploma in Audiology" or M.Sc. in Audiology for graduate with higher entry qualification.

University of Salford

A modular course leading to the M.Sc., usually extending over more than a year, which the student may follow as a continuous training or interspersed with work in a relevant occupation.

University of Southampton

In Part I of the M.Sc. course, which lasts six months, students will study, at an advanced level, audiological and vestibulometric investigation of patients, psycho-acoustics, statistics and experimental design, neurophysiology, psychophysical methods, electro-acoustics, hearing aids and hearing conservation. Additional lectures will cover speech pathology, problems of deafness in children and physics related to audiological instrumentation.

There will be daily audiological clinics and case seminars at the Institute, visits to E.N.T., neuro-otology and other departments in the Southampton University Group hospitals, and audiological and vestibulometric testing, under close medical and technical supervision, of patients referred by Ear, Nose and Throat Surgeons to the Institute for investigation. The course and its examinations is "to ensure that those graduating have a high level of 'para-medical' clinical competence so that they can correctly select, perform, interpret and report any such investigations."

The main feature of Part II of the M.Sc. course will be a research project, plus further practical training in the audiological investigation of patients.

There will be a more restricted course of 6 months' duration leading to the Certificate in Medical Audiology. "In general, but not exclusively, this is intended for non-graduate students seeking an advanced training and qualifications in audiology" (Departmental Prospectus, 1974).

Social Work Training

Although I feel that no audiology team is complete without an experienced social worker, I do not propose to include their patterns of recruitment and training within this section.

RESEARCH

The reader will find a most succinct and authoritative survey of research in the general field of hearing impairment in the United Kingdom contained in a report presented by Dr. Annette Rawson (1973) to the Department of Health and Social Security. The present summary owes much to that report and includes one or two additional areas designed to create a widening of the field of enquiry. Rawson's report illustrates the complexity of relationships, staffs, and specialties in the whole field of rehabilitation of people with hearing impairments. It also illustrates that, even with centralised government control of health and education services, it has not proved possible to ensure an even distribution of provision, nor to attract public or private support on the scale necessary to maintain research impetus at an ideal level. This last comment is particularly relevant to the areas which, although recognised as significant, have not yet commanded support from individuals or groups to whom government departments have tended to turn for advice in the past. During times of financial stringency or of centralised control, research tends to be whittled to levels which might be described as more gestural than ideal. Most funding bodies rely on panels of assessors; if such panels are limited for either financial or other reasons, it follows that new fields of research are unlikely to compete successfully with areas which are of more immediate interest to the assessors. As in the case of individual researchers, funding bodies find it essential to protect themselves from diffusion of resources and interest. Necessary although this attitude may be, it is also prudent to look beyond immediate fields of concern into areas which, at first sight, may appear less immediately relevant. An additional problem arises when educational, sociological, or philosophical research matters are planned. Unless there are the funding and the interest to promote investigations which will not yield "hard facts," there is a grave danger that much of their value will be limited.

Under such circumstances, there is a very real danger that superficial investigations may be described as research or that, because of lack of research information, there is a certain naïveté in readers which accepts findings too readily without examining the quality of work upon which they are based. In this way, opinions or intuitive conclusions are represented and accepted as facts, and whole areas of investigation or of provision may develop which, given more adequate research, might have been prevented.

Present educational and sociological research has tended to be fact-oriented, surveys of incidence of various phenomena (mental subnormality, cognitive structures (Watts, 1967) or of the extent and quality of provision of social services, (British Deaf Association, 1974) large-scale research on educational methodology or on the application of different communication systems has not yet occurred. Similarly, since the exhaustive genetic studies reported by G. R. Fraser (1970), there has been a dearth of long-range genetic research which would utilise new research techniques and facilities. Speculation is also common about the consequences of persistence of the live virus in rubella embryopathies. Statements have been made about the efficacy or otherwise of immunisation processes. On the one hand, reports confidently predict that rubella embryopathies will be eliminated. On the other hand, reports question whether present immunisation can give guaranteed protection for the whole of the potential childbearing years. Since a significant proportion of present deaf education and of provision for children affected by multiple pathology arises from rubella, there is obviously a good case to be made on administrative, as well as humanitarian, grounds for research in this topic. Major limitations on research in these countries arise from a combination of factors: shortage of trained staff; ethical considerations involved in certain educational or clinical investigations; shortage of accommodation or adequate facilities; shortage, with rare exceptions, of people of the right calibre to initiate, direct and analyse wide-ranging investigations of an interdisciplinary character; and shortage, above all, of funds and of the pattern of information likely to produce goodwill in those who control the national purse strings. Perhaps, too, there is a shortage of confidence that the present administration will be able to provide facilities to implement the findings of large-scale research projects.

Researchers in the field of hearing impairment in these countries have learned the sobering lesson that we cannot, at present, pursue knowledge for its own sake. The current climate of research tends, therefore, to pragmatism, short-term gains, and limited objectives. For an excellent history of research, see T. J. Watson (1969).

Major Organizations Supporting Research into Hearing Impairment

Government organizations include: (1) Medical Research Council (MRC); (2) Department of Health and Social Security (DHSS); (3) Department of Education and Science (DES); (4) Science Research Council (SRC); and (5) Social Science Research Council (SSRC). Voluntary and philanthropic organizations include: (1) Nuffield Trust; (2) Welcome Foundation; (3) National Deaf Children's Society; and (4) Royal National Institute for the Deaf.

The Medical Research Council and the DHSS share the major responsibility for funded research. The MRC has been assisted by a number of committees and working parties and was involved in otological research in 1944 when it established the Otological Research Unit with Dr. Hallpike as director. At present, it has one other major research unit on "Hearing and Balance" at the National Hospital, Queen's Square, London, with Dr. J. D. Hood as director. One of MRC's committees was concerned with electroacoustics. Dr. T. Littler, secretary to that committee, was also director of the Wernher Research Unit which collaborated with the General Post Office in the production of a specification of a National Health Service hearing aid (the term "Medresco," used to describe this aid, is derived from the title of the *Med*ical *Res*search *Co*uncil). As well as this work, the MRC has recently sponsored research into hearing impairment at the Universities of Manchester, Cambridge, and Southampton (to name but a few). The DHSS, either directly or through its funding of regional hospital board research, has supported, in whole or in part, a number of hospital-based projects, particularly at Whittington Hospital, Preston, Lancs (psychiatric problems of deaf adults), Royal National Throat, Nose, and Ear Hospital, Gray's Inn Road, London (hearing aids). In addition, it has supported a survey of audiological equipment and additional research into the development of specialised amplifiers by the technical department of the Royal National Institute for the Deaf.

Recent research reports on various aspects of infant testing from the Audiology Research Unit at the Royal Berkshire Hospital (Bench, 1970; Collyer, Bench, and Wilson, 1974a, 1974b) were made possible by a grant from the Medical Research Council.

The Rawson report makes interesting comments on rehabilitation (pp. 17–20). Most of the recent sociological surveys relating to hearing impairment published in the last 5 years, however, stress another fact that merits discussion. The community within which the person with any disability lives and works is also affected or "diminished" (Donne, 1535). Recent television programmes in the United Kingdom and the Republic of Ireland, designed as part of a national service for hearing-impaired people, have provoked a new kind of awareness of hearing loss and its effects on the individual. Insensibly, this should also create a new quality of concern for society's own deprivation in the presence of hearing loss. As concern for aged people develops, society should be able to recognise the duality of disability. On the one hand, it should see, and empathise with, the individual's disability and, on the other, society's own deprivation. Should this prove to be an accurate prediction, the time may come when help for the individual is seen to be equally important for the community. Sociological research will, therefore, need to concern itself more specifically with the anthropology of disability. Although, at first sight, such a suggestion might appear to be predominantly academic, I feel that much of the urgency for preventative medicine, whether it be in such areas as noise pollution, immunology, or mental health, will eventually be fueled by the community's concern for its own group well-being.

Future Research

At the present time, there are two working parties seeking information on various aspects of childhood disability. One, chaired by Dr. Donald Court, is concerned with child health (1971). The other, chaired by Mrs. M. Warnock (1971), is concerned with more general aspects of disability (particularly educational provision). Both of these are seeking comments and taking evidence at national and international level of matters which include rehabilitation. There is a ferment of suggestions for future research, and the reports of these two working parties will be of considerable interest. Taken in conjunction with the findings of the Rawson report and the MRC's own two working parties (1974), there will be no lack of material for future research. Suggestions put forward in this paper, therefore, can only represent a minute selection of the total and, hence, reflect the personal interests of the writer.

Research is needed into processes of alerting the community to the effects of hearing impairment, modes of prevention, therapy, or rehabilitation. This suggestion is made because research support is unlikely to be forthcoming unless the community can see a value to itself in such projects. Improvement of detection, diagnosis, differential diagnosis, and delivery of services cannot come about unless we know more about the accuracy of our investigations, can make reliable prosthetic provision, and initiate family counselling where needed (based on an accurate knowledge of the totality of the disability and of the residual skills of the disabled individual). The best hearing aid in the world is of no use until it is connected to the auditory pathways and switched on. Even then it is vulnerable to environmental factors which may be variably relevant at different ages or in relation to age of onset of impairment. More research is needed into the cosmetisation of hearing aids and the creation of an attitude of mind which will encourage their acceptance and, subsequently, their skillful usage. Personality factors are a significant part of the evidence which needs to be collected before an accurate assessment of prognosis can be made. More information is needed before individually tailored therapeutic programmes can be devised. Present tests of cognitive function, auditory or visual attention, intersensory function, bases of linguistic skill, relevant to the age, experience, and extent of hearing impairment, are not satisfactory for children or adults. Within the constraints imposed by ethical considerations, various facets of research into the perceptual, cognitive, and educational processes need developing. When they are developed, much of the present controversy about communication methods may well disappear. More information is needed on multiple disability, and this should take into account such factors as aging, cardiovascular insults, and muscular or ossicular degenerative disorders. New systems of delivering amplified, filtered, or transposed sounds are needed. If subcutaneous approaches are to be made, miniaturisation of components and power sources will be required, together with different systems for signal detection and delivery.

The last point that should be stressed is the pressing need for coordination of services, interdisciplinary cooperation, support, and communication. Less than 1% of the research into industrial communication and cooperation would be needed to apply present knowledge to the problem. However, we are faced with the intractable phenomenon that all rehabilitation demands goodwill. Research may not produce this, but it should serve to foster and preserve it.

At a meeting with the Minister for the Disabled, a panel of representatives from the four leading voluntary organizations in the field of deafness outlined a number of points of concern which included the following: "A serious lack of statistical information about deaf and hard of hearing people and the urgent need for a survey; multi-disciplinary assessment of deaf children; provision for children not admitted to, or excluded from, schools for the deaf; facilities for further education and vocational training; problems of employment; recruitment and training of specialist social workers with the deaf and teachers of the deaf; public recognition of the problems of deafness; essential medical research (viz., viruses, genetics, obstetrics, neonatal care and tinnitus)" (National Deaf Children's Society, 1974). Within these areas of concern, there are valuable pointers to research, and the quotation provides a useful summary.

It should be stressed that the suggestions outlined above relate to *more* research. Much research has already taken place, and funds are becoming more freely available through the statutory and voluntary bodies. A recent grant from the Leverhulme Trust to the Reginald M. Phillips Research Unit at the University of Sussex has facilitated a twin project into curricula for junior and senior schools for hearing-impaired children. The two working parties established by the Medical Research Council ((1) clinical and epidemiological features of sensorineural deafness and (2) social and rehabilitation needs of the deaf) should also illustrate needs and establish orders of priority upon which funding decisions can be made.

PROFESSIONAL AND LAY ORGANIZATIONS AND ASSOCIATIONS RESPONSIBLE FOR HEARING HANDICAPPED

Voluntary Societies

Local As Lyssons (1969) pointed out, national agencies grew from local services or "missions" and, hence, it is logical to begin this brief summary there. At the time of writing, Lyssons reported 57 local voluntary societies, a national coordinating body, and five regional associations which aimed to coordinate educational and welfare work for deaf people within their areas. (A survey conducted by the Royal National Institute for the Deaf in 1972 updated the figures to a total of 84 as follows: England–69, Scotland–9, Wales–2, N. Ireland–2 and Republic of Ireland–2.) They also "provided a forum for consultation and discussion between teachers and welfare workers, audiologists and representatives of local authorities. In 1962 all but three welfare societies for the deaf in England were members of a Regional Association." As well as these bodies, other voluntary organizations have developed at a local level to meet the religious needs of deaf persons which are not met by the existing voluntary organizations. Clubs, centres, and/or religious workers have been provided to meet the needs of such religious groups as Catholics, Jews, and Salvationists. Such organizations as The Spurs Club cater for deaf persons who do not wish to attend "missions" or clubs frequented by other deaf individuals. Middle class in ethos, they tend to emphasize the social and linguistic aspirations of their members and usually provide a pattern of social/cultural activity, often shared by persons of like interest who have normal hearing, which would not normally be of interest to the standard clientele of a "deaf club." Another interesting development has recently emerged. The existence of "The Breakthrough Trust" is, to a considerable extent, based on the fact that some highly intelligent, well educated, independent, deaf individuals want to have more influence upon welfare provision and to plan their own social and cultural activities. This association began in southeast England, but has developed with remarkable speed to a stage where it can now afford to support a full-time officer (Talk, 1974).

In 1947, the Royal National Institute for the Deaf (then the National Institute) drew up a draft scheme to assist voluntary societies in a united approach to Local Authorities for assistance under the National Assistance Bill. This scheme outlined six categories of activity and is still an accurate representation of their main functions. They are: interpretation, spiritual care, placement and industrial supervision, social services, visiting, and individual welfare. In addition, it suggested that societies with adequate staff and premises might extend their work to include: (1) "further education, increased facilities for sport and physical recreation and training in hobbies, handicrafts, housewifery, etc.; (2) "cooperation with organisation for the Blind in promoting improved arrangements for the deaf-blind;" and (3) "provision for the needs of the Hard of Hearing."

Following on the recommendations of the Younghusband Report, there has been a slow build-up of local authority services or, perhaps more significant, of local authority financial support of voluntary organizations employed on an agency basis. This has led to pressure for improved qualifications and to a considerable increase in a casework approach which has added considerable strength to the voluntary agencies and, to a certain extent, ensured the continuance for the time-being of the agency system by Local Authorities which all find themselves short of trained staff and adequate facilities.

National Bodies The foundation of the various organizations described below has already been outlined. The present summary is designed to illustrate their specialised roles and emphases:

1. The Royal National Institute for the Deaf (RNID), a national coordinating body with an internationally famous library and technical department which represents the needs of deaf people and their supportive agencies at a national and an international level.
2. The British Deaf Association (BDA), originally the British Deaf and Dumb Association, planned by deaf persons to present their needs and views to the authorities and to the general public, it now acts as a national organization designed to complement local welfare services in addition to promoting a better understanding of the problems of deafness.

3. The Council of Missioners to the Deaf and Dumb serves to meet the spiritual needs of deaf members.
4. The Church of England Council for the Deaf also serves to meet the spiritual needs of deaf members of the Anglican and Church of England communities.
5. The Deaf Welfare Examination Board was set up to provide training for, and to maintain the academic status of, missioners and welfare officers.
6. Royal Association in Aid of the Deaf and Dumb (the oldest of organizations for deaf people in these countries, established in close contact with the Church of England, with work concentrated in the south of England) it has recently begun to involve itself in work for deaf people with other disabilities although it is generally social and philanthropic in character.
7. The National Council of Missioners and Welfare Officers to the deaf was established to foster cooperation between workers in the two fields of spiritual and general welfare.
8. The British Deaf Amateur Sports Association is concerned with national and international aspects of sports management for deaf amateurs.
9. The National Deaf Children's Society acts as a coordinating body for matters relating to hearing-impaired children and their families.

The following list includes all the organizations known to the writer to be concerned with various aspects of hearing impairment: Association for Experiment in Deaf Education, Ltd.; Breakthrough Trust; British Association of the Hard of Hearing; British Association of Otolaryngologists; British Deaf Association; British Deaf Chess Association; British Deaf Drivers' Association; British Society of Audiology; Church of England Council for the Deaf; Commonwealth Society for the Deaf; Deaf Welfare Examination Board; Ecumenical Council of Christian Workers with the Deaf; Hearing Aid Council; Hearing Aid Industry Association; National Association for Deaf/Blind and Rubella Children; National Association for the Oral Instruction of the Deaf; National College of Teachers of the Deaf; National Council of Welfare Officers to the Deaf; National Deaf/Blind Helpers League; National Deaf Children's Society; Royal Association in Aid of the Deaf and Dumb; Royal National Institute for the Deaf; Royal National Institute for the Deaf (Scottish Technical Department); Society of Audiology Technicians; Society of Hearing Aid Audiologists; and Society of Teachers of the Deaf.

RNID regional associations include: Midland Regional Association for the Deaf; North Regional Association for the Deaf; Scottish Regional Association for the Deaf; South East Regional Association for the Deaf; Welsh Association for the Deaf; and West Regional Association for the Deaf.

Centres for training workers in the field of deafness include: Croydon Technical College, Manchester Polytechnic, and Polytechnic of North London for social workers for deaf adults and for the Certificate in Social Work with the Deaf. For teachers of lipreading, there is City Literary Institute. For teachers of deaf children, there are: University College, Dublin; Lady Spencer-Churchill College of Education; University of Manchester; Scottish Centre for Education of the Deaf, Edinburgh; University of London Institute of Education; and University of Newcastle upon Tyne. Additional centres offering higher degrees in audiology are the University of Southampton and the University of Salford.

ACKNOWLEDGMENT

The writer wishes to acknowledge the valuable assistance given by Dr. A. Rawson, the Library and Information Services of the Royal National Institute of the Deaf, and my secretarial staff.

SURVEYS OF WELFARE SERVICES FOR DEAF PEOPLE IN THE UNITED KINGDOM

British Deaf Association, 1974. Interim report of the working party review of developments in welfare services for deaf people.

London Borough of Hillingdon. 1973. The hearing impaired in Hillingdon: A report to assess the needs of those with hearing impairments and to make recommendations for the improvement of current services.

Suffolk County Council and Suffolk Mission to the Deaf. 1974. Report of working party on services to the deaf set up by Suffolk County Council and Suffolk Mission to the Deaf, Ipswich.

West Sussex County Council. 1973. Social services for the hard of hearing: A pilot study. West Sussex Social Services Department, Chichester.

LITERATURE CITED

Annual Hospital Return (England). 1973. HMSO, London.

Bench, J. 1970. *In* G. Fant (ed.), Speech Communication Ability and Profound Deafness, Stockholm, 1970. Alexander Graham Bell Association for the Deaf, Washington, D.C.

Bennett, M. J. 1973. Acoustic bridge measurement with the neonate. Presented to the Section of Otology, Royal Society of Medicine, March 2.

Boscak, N., and F. Dempster. June 1970. The incidence of additional learning disabilities in a group of 25 deaf maladjusted children. Unpublished report to Managers Larchmoor School.

Brain, Lord. 1965. Children with Communication Problems. Pitman Medical Publishing Co., London.

British Council of Rehabilitation of the Disabled. 1974. Foreword to International Conference on Rehabilitation London.

British Deaf Association. 1974. Interim Report of the Working Party Review of Developments in Welfare Services for Deaf People.

Brooks, D. N. 1971. A new approach to identification audiometry. Audiology 10.

Brooks, D. N. 1973. Hearing screening: A comparative study of an impedance method and pure tone screening. Scand. Audiol. 2(2): 67–72.

Broomfield, A. M., and G. B. Campbell. 1969. Guidance to parents of deaf children: A survey of a year's work. Teacher Deaf 67.

Burton, D. K. 1972. Services for deaf people in the new social service departments. Address to The Biennial Conference of the Royal National Institute for the Deaf.

Chittendon, C. 1974. The Paget-Gorman systematic sign language. Brit. Deaf News 9(12): 408–409.

Chomsky, N. 1968. Language and Mind. Harcourt, Brace and Company, Inc., New York.

Chronically Sick and Disabled Persons Act. 1970. HMSO (1957), London.

Clarke, B. R. 1957. Use of a group hearing aid by profoundly deaf children. *In* A. W. G. Ewing (ed.), Educational Guidance and the Deaf Child. Manchester University Press, Manchester.

Collyer, Y., J. Bench, and I. Wilson. 1974. Brit. J. Audiol. 8: 14.

Court Committee 1971. Written Replies Hansard. Col. 371. HMSO, London.

Critchley, E. 1967. Speech Origins and Development. Charles C Thomas, Publisher, Springfield, Ill.

Crystal, D. 1972. Brit. J. Comm. Disorders 7: 3.

Dale, D. M.C. 1967. Deaf Children at Home and at School. University of London Press, London.

Dale, P. S. 1972. Language Development. Dryden Press, Hinsdale, Ill.

Darbyshire, J. O. 1971. Sociology and children with impaired hearing. J. Soc. Teachers Deaf 8: 33–39.

Davie, R., N. Buttler, and H. Goldstein. 1972. Reports of the National Child Development Study, Longmans, London.

Department of Education and Science Circular 352. 1959. HMSO, London.

Department of Education and Science. 1967. Education Survey No. 1. Units for Partially Hearing Children. HMSO, London.

Department of Education and Science. 1968. The Education of Deaf Children: The Possible Place of Signing and Finger Spelling (Lewis Report). HMSO, London.

Department of Education and Science. 1969. Education Survey No. 6. Peripatetic Teachers of the Deaf. HMSO, London.

Department of Education and Science. 1974. The Health of the School Child (1971–72). HMSO, London.

Department of Health and Social Security. 1969a. On the State of Public Health. HMSO, London.

Department of Health and Social Security Survey. 1969b. Screening of Hearing. HMSO, London.
Donne, J. 1535. Devotions.
Douek, E., W. Gibson, and K. Humpries. 1974. The crossed acoustic reflex. Dev. Med. Child. Neurol. 16: 32–39.
Ewing, A. W. G. 1973. *In* W. Taylor (ed.), Disorders of Auditory Function. Academic Press, Inc., London.
Ewing, A. W. G., and E. C. Ewing. 1967. Hearing Aids, Lipreading and Clear Speech. Manchester University Press, Manchester.
Ewing, E. C. 1967. Parent Guidance. Proceedings of the International Conference. Alexander Graham Bell Association for the Deaf, Washington, D.C.
Ewing, I. 1957. Screening tests and guidance clinics for babies and young children. *In* A. W. G. Ewing (ed.), Educational Guidance and the Deaf Child. Manchester University Press, Manchester.
Ewing, I. R., and A. W. G. Ewing. 1947. Opportunity and the Deaf Child. Univ. London Press, London.
Ewing, I. R., and A. W. G. Ewing. 1958. New Opportunities for Deaf Children. Univ. London Press, London.
Fisch, L. 1964. Hearing Tests as Practised at Present. *In* L. Fisch (ed.), Research In Deafness in Children. Blackwell Scientific Publications, London.
Fisch, L. 1964. The contribution of audiology. *In* C. Renfrew and K. P. Murphy (eds.), The Child Who Does Not Talk. Heinemann Medical Books, London.
Fraser, B. 1970. Initial Stages of Parent Guidance. Talk 1970. Vol. 57. National Deaf Children's Society, London.
Fraser, G. R. 1970. The causes of profound deafness in childhood in Wolstenholme. *In* G. E. W. Knight and J. Knight (eds.), Sensorineural Hearing Loss. CIBA Foundation Symposium, Churchill, London.
Friedlander, B. Z. 1970. Merrill-Palmer Quart. 16: 7.
Goffman, E. 1968. Stigma. Pelican Books. Middlesex.
Gorman, P. P. 1960. Certain Social and Psychological Difficulties Facing the Deaf Person in the English Community. Unpublished Ph.D. thesis, University of Cambridge.
Green, P. 1972. Identifying emotional disturbances in hearing impaired children. Teacher Deaf 70(415): 380–388.
Groves, J. 1974. Services for the Elderly Deaf. Modern Geriatrics, London.
Guthrie, D. 1973. The implementation of the chronically sick and disabled persons act. Report by Social Policy Research for The National Fund for Research into Crippling Diseases, London.
Health and Personal Services Statistics for England, Wales and Scotland. 1973 (1974). DHSS Report. HMSO, London.
Health of the School Child. 1962–63 (1964). HMSO, London.
Health of the School Child. 1966–68 (1969). HMSO, London.
Health of the School Child. 1969–70 (1972). HMSO, London.
Health of the School Child. 1971–72 (1974). HMSO, London.
Ives, L. A. 1967. Deafness and the development of intelligence. Brit. J. Dis. Comm. 2: 96–111.

Ives, L. A. 1974. A Screening Survey of 2060 Hearing Impaired Children in the Midlands and North of England. (Published) Cheadle Hulme Royal Schools for Deaf Children, Manchester.

John, J. E. J. 1957. Acoustics and efficiency in the use of hearing aids. *In* A. W. G. Ewing (ed.), Educational Guidance and the Deaf Child. Manchester University Press, Manchester.

Jones, M. C., and V. W. Byers. 1971. J. Learn. Disab. 4: 46–49.

Joseph, Sir K. 1973. Parliamentary Reply, June 26, Hansard, HMSO, London.

Joseph, Sir K. 1973. Parliamentary Report, July 9, Hansard, HMSO, London.

Katz, J. J. 1966. The Philosophy of Language. Harper & Row, Publishers, New York.

Lewis, M. M. 1965. Children with Communication Problems. Pitman Medical Publishing Co., London.

Ling, D. 1959. The Education and General Background of Children with Defective Hearing in the Borough of Reading. Unpublished research. Dissertation, Institute of Education, Cambridge.

Lloyd, L. L., and R. D. Frisina. 1965. Proceedings of the National Conference at Parsons, Kansas. Parsons State Hospital and Training Center 205.

Local Authorities Social Service Act. 1970. HMSO, London.

Local Government Act 1974. HMSO, London.

Lyssons, C. K. 1965. Voluntary Welfare Societies for Adult Deaf Persons in England 1840–1963. Unpublished Master's thesis, University of Liverpool.

Lyssons, C. K. 1969. Proceedings of Conference of International Society for Rehabilitation of the Disabled, Dublin.

Markides, A. 1971. Pre-school audiological services. Sound 5: 65–69.

Markides, A. 1972. Home atmosphere and linguistic progress of pre-school hearing-handicapped children. Teacher Deaf 68: 323–330.

Martin, J. A. M. 1971. Problems of diagnosis of hearing loss in the young child. Proc. Royal Soc. Med. 64: 571–574.

Martin, M. C. 1975. Audiometers. *In* D. Harrison and R. Hinchcliffe (eds.), Scientific Foundations of Oto-Laryngology. William Heinemann, Ltd., London.

McNeil, D. 1966. Psycholinguistics Papers. Edinburgh University Press, Edinburgh.

Midgeley, J. 1957. Screening tests of hearing in primary schools. *In* A. W. G. Ewing (ed.), Educational Guidance and The Deaf Child. Manchester University Press, Manchester.

Ministry of Education. 1945. Handicapped Pupils and School Health Service Regulations. HMSO, London.

Ministry of Education. 1946. Special Education Treatment. Pamphlet No. 5. HMSO, London.

Ministry of Education. 1953. School Health Service and Handicapped Pupils Regulations. HMSO, London.

Ministry of Education. 1959. Handicapped Pupils and Special Schools Regulations. HMSO, London.

Ministry of Education. 1962a. Amending Regulations. HMSO, London.
Ministry of Education 1962b. Circular 10/62. Children with Impaired Hearing. HMSO, London.
Ministry of Health Circular 32/52. 1951 (August). HMSO, London.
Ministry of Health Circular 15/60. 1960 (July). HMSO, London.
Ministry of Health Circular 23/61. 1961. HMSO, London.
Ministry of Health Form. 8M (IV) 1971.
Mohay, H. 1972. Counselling the Parents of Deaf Children. Presented at the Fifth International Round Table for the Advancement of Counselling, Paris.
Murphy, K. P. 1972a. *In* M. Rutter and J. A. M. Martin (eds.), The Child with Delayed Speech. William Heinemann, Ltd., London.
Murphy, K. P. 1972b. Learning and learning disorder. *In* W. B. Crouch (ed.), Overcoming Learning Difficulties, pp. 24–39. Benn, Tonbridge, Kent.
Murphy, K. P. 1973. Deaf children with additional difficulties. *In* E. Kampp (ed.), Evaluation of Hearing Handicapped Children, pp. 9–21. Fifth Danavox Symposium.
National Association for the Deaf. 1973. Young Adult Deaf Population of Ireland. A General Survey. National Association for the Deaf, Dublin.
National Deaf Children's Society. 1966. NDCS Yearbook 1965–66. National Deaf Children's Society, London.
National Deaf Children's Society. 1974. NDCS Yearbook 1973–74. National Deaf Children's Society, London.
National Health Service Reorganisation Act 1973. HMSO, London.
National Institute for the Deaf Booklet 485. 1947. Royal National Institute for the Deaf, London.
National Rehabilitation Board Survey. 1970. Characteristics of the Adult Deaf Population of Limerick City and County. National Rehabilitation Board, Dublin.
National Summary (All England). 1974. Hospital Return (SH3)–Department of Health and Social Security, Year ending December 1973. HMSO, London.
Neate, D. 1974. Oralism. Brit. Deaf News 9(12): 411–414.
Parliamentary Reply to Questions. 1973. Hansard. HMSO, London.
Pickles, A. M. 1957. Hearing aids. *In* A. W. G. Ewing (ed.), Educational Guidance and the Deaf Child. Manchester University Press, Manchester.
Rawson, A. 1973. Deafness: Report of a Departmental Enquiry into the Promotion of Research. HMSO, London.
Reed, M. 1974. The Education of Handicapped Children. Supplement to "Education." London.
Reed, M. 1974. Unpublished paper read at RNID Conference at Bath.
Renfrew, C., and K. P. Murphy (eds.). 1964. The Child Who Does Not Talk. William Heinemann, Ltd., London.
Report of the Committee on Social Workers in the Local Authority Health-Welfare Services (The Younghusband Report). 1950. HMSO, London.
Rimmer, G. 1974. The Hard of Hearing in Britain: Are Their Needs Being

Met? *In* D. M. Boswell and J. M. Wingrove (eds.), The Handicapped Person in the Community. Tavistock Publications, London.
Robinson, J. B. 1958. Care of the Deaf. Report for the National Deaf Children's Society.
Royal National Institute for the Deaf. 1974. Information File.
Rutter, M., and J. A. M. Martin (eds.). 1972. The Child with Delayed Speech. C.D.M. 43. Spastics International Medical Publications. William Heinemann, Ltd., London.
Scottish Education Department. 1967. Ascertainment of Children with Hearing Defects. HMSO, Edinburgh.
Seebohm Report. 1968. Report of the Committee on Local Authority and Allied Personal Social Services. HMSO, London.
Sheridan, M. D. 1960. The Developmental Progress of Infants and Young Children. Ministry of Health Report 102. HMSO, London.
Sheridan, M. D., 1962. Infants at risk of handicapping conditions. Monthly Bull. Min. Health Pub. Health Lab. Service 21: 238–245.
Sheridan, M. D. 1973. Children's Developmental Progress From Birth to Five Years: The Stycar Sequences. N.F.E.R. Publishing Company, Windsor, Engl.
Simon, G. B., I. Tempowski, and H. Selstead. 1974. Deafness and the mentally retarded. Apex 2(2): 4.
Slobin, D. I. 1966. *In* F. Smith and G. A. Miller (eds.), The Genesis of Language. M.I.T. Press, Cambridge, Mass.
Society of Teachers of the Deaf. 1970. Parent Guidance. Report of a One Day Conference. J. Soc. Teachers Deaf 7: i–xxxii.
Swannie, E. M. 1966. Impedance Audiometry in Clinical Practise. Proc. Roy. Soc. Med. 59(10): 971–974.
Talk. Summer 1974. National Deaf Children's Society, London.
Toomin, S. Winter 1974. Talk. National Deaf Children's Society, London.
Toomin, S. Spring 1975. Talk. National Deaf Children's Society, London.
Tumin, W. 1971. Parent Counselling (Part I). J. Soc. Teachers Deaf (No. 10).
Tumin, W. 1971. Parent Counselling (Part II). J. Soc. Teachers Deaf (No. 11).
Tumin, W. 1972. Parent Counselling (Part III). J. Soc. Teachers Deaf (No. 12).
University of Southampton Prospectus. 1974. Training in Audiology. Southampton.
Warnock Committee 1971. Written replies, Hansard V864, Col. 511. HMSO, London.
Watson, T. J. 1957. Speech audiometry for children. *In* A. W. G. Ewing (ed.), Educational Guidance and the Deaf Child. Manchester University Press, Manchester.
Watson, T. J. 1967. The Education of Hearing Handicapped Children. University of London Press, London.
Watson, T. J. 1969. Teacher Deaf 67(398): 459–478.
Watts, W. J. 1967. Teacher Deaf 65(385): 351–358.
Wells, J. 1970. Address to Reading Branch National Deaf Children's Society. Unpublished report.

Whetnall, E., and D. B. Fry. 1964. The Deaf Child. William Heinemann, Ltd., London.
Williams, R. Hunt. 1968. The Prevention of Conductive Deafness. International Audiology. Vol. 7, p. 3. Karger, Basel.
Williams, S. C. 1970. Some psychiatric observations on a group of maladjusted deaf children. J. Child. Psychol. Psychiat. 11:1–18.
Wilmot, P. 1971. Consumer's Guide to the British Social Services. 2nd ed. Penguin Books, Harmondsworth, Middlesex.
Worthington, S. M. 1974. Talk (No. 73). National Deaf Children's Society, London.

chapter 7

Communication for Hearing-handicapped People in France

Guy Perdoncini, M.D.,
and Marie-Claire Barbera, M.D.

First of all, we shall divide the hearing impaired into two categories: adults and children.

Adults who have suddenly or progressively become deaf are familiar with language. It is best to equip them so that they retain auditory communication and eventually to teach them lipreading only if the auditory pathway becomes inadequate. The adult who has become deaf deserves our consideration and our help because it is a terrible social handicap whose adverse effects upon the individual are always present.

For children, it is somewhat different. We will consider, in the main, the problem presented by children born deaf.

Contrary to what may have been written, especially in France, our experience leads us to consider the child born deaf as belonging to a group whose intelligence is comparable to that of children with normal hearing.

There are, of course, retarded children who will remain retarded with no possibility of improving regardless of the quality of their education. The majority of deaf children, however, are normal in other respects.

The child who hears normally, and is of normal intelligence, needs guidance from birth on to become an adult who corresponds to the standards of normality as they are commonly defined. Similarly, the child born deaf also needs training, but a training which is highly specialized. Thus, our position concerning the child born deaf is defined by the following considerations. The deaf child, otherwise normal, needs all the development as a child who hears normally, but, in his case, special training is required for social development. Really, what is it to be normal? Is it to be the most intelligent, the most skilled, the strongest, to have the most pleasant voice, the best language, and the best hearing? To be normal is to have a certain capability in the various functions just mentioned, such that it permits the individual to lead a normal life in society.

Once this definition is accepted, it is easy to understand the position we have held concerning deaf children for over 25 years. They have a capacity to become normal. We must put to work our multidisciplinary knowledge to obtain this result which, once obtained, allows the integration of educated deaf subjects into normal life to compete with people who hear normally.

Our philosophical position is, thus, determined by the fact that deaf children, who are otherwise normal, can and must be integrated with those who hear normally. We must, thus, consider the deaf child as temporarily unadapted, while avoiding any action which might transform him into a permanently unadapted person (lack of normal communication, psychological characteristics inadequately evolved, family environment insufficiently developed, society not prepared to receive the deaf child).

These considerations define the principal bases of various sections within this chapter.

DEFINITION OF AURAL HABILITATION AND REHABILITATION

One must consider separately the case of the adult and that of the child. An adult might become deaf suddenly as the result of an accident or might show progressive deafness caused by age (presbyacousis). In the former case, deafness can be total because of internal lesions; or it might be only partial; remnants of hearing might exist basically for the low frequencies. One must keep in mind that, in this type of case, the auditory sensations of the subject, even aided by a good hearing aid, are different from those which his memory has recorded. It is, thus, best to provide auditory education, to record the new sound forms of the message heard, and to add to this sensory and memorial training and counseling aimed at acceptance of the realities of the handicap, recognizing that the messages received will always be partial and often inadequate for complete understanding.

In this case, it is best to teach lipreading, but always as a complement to auditory reception, never as the major method or even as the only method of communication. Indeed, one of our basic rules, proved by experience, shows that in all cases of profound deafness in both adults and children, an auditory education must always be the basis of reception, for in this case the eventual association of it with lipreading gives highly superior results from all points of view to those obtained by lipreading alone. This auditory education needs educators who are well trained and who believe in the result of the training.

Auditory education of the adult subject suffering from presbyacousis must be done under the supervision of a medical specialist in audiology, so that the beginning of the two following stages can be defined: the basic one wherein the subject begins to need a hearing aid so that he can train himself to accept it psychologically and, on the physiological level, so that he can adapt himself to the transformation of the message inherent in the hearing aid. Indeed, one must not wait until the subject absolutely needs this equipment. It is then often too late to effect the necessary adaptations.

The second and later stage is defined by the unrelenting progress toward more and more complete deafness, which, in addition, requires lipreading training. Medical audiologists must be sufficiently trained to recognize this type of deafness (*presbyacousis*) in order to prescribe medical treatments which often may improve the functional capacity of the individual, thus improving his auditory reception capacity. Medical supervision will, thus, be beneficial, both psychologically and physiologically.

Deaf children present varying degrees of deafness, divided into two large categories, with a border between them hard to define because of differences of intelligence, family and social situation, and psychological ability among each individual in each group.

The first group comprises those only slightly deaf and those moderately deaf; the second group includes the severely hard of hearing and profoundly deaf.

The performance of the *phoniatric* team will differ according to the group. In the first group, children born deaf have certain auditory sensations from birth. The number of these and their quality of reception are essentially a function of the degree of deafness. But, in this case the auditory sense exists, and the auditory function, which stems from the auditory sense, exists naturally as for normal children.

In these cases, the *phoniatric* team, after having discovered and diagnosed the exact extent of deafness, and having determined the mental and affective value of the subject and of his family, will prescribe a good hearing aid adapted to the individual; in most cases stereophonic. By this means the subject, helped by lessons from an orthophonist, will be able to attain normal audiophonic communication, go to school with those of normal hearing, and live like young people with normal hearing.

In the second group, the subject has had only infrequent auditory sensations; in the case of profound deafness, he has no sensation at all. In any case, with the auditory sense having functioned very little or not at all, one may assume that it does not exist in the psychosomatic image which the subject has of himself.

As a consequence of absence of auditory sense, obviously, auditory structures do not develop, and the auditory function in general is lacking.

It is not enough to adapt a hearing aid to these patients because the amplified sounds as heard by the subject are inadequate to carry a semantic value, which is indispensable to motivating the subject to hear and to communication by this means.

It would seem that the auditory function is defined by the existence of differential thresholds of duration, of intensity, and of frequency which are not inherent in the equipment used by the subject, but which are the result of social interaction resulting from spoken language and the soundfield of those who hear normally. We have shown this possibility in a joint publication with Dr. Robert McCroskey at the American Speech and Hearing Association Convention in 1969. In this work we showed that, before any aural rehabilitation is attempted, the differential thresholds are practically nonexistent, but that they progress more or less rapidly, and also increase in quantity when a systematic aural habilitation approach is employed.

Thus, in cases of severe and especially of profound deafness, the deaf child cannot attain auditory function unless a long process of specialized education creates and structures this function.

It is interesting to note that, for the extreme cases where the hearing remnants do not go beyond 1,000 Hz, one can and must effect a systematic and well programed auditory re-education, while believing firmly in these results. Auditory re-education does not immediately pay off, and one must frequently wait months, even years, before seeing beneficial results not only in the subject's communication, but also in the normalization which this causes.

An error frequently seen in France, and in many other countries, is that of believing that the hearing aid will never work, since it gives no results after days and weeks of work. Profoundly deaf persons have a very narrow auditory passageway which allows re-education to enter only very slowly. Nonetheless, it is certain that these slowly acquired results accumulate and lead to the favorable results previously mentioned. In most cases, in this second group, it will be necessary to formulate a rigorously applied re-education plan. After a preliminary examination and a preliminary diagnosis—during the first year—a hearing aid will be fitted as soon as diagnosis of the degree of deafness is sufficiently certain. This equipment will consist of either a single aid for both ears or a stereophonic aid.

The phoniatric team will give the family the support necessary to understand and accept the child's deafness, in order to fully play its role in his re-education, with a family effort counseled and helped by the different members of the team, basically psychologists and especially orthophonists.

The subject will go to a specialized kindergarten as soon as possible, then into a special school to undergo systematic education in hearing and the use of voice, words, and language in general. His psychological growth will be the object of special care.

It is best that the stay in a specialized establishment be done with the student living there part-time. Full-time residency at the establishment should be reserved for cases where the family is dispersed, or where the educability of the child is dubious or nonexistent, or where the family lives too far from a part-time boarding school. Contrary to what one might think, a good and not-too-large boarding school (50–100 students) can be an excellent milieu of great psychological and even psychotherapeutic value by the simple fact that the deaf child is understood and loved there. He can communicate with the milieu, and the milieu with him.

By this means of communication, most of the elements of maladjusted reactions, which are a usual consequence of his deafness, are done away with in his first year of boarding school. This is because the maladjusted reactions of a deaf child are based upon inadequacy or absence of communication between the family milieu and the child, and vice versa.

With the considerations enumerated above taken into account, auditory education must be used in all cases of deafness, with the assistance of advanced technology, and with unshakeable confidence in the results.

HISTORICAL OVERVIEW

One must await the 18th century in France before finding evidence of the first teachers of deaf children, and even then we were without a written record of a work method. Those teachers, having limited themselves to a materially privileged few pupils, did not desire to spread their procedures. The names of J. R. Pereire (1715–1780) and of Father Deschamps (1745–1791) are those reported. These teachers, inspired by Ponce de Leon, who was born in Spain in the 16th century, taught the oral approach, and the results of these efforts are unknown to us.

It was around 1760 that Father De l'Epée, moved by the neglected situation of the deaf of less privileged background, created the first free school in his own Paris apartment. Totally unaware of methods of oral education existing in France and elsewhere, he thought up, from bits and pieces, a precise code of hand gestures, departing from the idea that spontaneous gestures constituted the only natural mode of expression and, thus, of communication for a deaf person. He, thus, conceived a whole methodology of gestures, expressing objects, action, type, number, verbal forms, etc. . . . based on imitation (the gesture imitating the object and arriving at a very elaborate pantomime based on a whole system of conventional forms; i.e., for black, one pointed to the eyebrow; for red, to the lips). Written language was taught at the same time. Even if this language of gestures is no longer taught in France, it subsists in various groups of deaf people of all ages, and the transmission of this language is carried on by "old-timers."

Tremendous merit is due to Father de l'Epée for having awakened the whole of society to the idea that education of the deaf was possible and that the creation of free schools was a necessity. His opinion resulted in the creation of the four National Institutes of Paris, Cognin, Metz, and Bordeaux. Numerous private schools, the majority opened by religious groups, are controlled and grouped under the Ministry of Health, and, thus, benefit from free medical aid while also under the Ministry of Education.

Nonetheless, under the influence of German pedagogues, little by little, the aural method resurfaced and, caused by the influence notably of Itard (1774–1838), a class on articulation was created at the Institute of Paris. A sketch of the "Méthode Auriculaire" is also found in his writings, which reveals him to be a distant precursor in this domain. His results, obviously mediocre because of a lack of technology, did not permit him to spread his ideas rapidly, and it was not until 1880, following the International Congress on the Teaching of Deaf Mutes, that the oral method was officially and definitively introduced in France.

The educational structures having been established, and the techniques of the oral approach having been admitted into usage, there began an effort about 1950 to relate isolated, modest trials of auditory education, solely to subjects who were only partially deaf.

Progress having been made in the development of amplification devices, use was made of amplifiers here and there during a limited time in classes attended by the partially deaf.

It was at this time in 1951 that Dr. G. Perdoncini began a class for the profoundly deaf at Nice and published a very rigorous methodology of auditory education strictly for the profoundly deaf. These efforts led to the creation of two medical centers of Phoniatry and Auditory Reeducation at Nice-Villefranche and at La-Norville (Paris). Many students came and still come to Nice-Villefranche from foreign countries to learn the general methodology and techniques to educate those with severe and profound deafness. After their stay in France, some of the students have created similar medical centers with the same methods, the same techniques, and the same philosophy in their own countries: Lebanon, Spain, Canada, Brazil, the U.S.A. (Wichita, Kansas), etc. Since then, the techniques of auditory education have spread to and have been incorporated in all existing schools of re-education.

It has been necessary to overcome skepticism concerning the difficulty of admitting to the possibilities of using any kind of residual hearing. And, even though at the present time in 1975 in France all professional educators of deaf children agree to the fact that auditory education is part of the global effort to educate the hearing impaired, they do not all subscribe to it with the rigor and steadfastness necessary for its fully expanded application.

GENERAL DESCRIPTION OF CURRENT PROGRAMS OF AURAL HABILITATION AND REHABILITATION

There is no official program for deaf adults. Each case must be treated individually, in accordance with the indications defined previously.

Many establishments in France administer auditory re-education. We shall group them in chronological order of their establishment.

The National Institutes for Deaf Children

These are part of the Ministry of Health and are the successors to the establishments created by Father de l'Epée. They are in Paris, Metz, Cognin-Chambéry, and Bordeaux-Gradignan. The students are either full-time or part-time boarders. They are admitted from 3 to 4 years of age up to the age of 18. They take elementary school courses until they obtain, if possible, a Certificate of Professional Aptitude (for manual labor).

Private Establishments for Deaf Children

These are part of either the Ministry of Health or the Ministry of Education.

The students are either half-time or full-time boarders.

The length of studies is variable, depending on the results obtained. Indeed, some students are directed to the Certificate of Professional Aptitude. Others reach a different educational level.

It is necessary to mention that a certain tendency shows in these two types of institutions or establishments; a tendency to send out certain sufficiently re-educated students who are capable of communicating with the hearing environment.

Special mention must be made of the Medical Centers for Phoniatry and for Auditory Re-education in Villefranche-sur-Mer and in La-Norville. Their philosophy, as we have already said, is to keep the deaf child for as short a time as possible, to teach him the structures of hearing, voice, words, and language, and to integrate him into the educational milieu of normal children. This philosophy will be defined in the course of following sections of this chapter. The reintegration of deaf students from the Medical Centers for Phoniatry and for Auditory Re-education was first tried 21 years ago.

Appended Classes

These were created a few years ago under the influence of the Association Nationale des parents d'Enfants Déficients Auditifs (ANPEDA).

In an educational group for normally hearing children, a special class is created for deaf children, functioning as a single class which mixes young children not yet educated with older children already educated. The deaf children, thus, have common activities with the normally hearing children during recess, at meals, in physical education, etc. The deaf children acquire a certain educational level, but most of them are directed toward the National Institutes to obtain professional training. The first appended school was created in Lyon, about 15 years ago.

Integrated Classes

The integration difficulties in appended classes led to a new form of association of classes for deaf children with classes for normal children. This new action was brought about by the activity of the Association des Parents des Jeunes Handicapés (APJH) (The Association of Parents of Handicapped Children) and under the auspices of the Ministry of Education and the Ministry of Health.

Within the APJH, a specific committee on the handicap of deafness was created, which was called the "Committee on Language and Integration."

Integration is attained in various ways: (1) either a homoegeneous class of deaf students in a school for the normally hearing, with common activities, as with the appended classes; (2) or a homogeneous class of deaf students, but with the possibility of an individual schedule determined by the physical, intellectual, and psychological capabilities of each subject; (3) or a class of normally hearing students which receives a deaf student, either full-time or part-time.

In all these cases, there are two types of teaching: one for the normally hearing and one for the deaf. This dichotomy does not cause embarrassment for the deaf child since relationships between the two types of teachers are there from the beginning.

The first school of this type, created 3 years ago, is the one in Argenteuil (Dr. Denise Busquet).

Integration is intended to eliminate all segregation. The child does not live at the school. Each evening the deaf child goes back to his family or to a foster family.

Family Re-education

Some establishments keep deaf students too long, and this segregation leads to definite maladjustment of the subject toward the normal hearing milieu. To remedy these errors, a certain current of thought has created opposition to programs with full-time or part-time boarding.

Some families try to educate their deaf child themselves. Certain teachers of the deaf (*orthophonistes*) think they are capable of re-educating the deaf child within the family, by placing the child in a kindergarten, then in a school of normal hearing children, and by working on re-education two or three times a week.

This practice is possible in cases of slight deafness, and even sometimes in deafness of average severity. But it gives catastrophic results when applied in cases of severe hearing loss and profound deafness.

To draw a conclusion among the different forms of re-education proposed, one must consider not only the structures offered here, but also the deaf child himself. One must also follow the schemas given later in this chapter.

DIAGNOSTIC PROCEDURES

With adults, audiometric tests are *threshold* and *subthreshold*, using pure sounds and tapes of *filtered white noise. Speech audiometry* plays a very important role since it measures the intelligibility of words and since it permits study of the practical gains made when a hearing aid is employed.

With deaf children, the evolution of ideas concerning their learning capacities has permitted an evolution of techniques adaptable to preliminary education (0–3 years of age) and preschool education concerning children from 3–6 years of age.

Since this early education rests largely on auditory education, it is necessary that the means of diagnosing the exact level of hearing impairment evolve in order to permit the use of an effective hearing aid without danger. It is, thus, especially to meet the needs of early education that the diagnosis of deafness must be made early, and the means for this is *audiometry*.

Audiometric research for a hearing deficiency must be able to permit the pedagogical orientation of students who are suspected of having one, and, thus, tends to become of general use: it then is called *dépistage* ("to uncover what is hidden, as disease").

This dépistage is becoming common in France because a recent law requires hearing examinations at the ages of 9 months and 24 months.

But even earlier, from birth, systematic examinations are beginning to be done in certain maternity wards and in wards for premature children.

We already have so-called "subjective" means of investigation, that is: simple observation of the child's reflexes, either conditioned or not by the emission of a particular sound, which are (sic) extremely valuable in the hands of an experienced specialist. These are: Baby Test; Réflexe d'Orientation Conditionné (ROC); Peep Show Box (PSB).

We also have objective means at our disposal which are useless generally because they require extensive equipment and which are used as a complement in cases where doubt as to true hearing level still exists. These are electroencephalography and electrocochleography.

Audiometric examination of a deaf child must be carried out by qualified personnel in order to avoid psychological trauma; for example, wearing a white blouse may bring to mind an unpleasant experience in the hospital.

The observation of a deaf child's reaction to a sound stimulus requires extensive practical training on the part of the audiometrist. Indeed, one must take into account latency time, movement of the eyes, of the face, of the head, reactions of stopping or of irritation, and the shape of movements of fingers and hands. The audiometrist must sort out the real reaction to a proposed stimulus from a number of gestures or movements.

Subjective Methods

Chronology of Audiometric Examinations

Baby Test at Birth (Veit-Bizaguet). This test can be done in the maternity ward in the first 48 hours. It is a systematic test for abnormality, intended to permit an early diagnosis of deafness and the application of education techniques.

The Principle The normal newborn child, exposed in favorable conditions to an acoustic signal of appropriate quality and intensity, responds by muscular, visceral, and psychological reactions, interpreted by a modification in his behavior.

The absence of response, if it is confirmed by the repetition of the tests, points to the possibility of a hearing impairment and justifies the administration of appropriate clinical and audiological examinations.

The acoustic signal must be effective (that is, sure to cause reaction) and without danger.

The reactions observed are not all specifically from an auditory stimulus, that is, they may appear because of a stimulus such as cold, light, a visceral spasm, etc.

In order for them to be attributed to auditory origins, it is necessary that the reaction be in definite temporal relation with the sound stimulus and that there be no concurrent stimulus.

We can classify these reactions in four large categories: alert reactions;

postural reactions; psychological reactions; modifications of autonomous functions (change in respiratory rhythm, in cardiac rhythm, etc.).

This early pedoaudiometry can be administered in the first 48 hours. The most favorable moment seems to be one when the newborn child is in a state approximating vigilance (watchfulness), most often a half-hour before meals.

The stimulus will be presented from a selection of tapes of low, medium, and high sounds.

Meaning of Responses The examiner will be a trained observer, capable from his experience of appreciating the pertinence of a response in relation to the existing temporal link between stimulus and response.

The results will be noted: (1) Normal–when clear responses are obtained for stimulus at a level below or equal to the detection threshold (background noise plus 30 decibels); (2) Questionable–clear responses only to a stimulus higher than the detection threshold: development should be watched in pediatric consultation; (3) Suspicious–absence of response to intensities of 100 decibels. A clinical and audiometric examination should be prescribed.

Signs of abnormality or warning signs can also be discovered by the family and the pediatrician, which is often the case.

But this detection at birth, which will certainly one day become used more generally, is at present still limited to a few privileged maternity hospitals and is still in the experimental stage.

Examination at 9 Months Dr. L. Moatti (Paris) has formulated a clinical hearing test made up of four sound-producing objects, imitating the cries of animals: the frequencies of their cries are well defined.

These sound-producing toys, attractive to all and which all can handle, allow one to note the existence or absence of raction to sound very early. As a last resort, an examination in a soundproof room will be tried; the baby sits on its mother's knee, and the threshold range will be explored in free field with filtered white noise. The experienced audiometrist will be able to note the smallest changes in posture or in mimicry, showing a reaction to the sound. This examination allows the establishment of a qualitative value of the baby's hearing capacity, enough to bring about therapeutic suggestions.

Examination at 12 Months to 4–5 Years The ROC and peep show box tests permit a rather precise investigation of the young child.

When considering the equipment and the conditions of examination, it is of great importance that the audiometer, where chrome, buttons, and dials gleam attractively, be away from the child's attention and that he have before him only a table and a screen.

The audiologist takes time to reassure the child and even to charm him. The baby can stay on its mother's knees, but absolute neutrality must be asked of the mother. For an ROC, the sound is emitted by speakers placed here and there around the child. Simultaneously, a window under these speakers lights up and shows an attractive toy. The deaf child is, thus, conditioned to turn his head left or right toward the sound source, since he wishes to see the fascinating object. Here again, the experience of the audiometrist will permit him to assign a response value to the movements of the eyes, to the form of rotations of the head, and to an imperceptible start.

The peep show box is designed for children from 3 years of age on, since it calls for their voluntary motivated response; when a sound is heard, the child must press a button in order to cause an image to appear on the screen.

Without the sound, pushing the button produces no image. The audiometrist, sitting beside the child, will activate only a single button with his hand or foot, to produce the sound (a technician will regulate the intensity and frequency of the sound as required). He may, thus, observe the entire child without interruption, and note all mimicry, blinking, startle reactions, vague movements toward the response button, and many other different small and expressive manifestations only meaningful to the experienced clinician.

The audiometric examination of a child conducted in this manner will permit the establishment of a curve, whose level, while still above that of the threshold, is exact in form, and which permits the fitting of the most suitable hearing aid immediately, an essential tool for a good auditory education.

Objective Methods

These methods cannot be used regularly because of the extent of the equipment, because of its cost, and because of the highly specialized personnel needed to operate it.

These are: (1) electroencephalography; recording the evoked potentials; and (2) electrocochleography. This second technique requires anesthesia and, thus, a hospital environment, to permit the introduction of an electrode to the cochlea through the tympanum.

Consequently, these two methods are reserved for cases where an examination, difficult because of the child's behavior or because of another handicap, does not permit one to ascertain deafness.

HABILITATIVE-REHABILITATIVE PROCEDURES

Procedures for the re-education of the deaf adult were the subject of a special paragraph in an earlier portion of this chapter.

The re-education of the deaf child no longer involves gestures of the *dactylologique* alphabet in France. Nonetheless, it is curious to observe that, following the human tradition of transmitting teaching from the old to the young in numerous institutions, the knowledge of a language of gestures is taught and used to the detriment of all other means of communication, especially hearing and phonation.

Lipreading is considered by many educators as something which should be systematically taught to every deaf subject. It is, unfortunately, a common phenomenon that many deaf persons, who could have been re-educated solely by auditory methods, have had their progress limited by the inopportune use of lipreading. On the other hand, it is certain that, at the present state of development of our knowledge, severely deaf subjects must augment their hearing reception with the observation of visual signals. This audiovisual reception must always be primarily auditory, with the subject learning to understand and use visual signals by himself.

As to total communication, it comes generally to a subject using mainly lipreading to receive the message and a language of gestures to transmit it. Total communication seems sometimes to contradict the latest discoveries in neurophysiology.

The use of hearing aids is quite widespread in France. Nevertheless, too many educators only marginally know how they function and how to use them. The motivation of these educators, of their pupils, and of the pupils' families is not sufficiently directed toward aural education, and, as a result, the wearing of the hearing aid is often forgotten. Our present knowledge leads us to generalize the use of stereophonic equipment.

It is regretable that many educators of the deaf are not sufficiently convinced of the indispensable nature of the permanent hearing aid, which must become an integral part of the deaf child's body. We advise, therefore, the use of good hearing aids which are now available on the market, but with the stipulation that, generally, those hearing aids were made for deaf adults and not for children (because of the fragility of the hearing aids), and that, while there are competent hearing aid specialists, there is also a group interested only in selling equipment.

It is not just a question of bettering absolute aural thresholds—which is, at present, impossible—but of developing, by training, differential thresholds or levels, by making use of residual hearing so as to hear sounds and identify the acoustical character of the spoken word. In the child who is either minimally deaf or who has an average disability, one must arrive at an understanding of spoken language by hearing alone. In the severely or profoundly deaf child, one must arrive at the perception of a certain number of acoustical indicators which permit a better adaptation and add to comprehension in association with lipreading.

A simple analysis of Table 1 shows that our act of re-education (rehabilitation) must serve three functions: (1) an auditory function with the re-education of hearing; (2) phoniatric and phonological function; that is, the education of voice and the spoken word; and (3) a verbal function; that is, education in spoken and written language with a particular emphasis on conceptual and structural memorization.

With a didactic goal in mind, these three points will be studied separately, but it is obvious that the education of a deaf child incorporates all three both successively and simultaneously.

As we have already said in the section concerning history, all those involved in the re-education of deaf children know that one must use remnants of hearing. Their use, as it is practiced in the Medical Centers for Phoniatry and Auditory Reeducation at Villefranche and at La-Norville and by their students in France and around the world, gives a concrete exemplary model. The other re-educators (in France) of infantile deafness apply it more or less.

In order to be convinced of the merits of auditory education, and in order to apply it strictly (the only guarantee of results), one must keep in mind, on the one hand, the histophysiological development of nerve fibers

Table 1. From the normal child to the deaf child

Age	Not deaf	Deaf
Birth–3 months	Babbling, repetition of a phoneme Pleasure motive	Babbling, repetition of a phoneme Pleasure motive
6 months	Feedback→imitation of himself then consciousness of others Substantial auditory control ↓ Jargon→understanding which precedes sound emission (first name +++)	Does not hear ↓ No feedback No imitation No repetition ↓ No words–no auditory structure No language ↓ Perhaps does not think ↓ "Mentally retarded"
18 months	20 words	
24 months	200 words	

of the hearing organs, and, on the other hand, the stages of development of hearing in the normal hearing child.

Indeed, our re-educative efforts run parallel to the successive states of hearing evolution in the normal hearing child.

Maturation of Nerve Fibers

The nerve fibers of hearing are capable of functioning long before those of voluntary phonation. (The first vocal manifestations are of a reflex type, but the child shows that he identifies various sounds: the bottle, the voice of his mother, her different intonations, etc.). This period of myelinization of the nerve fibers is favorable to training. There is, thus, a necessity for a very early auditory education, especially for the subject who tends toward normal development.

Stages of Development of Hearing

Whatever the lapse in time, we will always try to respect these stages in the development of hearing.

Acoustical Hearing From the first days of life, the child is plunged into a world of sound; he discerns the sounds which are related to concrete situations, which quickly take on significance. The child shows by non-verbal reactions that he has understood the meaning of these sound messages. These signals are interpreted simply by their acoustical character: intensity, loudness, and duration.

In the same way, he recognizes his parents by the pitch of their voices. Later he can reproduce the rhythmic scale of a sentence which he hears. There is, thus, no possibility of beginning auditory training by words and sentences, which would be much too difficult. The acoustical aspect of hearing will be emphasized at first. On a parallel level, we will emphasize familiar sounds, music, etc.

Verbal Hearing From the time of his birth, a baby is spoken to frequently. Little by little he becomes conscious of the information value of language. The sounds of a language are of significant value to him. The child then becomes less interested in individual acoustic characteristics and more interested in picking out phonemic categories. The order of the acquisition of phonemes follows certain general rules. The order of use does not exactly follow the order of comprehension, one of the factors which contributes to difficulties of articulation.

Vowels and consonants develop simultaneously. Vowels are better heard because they are of greater intensity; but consonants have greater informational value. There is, thus, an equilibrium which establishes itself in the system.

Special Techniques

The goal to be achieved is in three major stages:

1. The child first learns to listen; there is a sudden consciousness of the world of sound—a difference between sound and silence.
2. The child learns to differentiate the sounds he hears; recognition of the sound's source and the significance of a noise (an animal's cry, a door shutting, etc.).
3. The child learns to analyze and understand the spoken word; distinction of words from other sound-messages. Attribution of significance to the perceived sound impression. Exploration of the different elements of spoken language, as with the child who hears: recognition of phonemes as to their acoustic individuality, then as symbolic wholes.

Results vary and certainly depend on the auditory curve, but they depend even more on the deaf child and on his interest in hearing. This phase is frustrating for the teacher and for the child, since the latter is not yet motivated and hearing does not bring him a means of communication which would justify his past efforts.

Stages of Auditory Training for a Young Deaf Person

Material Used Sounds and criteria on their use.

In the newborn child, until about 3 years of age, auditory training can only be passive, a "bathing" in sound and in language.

Since the hearing aid is not immediately usable, it seems that the most efficient and least dangerous method is speaking. According to the Perdoncini technique using the voice *en champ libre*, the mother or father speaks in a loud voice, cheek to cheek with the child, with the mouth at two fingers breadth from the child's ear. Under these conditions, the deaf child receives the parent's voice at an intensity of 90–100 decibels. By this method, he becomes aware that the mouth's movements are not just movements, but vectors of the sound-producing element. There will be no stages of transition if the child, from the time of his birth or soon after, has lived in a world of amplified sound, adapted to his deficiency and in which he does not realize what is missing. That deaf child will pass unaware from a passive auditory education to an active one. But most often, even in the best conditions, we are dealing with a young child of about 3 years of age, having completely deleted the little bits of auditory information which might have come to him spontaneously, having no understanding of his auditory sense, and having concentrated all of his attention on the ability to see, which is the only source of learning for him.

The material for work undertaken must then be very easy to handle; that is, emitted at the discretion of the educator and always at an appropriate level for training. It must be rich in possibilities for variance of the parameters to be worked out: intensity, frequency, and duration, for example, pure sounds, pulsated, emitted by a frequency generator (called a "pulsatone"), bringing into play only the identification of acoustical parameters, without visual or verbal interference.

Nonetheless, if the child works with an orthophonist who is not trained for the pulsatone, the principle of auditory work and its programs should be the same, namely: (1) the awakening of awareness to sounds–identification of sound versus silence; (2) differentiation of duration–short sounds versus long ones; (3) differentiation of frequency–low sounds (250) versus high ones (1,000); (4) differentiation of intensity–loud versus soft; (5) mixture of these parameters; (6) rhythmic groupings to be reproduced either by gestures or by graphic representation, always respecting the length of silences, which are as important as sounds; (7) auditory memorization exercises–reproduction by the pupil of the schema dictated by the teacher; (8) sequences of impulses to memorize, which become longer and longer.

But pure sounds are rarely present in the sound environment, and at high frequencies there is a risk of high intensity trauma. Thus, if the impulses are necessary as a basis for true, repeated auditory exercises, the impulses cannot and must not be the only material used. We regularly hear complex sounds (of several elements and their harmonies), and we must try to have the deaf child hear them. Thus, the schema for auditory work will always be parallel to the spoken sounds; syllables pa for the low sounds and pi for the high ones.

These exercises will be done with the lips of the trainer hidden, so as to remain purely exercises in auditory training, without any visual interference competing for the attention.

The small child has a short attention span. As a result, these auditory exercises will never be longer than 5 minutes in the beginning; and later, rarely longer than 10 minutes. But they will be repeated two or three times a day. These exercises will always be followed by easier and more pleasant ones for the child–vocabulary exercises with the lips visible. Psychomotricity exercises which relax and the use of educational material, in a passive "sound-bath" through the radio or recording, are also important.

To this work base, which must be strictly carried out, will be added a number of other auditory exercises much less rigorous and often more attractive, presented in the form of games, depending upon the imaginative genius of the educator, such as vocabulary games calling for word recognition, language games calling for sentence recognition, and recognition of different familiar sounds and recorded words. Remember that, in the beginning (and always with a profoundly deaf person), auditory work on recognition must be presented ahead of time, and the child should be alerted to that which he will have to recall. One cannot recognize what one does not know. And there we see the intervention of language building as not being separated from building of the auditory sense.

At this stage it is necessary to review all the factors which make possible the intelligibility of language. We have already treated objective factors which permit the identification of acoustic characters belonging to sounds with appropriate auditory examples. It is essential to remember that with consonants certain indices will not be usable—the shrill components of the occlusives and the unvoiced constrictives. But, on the other hand, others will be perceptible: low frequencies of the voiced consonants b, d, g, v, z; the nasal formation of m and n; the very brief duration of the occlusives as opposed to the much longer duration of the constrictives; and the attack of the vowel, much softer for the voiced than for the unvoiced.

Among all the acoustic signs which can serve to differentiate the phonemes, there are many redundant elements which may seem superfluous for those who hear normally, but which are essential to the education of the deaf. The perceptions of the deaf child are different from those of the child who hears normally. But the main point of auditory education is to permit him, via a different code, to distinguish many tiny acoustic nuances which exist, but of which the normal of hearing are not aware because they do not need them.

It has been suggested that auditory education consists of using residual hearing and calls for the deciphering of sounds of language by using symbols that might be secondary in normal hearing.

Speech Training

In what concerns speech, we will stay on the level of the significant. When we later study language training, we will treat the "Signifié," as well as the link between *signifié* and *significant.* Language is acquired in a rather collective way, and speech (phonation, articulation, rhythm) in a rather particular way.

To summarize what is to be remembered during the deaf child's speech training: imitation is very important during the first and especially during the second year. As with every activity which requires training, it demands autocontrol. This is the role of auditory feedback (the closed audition-phonation circuit).

During the first months, there is babbling; frequent repetitions of the same sound, generally of a single syllable. The child carries on this activity for pleasure; he discovers the possibilities inherent in the phonetic and articulatory system. He learns, thus, to master and combine the movements of the participating organs in the phonatory act (lungs, larynx, tongue, velum, and lips).

Around 6 months, hearing and the feedback circuit take on great importance. Because of the constant repetition of sounds, a circuit is established between the kinesthetic and tactile impressions on the one hand and the corresponding sounds on the other. For each sound produced and "heard," there is a corresponding articulatory arrangement. It is thus that the child learns to modify the arrangement to modify a sound; he learns to master his vocal emissions.

Hearing permits him to direct his vocal attempts to make them similar to models furnished by adults.

Imitation is at first awkward (jargon), but becomes more and more similar to the model because the child needs to make himself understood; he better analyzes his perceptions; and he more thoroughly masters his motor activity.

Speech being the phonatory and articulatory aspect of language, vocal emissions become significant (in the linguistic sense), and articulations become phonemes. This is possible because speech is linked to real situations and the child learns the sign and its significance at the same time.

Behavior of the profoundly deaf child is characterized by babbling like a normal child, since in the beginning it is only a motor game.

If both internal auditory stimulation (coming from his own babbling) and external auditory stimulation (coming from the environment) are deficient or entirely lacking, it causes the vocal emissions of the deaf child to disappear.

Later, since speech as an instrument of communication is not accessible to him, the child does not want to speak, but, even if he wanted to, he could not. Having no auditory feedback, he could not direct his vocal emissions to make them more closely resemble models which he does not perceive. The deaf child cannot spontaneously arrive at the spoken word. Thus, in order for speech to develop in the deaf child, it is necessary: (1) to begin education as early as possible so that the passage from babbling to the spoken word is made without interruption; (2) to use residual hearing very early to create a feedback control, be it imperfect or partial; and (3) to augment auditory information with other information from other sensory channels: sight and touch (lipreading, feeling vibrations, machines to translate acoustic signs).

Classically, education for the spoken word has two stages: (1) *démutisation*: the first part of speech education consists of drawing the child out of his muteness, giving him a taste of speech and the means of doing it, giving him a consciousness of its usefulness and of its use by everyone; and (2) *orthophonie*: when the child has acquired a phonemic system, it is a question of perfecting his speech and making it intelligible. Really, there is no clear obstacle to this since, as we shall see, there is no possibility of teaching a child isolated phonemes and then later grouping them to form a word (Table 2).

As French and English do not use exactly the same terms, it is best to be precise: (1) during the period of *démutisation*, one takes the child out of his silence and has him emit sounds belonging to a certain elementary phonology; (2) during the orthophonie period, work is directed above all toward exactness of articulation, language being taught progressively during the two periods.

Use of Babbling When dealing with young children of slight or average deafness, babbling is spontaneous. One must know how to capture this spontaneous behavior to make the child conscious of it: he often says "mama," or produces sounds which resemble (a), (o), or (i). These sound emissions are unconscious.

One must make use of the basic consonant of these repetitions to produce words such as "papa" and "mama." Then, an effort must be made

Table 2. The logic of re-education programs

Problems to resolve	Methods to follow
To learn to hear	Auditory consciousness Attention to hearing To understand what one hears, to then be able to recognize it Auditory structure-building (rigorous training +++–hearing aid +++)
To learn to speak	Inadequate auditory feedback, but criteria +++ (acoustic clues, durations, rhythm)
To learn to understand	The words of others→lipreading and auditory control
To create a language	Lexical education (vocabulary) and structural education (sentences) with spontaneous use of the spoken language as the goal

to make the child consciously aware of the relationship between sound, hearing, and phonation.

When there is no babbling in the profoundly deaf child, the awakening of consciousness takes longer (several months). The auditory training must be intense before obtaining phonation.

The child must be plunged literally into a "bath" of spoken words, be spoken to frequently (the parents' role), with enough amplification (the role of the hearing aid) so that he becomes aware of the adults' emitted speech and so that he has a desire to imitate it. In the child of average deafness, one notes a reaction to amplification from the first year on.

The child is playing and his vocal emissions are spontaneous. If one stops amplification, the emissions stop. In other cases, we do not realize that the hearing aid is broken and often, in this case, one observes a lowering in the intensity of the child's voice.

Auditory training is associated with complementary means such as: tactile ones; concomitance of sounds and vibration of the larynx; visual ones; and signal lights. In the beginning, the sounds produced by the profoundly deaf child do not resemble any phoneme. One, therefore, creates a sound-sight association; in front of a mirror he is shown the placement of the lips to form an *a* and *o* (those phonemes most easily learned). Structural organization of phoneme groupings follows but always with auditory recall at the end of each exercise.

Phoneme training will incorporate the knowledge put forth by modern theories of linguistics which, nonetheless, must not be applied without correction, because the acquisition of the first phonemes must permit the acquisition of the first immediately useful words for the child. Without our being able to confirm it, it seems that the deaf child does not have the same criteria for acquisition of phonemes as the child who hears.

In the acquisition of each new phoneme, one uses all possible means: (1) pure hearing is of highest priority; (2) visual means (a mirror, signal lights); (3) tactile means; (4) as a last resort, the tongue guide, a very artificial means which will only be used with discretion and a light hand.

Having come to this stage, the goal of our education is to give the child an exact phonology, because, from its strict observance, will come the bases of intelligibility for his spoken language. We know that there is practically antagonism between the best articulation and the indispensable regard for rhythm and melody, whose physical bases are duration and intensity. Orthophonic behavior will always be perilous with the constant risk of a bad overall utterance or of defective articulation.

It is advisable to observe that the auditory feedback, which we have described as going from hearing to phonation, is joined by another opposing current, which goes from phonation to hearing. Indeed, the child pronounces because he hears, but, at this state, he hears better because he knows how to pronounce.

Language Training

Language is a means of both expression and communication. In the child who can hear, evolution is in slow states. The linguistic period begins at about 7 months. He understands at that time that sounds associated with a gesture or mimicry have meaning. Between 7 and 9 months appear the first words: "papa," "mama," then "no" (opposition to the outside world, a refusal of undesired things); "yes" comes later.

He understands simple orders and associates several words by about 18 months. He says sentences at about 2 or 2½ years. During this period the child plays with words, he says them, repeats them, creates neologisms, tries them out on those around him.

At about 3 years, he expresses himself easily concerning concrete facts and uses a rudimentary syntax. He says "I" and considers himself separately relative to the rest of the world. He uses the word "why."

Between 5 and 7 years, he begins abstraction and efforts at logic.

Deaf children who come to us at about 3 or 4 years of age are at different levels of this evolution, according to the degree of deafness. The profoundly deaf only make noises without modulation, rhythm, or response value. Those of average deafness speak words, but sentences are not shown. The slightly disabled speak in sentences, but with speech difficulties.

The development of the taste for spoken language must be worked upon. The deaf child does not know what language is and, in the beginning, it takes a long time with a great deal of difficulty to teach him that language serves to express oneself. He has become accustomed to communicating with gestures and mimicry and finds those means sufficient. If language education is not begun early, his thinking will remain of an elementary nature. We, therefore, provide him with this mode of expression and make him understand that language is a means of expression.

To help him in transferring from his original language, we first make this spoken language interesting for him and later make him consciously aware that it is necessary for communication.

This training is at present being applied in the Medical Centers for Phoniatry and Auditory Reeducation in Villefranche and La-Norville. It is a model more or less followed by other French professors.

In order to show the interest in language, we are interested in all of the child's vocal productions, even if mimicry is still necessary to communicate effectively with him.

Language training exercises can be accomplished in the form of games. Subsequently, all those who surround him must express a great deal of interest in all that the child says to encourage him to speak. That is the principal objective of all activity. We try to take advantage of every little event of daily life, encourage chattering about all that the child encounters and about everything that interests him. We interrupt class to look at a passing airplane, or a cat climbing a tree, and talk about it for a moment: "Look at the plane, it's going fast, it's gone, etc."

This demands a very flexible class discipline, and one must not be afraid of noise—one must create a "language-bath." For the older children, one must get out of the boarding school structure, break with routine to encourage the child to talk, encourage those who go outside the school to tell the boarders what they saw in town the night before. The boarding students will recount their Thursday and Sunday outings to the zoo, aquarium, their walks, their activities such as manual work, and even tell about the television movie for those who have not seen it. That can take up a good deal of time because it requires a great effort at articulation and for the construction of sentences, and we will see later that this is a means of acquiring vocabulary.

But this is not sufficient, and we use, along with audiovisual techniques, the following: very easy sequences on slides (or photographs) where there is a beginning of dialogue, drawings recounting a little story which incorporates vocabulary words. At present, in first and second grade, the method used is that of the Center for Applied Linguistics at Dakar (CALD)—a method used to teach French to Africans, and adapted to deaf children.

All these activities stimulate interest in language, and all favor dialogue among the pupils.

To show the necessity of language, we make the deaf child understand that language is necessary in communicating with others. Because they are grouped together, deaf children tend to retain the easier language of gestures and a jargon which demands less effort of them. It is, thus, necessary for educators to know exactly what each child is capable of saying, to be able to exact from him constructed sentences, articulated in the most intelligible fashion possible.

One must be prepared to react in such a way as to pretend not to understand a sentence lacking a word or where a word is replaced by a gesture. The child must feel obligated to use words and structures which he knows, to make the effort which this demands of him. For example, at the table it is much easier to immediately serve a child who says "drink" with a supporting gesture, but one must force oneself to "not understand" and await the sentence: "Please may I have something to drink," or "Give me some water."

Programing

We find it necessary to quickly provide the deaf child with verbal expression on two levels–lexical and syntactical.

Lexical Level

Choice of Words In the beginning, words are chosen according to the extremely limited articulation possibilities of the children. But later, this is done according to the interest and frequency of the words.

In kindergarten, one chooses very simple words–daddy, mommy, the pot, the doll, the boat–to show a link between the sound which is heard, an articulated sound, and the label put on an object. This difficulty is hard to overcome. The children, in the beginning, do not have any reference points. One must create the function of word-object association. For several months they point to anything on hearing the word "doll," for instance. At about the 5th month, the profoundly deaf begin to recognize about four or five words.

When the first means of coding is created, one can extend the vocabulary much more quickly. Then, one chooses words which are useful in daily life, those which correspond to the interests of the children–bread, water, the names of toys, car, etc. Later, words will be chosen according to the frequency of their use in the French language (with reference to fundamental or basic French).

Method of Acquisition At the end of the second grade, children know about 10 subjects, about 30 verbs, and a varying number of objects.

1. Words have been proposed by the teacher according to need, first in reality (objects, actions), then in photographs, from images.
2. In first and second grade (after kindergarten), acquiring of vocabulary is done in settings of interest, after concrete observations in different rooms of a house and on walks. Vocabulary builds considerably. Acquiring of vocabulary is at a maximum in real life situations.
3. In the third grade, vocabulary is acquired differently. The children already have a vocabulary base; there are no longer systematic lessons of vocabulary proposed by the teacher, but words will be learned in free conversation. On attempting to express himself, the deaf child realizes that he lacks certain words. He uses those he knows, but, all of a sudden, he

stumbles over objects or actions of which he wishes to speak and whose significance he does not know. He then uses mimicry or drawing.

Memorization All learned words are rapidly reused in different situations so that they will be understood without a particular or restricted meaning. Memorization exercises follow, always with images, where the meaning of a word is well understood (more work in pure hearing and articulation). In first grade, written exercises are begun and, in the second and third grades, one collects acquired vocabulary in a little dictionary or lexicon.

Next, we think of reusing learned words frequently or they will be quickly forgotten. One must be on the watch for every propitious occasion to use this or that word.

Structural or Syntactical Level If the deaf child succeeds in memorizing words after numerous exercises, he still has much difficulty in constructing sentences. Among the bits of information he receives, he picks out certain words he knows, but pays little attention to morphological variances in words; he does not generally hear little words (articles and prepositions); and the order of words in a sentence is of little importance to him.

The syntactical order in French, subject-verb-object, is not a logical necessity, but a convention. To do this, one uses several methods: (1) first, one always mimics the action in speaking: "I give the doll," "Mommy gives a little car," to make him discern the order, subject-verb-object; (2) afterward, one uses the *organigramme* as a means of memorization.

The structure and organization of the organigramme are well known by all student teachers at the Medical Center for Phoniatry and Auditory Reeducation at Villefranche. The organigramme is universally applied by them. It has been described several times, and it seems unnecessary to do so here. Suffice it to mention its interest and importance.

It is only in the last grade that deaf children have been taught grammatical terms, because they will need them in real life; but they do not pose any special problems because their significance is already acquired and all that is left is to add a label. Next, it is necessary to use this acquired vocabulary in spontaneous speech.

The CALD method is very interesting, even though it was not planned for deaf children (indeed, the case of foreign children is different; they have already learned a mother tongue and a first system, while for the deaf child there is no previous model and one must, thus, create a model). Using an audiovisual method, perception and understanding of this model are made easier by situational indicators.

Furthermore, children are motivated by its resemblance to movies, its scenario, and by mimicry which interests them greatly. They acquire, as well, a desire for dialogue (especially important, because it is so difficult for deaf children).

Afterward, one can exploit this technique on the level of writing; this is the beginning of putting into words (a recounting of the story they have seen). The logical order of a written story is learned more easily. On the other hand, where deaf children are concerned, programing can follow too quickly upon this method, and it cannot be used integrally until the last year of re-education. This situation is created by presenting figurines on a felt board. The figurines are mobile and this permits changing the action. Using this method, language is acquired through dialogue, which corresponds to our goal in teaching deaf children, to give them a tool for communication. Indirect discourse comes next; it is necessary, but less important. Nonetheless, the same notions are reworked on two levels: direct discourse—"Are you going to play?" and indirect discourse—"Is Michael going to play?"

Written expression plays a less important role in this training. It permits checking and reinforcing vocabulary (when vocabulary becomes larger, there are numerous opportunities for confusion). But this does not come until the end of a series of oral exercises (compositions, summaries, dictations, and grammar exercises).

Whatever the training method, we keep a watchful eye to see that the acquired knowledge or vocabulary is used in everyday life. Language must not remain solely a scholarly activity for the deaf child. In order for acquired knowledge to become fixed, there must be frequent repetition in different frameworks.

Close collaboration must be maintained with the parents and the supervisory personnel of the boarding schools. (The little lexicon of acquired vocabulary can serve as a link, showing the persons who are responsible for the child outside of class what can be expected of the child on the language level.) After 5 or 6 years of training, the successful deaf child has acquired a minimum vocabulary, the structure of sentences which are simple but correct, the various uses of most common words, and the most common idiomatic expressions.

It remains for the child to enrich his vocabulary and, thus, his means of expressing himself. To do this, he needs to be among those who hear; a more enriching experience than the specialized residence school. In France we try to avoid prolonging this segregation even if the oral expression and reception capabilities of the deaf child are far from perfect.

It is necessary, consequently, to introduce this child into an open milieu, into normal scholastic environment if his intellectual coefficients permit. The role of teachers (those who teach elementary classes for the normal hearing) will be to provide a favorable climate for his social integration. The role of the parents will be to help perfect linguistic and scholarly acquisitions. But the child must nonetheless continue orthophonic re-education for several more years.

INTERPROFESSIONAL RELATIONSHIPS

Relationships between the different people who take care of deaf children are complicated by the fact that two Ministries, Health and Education, are concerned with deafness. They have, thus, created bureaucracies with different personnel.

There are a number of private establishments whose personnel come from one of these Ministries or the other. Orthophonists and medical phoniatristes come into this as well. It also sometimes happens that those who take care of the deaf child are unqualified doctors, educators, and orthophonists who have complete liberty in their private practice (although technically supervised by physicians). Psychologists who are often not competent in child deafness, or child psychologists, who are very competent in diagnosis but not in re-education, often serve the deaf. The life of a deaf child is often parceled out, being entrusted to this and that qualified person or organization with no continuity between them in methods or even in goals. It follows that each individual or organization usually works alone, with no link to the others.

The Union of European Medical Phoniatristes has studied the importance of the problem of establishing communication between individuals and organizations who care for deaf children. We have presented the organizational schema as it exists in the Medical Centers for Phoniatry and Auditory Re-education, and which, without claiming to be perfect, assures that work will be organized by basing everything on the deaf child's needs and interests, rather than on the capabilities of individuals and organizations.

We, therefore, have proposed that a wider phoniatric team undertake the totality of education for the deaf child, from the initial diagnosis to his establishment in normal life as an adult. Obviously, when such a team is formed, each of its members freely accepts being part of it and, thus, accepts the structure of the team, its organization, and its modes of action. Relationships between team members are consequently guided by each member's motivation to the supreme goal: the eventual integration of the deaf child as an adult into society. But in order for the team to be homogeneous and to work in harmony, it must define its action on the basis of the deaf person.

Total Phoniatric Team

It is essentially made up of medical phoniatrists, medical audiologists (who may also be otorhinolaryngologists), medical child psychologists specializing in deafness, orthophonists, linguists, and certain other specialized professors.

To this intrinsic group, one can add hearing aid specialists, teachers, and professors in schools for the normal of hearing, who, after their specialized education, have the task of accepting, understanding, and teaching deaf subjects. We also have laboratories specializing in research on deafness, with mathematicians, information specialists, electricians, and mechanics.

This group of people is a complete normal team, such as we have formed within the frame of the University of Nice and the Medical Centers for Phoniatry at Villefranche-sur-Mer and at La-Norville.

Activity of Phoniatric Team

Dépistage (detection) and preliminary diagnosis are under the direction of a medical-phoniatrist. A paramedical team must detect suspected cases of deafness, but the phoniatrist must confirm the diagnosis in the first year of life.

From 0–3 years of age, family pre-education is given, directed toward two principal areas: (1) psychological behavior and relationships and (2) early auditory education. This period in the life of a deaf child is created by the family, with the help and advice of the orthophonist, and the intervention of the medical-phoniatrist if required.

From 3 years of age on, the diagnosis of deafness is solidified, and the degree of deafness is measured. There are two different cases. In the first, the deaf child does not need specialized education and will go to a normal kindergarten for a normal education to which the help of the family and orthophonic lessons will be added. This is essentially in cases of mild deafness or of moderate deafness. In the second case, the deaf child suffering from severe or profound deafness needs specialized education. For a period of 4 to 5 years, preferably as a half-time resident student, he goes first to a kindergarten for 2 years, then into specialized classes for 2 or 3 years. The deaf child is then under the charge of the establishment's physician, specialized professors, and orthophonists. A close relationship is maintained with the family, the physician, and the orthophoniste who originally cared for the deaf child.

When he leaves the specialized center, the deaf child returns to the normal system under the supervision of physicians and orthophonists. Even if educational results seem to show that he does not understand, the deaf child undergoes an evolution psychologically by making a number of friends in the normal milieu, thus preparing himself for life among the normal of hearing.

One must remember that educational results are not those which the future adult will obtain in real life; they are not criteria by which to judge if the deaf child should be kept in a normal school as a normal child and not as an outcast.

After finishing elementary school, the deaf child, depending on his intelligence, will either terminate his studies and begin professional training or continue his studies to obtain the *Brevet Elémentaire du Premier Cycle* (a secondary education certificate), the *Baccalauréat* (similar to two years of college), or even a university degree, depending upon the psychological motivation of the subject's family. During this period, the phoniatric team will observe closely the development of the deaf student.

The Deaf Child Is an Adult We have created a program for him entitled "Social Adaptation for Young Handicapped Workers," under the law concerning Continued Development passed on July 16, 1971. This is intended to give the handicapped subject a better understanding of human relationships, both on the psychological level of communication (audiophonatory and language), and on the social level (relationships with the employer, government organizations, professions, Social Security, retirement, etc.). Those who teach this educational program are specialists in the pathology of communication and in its treatment, using all audiovisual means and group psychology techniques.

The entire phoniatric team, well organized in a manner accepted by all of its members, creates an harmonious milieu in which each individual concerned with the deaf child makes a most meaningful contribution within the context of optimum interprofessional relationships.

As for deafness in the adult, the medical phoniatrists who are also audiologists maintain relationships with trained hearing aid specialists. They also use the services of orthophonists where auditory education is concerned, where there is a question of preserving voice and speech, or in teaching lipreading to adults in cases of profound deafness.

FAMILY INVOLVEMENTS

Deafness, the common characteristic of all deaf children, is often chosen as the only variable in groups studied. Left hidden is the preponderant influence of other factors in development. The child could benefit from these other factors even though deaf, and the lack of these often deprives the child even more than deafness deprives him.

The quality of verbal exchange between the child and the family during early childhood, and even later, can be disturbed by family reaction to the child's deafness, by the separation of the child from the family, by the lack of nonverbal stimulation in the milieu, etc. The family, as well as the child, must be "treated" because it is endangered by an abnormal event: the presence of an abnormal child.

Specialists must, thus, act therapeutically toward the family, so as to reduce the risks of rejection and to orient the parents toward efficient reparative attitudes.

Guidance of the parents changes as the age of the child changes, but in all cases it must be principally directed toward re-establishing communication between the deaf child and the different family members. It, thus, presupposes considerable knowledge of the mechanisms which block communication in the various networks where it should exist and a practical therapy capable of acting upon the defenses brought into play. The means used for this can be classed in two large categories: information and psychotherapeutic action. Each can be brought to the parents in individual and group format, individual action being reserved for those parents who ask for it.

Information

In all institutions, meetings are held on a theme chosen by one of the team members or by the parents and are intended to provide collective information on deafness and on the general problems of the deaf child.

These meetings, apart from the useful information which they impart to parents, are intended to dedramatize the conflict situations concerning certain myths about deafness (equipment, operations, miracle cures, etc.). Being better informed, parents more easily abandon their scattered attempts at useless searching to find more efficient courses of action. To the individual, information is imparted by all of the team members and especially by the re-educator who is responsible for the child and who shows the parents by his example what can best be done for the child, or what not to do. The parents should not be different at home as re-educators of the child.

Libraries and parents' discussion groups under the guidance of a moderator, based on information or on a reading, are also forms of therapeutic action based on information. These different types of action, which parents often use to put off awareness of more important things for the child's re-education, are nonetheless necessary and prepare the ground for an eventual individual or group activity aimed at an in-depth approach, and of which we will now speak.

Psychotherapeutic Action The parents' first reaction to a child's deafness is anxiety. In a research project done by Mottier on the reactions of parents of deaf children to childhood deafness, 84% described their feelings in depressed terms, going from "sorrow" to "catastrophe," and from "anguish" to "despair." After these reactions to the initial shock, worry shows up in answers concerning individual and social development of the child. These responses are given here in the order of their importance: fears of a difficult scholastic and professional life, fears of accident, fears of emotional instability, etc.

Thus, it seems, and the reactions of young parents prove it, that part of the reactions of anxiety to deafness can be reduced by a less somber picture of the future presented by those who have become deaf.

Even when the real world no longer legitimizes a paradoxical anxiety, it is easier to help parents to discover by themselves the deepest reasons for their uneasiness toward their children and the best ways of fighting depression. Development groups and individual psychotherapy are intended to permit parents to elucidate by themselves the personal problems into which the deafness of their child has placed them. Frustration engendered by the handicap only reactivates deeper anguish, and it is in the old processes of adaptation to the surrounding world that adults will find a possible clarification of their present malaise.

Every child is the object of projection of the parents' fantasies and desires, by which they atone for that which they once considered their own deficiencies. Scholastic valuation comes in part from the fact that access to knowledge is done through another. To live in this child who succeeds is a narcissistic pleasure which many parents find satisfying. But how can one project oneself into an imperfect body? What revaluation can one expect from this child, who will perhaps not have access to this knowledge since he is lacking the principal instrument for it, namely, language? The narcissistic wound is open, and it awakens other, older ones. To escape or to atone, the parents have no choice. Therapeutic action will try to make the parents understand these atonement and escape forms of behavior into which they rush in order to combat depression, anxiety, and guilt.

Of course, attempts at atonement, although they show parental immaturity simply by the need for them, are better for the child than attempts at escape. But it is best to change these forms of behavior in depth, for active rejection can take place in what appears to be an attempt at atonement. For example, the mother transformed into a re-educator, apparently brave and efficient—which she is: she does all that the re-educator does; but her relationship with the child no longer goes beyond this way of mediating attitudes, the vehicle for her rejection. Another form is in overprotection by parents, who destroy all possibility of autonomy, while wanting to protect the body, and believing that they are.

To reject deafness, to fight it, to defeat it, while giving the child the maximum possibilities for communication, without rejecting the child who suffers from deafness, presupposes an understanding both of the child's problems and one's own, an understanding rare in a so-called "normal" subject. But all this presupposes a competence which depends on a highly specialized training in psychology on the part of the team that takes care of the parents.

Centers which can undertake all of parental guidance are rare. Education may be done at all levels in most specialized centers for the hearing impaired; parent groups may work very usefully as meeting places where common feelings are aired. But psychotherapy and development groups (or training groups) which require more specialized personnel are often confused with the aforementioned groups, from which they differ greatly, in many institutions.

The deaf child, like any child, is caught up from the moment of birth in a network of relationships which creates a significant structure, well before language comes into being. The deaf child will not be involved in verbal communication unless, before this, his subconscious is slowly structured like a language, and this must be done in the basic environment of the family. It is, thus, the family, perhaps even before the child, that must be helped to assume a paradoxical relationship, as a normal relational phenomenon.

Psychological Examination The psychological examination of a hearing-impaired child is no different from that of a normal child, except in the interpretation which is given to the language tests, which are always the last given. Apart from these few points of technique and interpretation, the psychological examination of a deaf child has the same goals as that of a normal child: (1) to aid in the establishment of a diagnosis of the problem presented by the child and his family; (2) to analyze the specific mental processes of the child and to compare them, if possible, to those of children with normal hearing of a given age; and (3) to analyze the system of family and pedagogic relationships which have been established around the child, in order to evaluate possible modifications of the environment for optimal re-education.

Methods of Psychological Examination: Tests and Interviews Tests, whose value rests on their standardization, allow one to situate the different sectors of the child's development (intellectual, motor, psychosocial, emotional, etc.) as compared to the norms of development. They also permit orienting therapeutic activity toward those areas which show that the child is behind.

Interviews with the family and with educators allow one to evaluate the ways in which the environment reacts to deafness, and the developmental possibilities of the relationships already established. Interviews with the child, whether or not verbal communication is established, allow one (often by games or by drawing) to broaden the psychological approach begun with the tests.

Thus comprised, psychological examination is part of the activity of the therapeutic team which takes the family under its care. The education of the child's deafness is in strict relationship with the network of communication which he can establish within his family. As a resident student at a special school, the psychotherapeutic value of the milieu is undeniable. As a child living with his family, the psychological relationships among the child, his parents, his teachers, and the outside world must of necessity be normalized. No re-education is worthwhile unless psychological normalization is effective.

TRAINING OF PROFESSIONALS FOR THE FIELD OF HABILITATIVE-REHABILITATIVE AUDIOLOGY

In France, there is no single group of people qualified in auditory re-education. This is, of course, an integral part of the education of young deaf people. Four types of educators, trained at different places, but with a more or less similar training, are concerned with the education of the deaf child.

In France, because of the two types of existing structures of education, several types of training lead to: (1) a professorship in the national institutes for young deaf people and (2) a professorship in private institutions for young deaf people.

The programs of study are made up of the following fields to include anatomy, physiology, and pathology of the organs of hearing and speech, the physics of hearing, bioacoustics, descriptive phonetics, teaching of speech and lipreading, orthophony, hearing education, elements of physiology of the nervous system, and the physiology of sensations, elements of child neurophysiology, child psychology, psychology of the deaf child, and general pedagogy. (3) Specialized personnel from the Ministry of Education teach in establishments for the hearing impaired. Regular public school teachers, after a 1-year training program, can obtain the Certificate of Qualification to teach handicapped children (with the option of either auditory or visual handicap), and teach in the special classes which come under the Ministry of Education. (4) Orthophonists, during their 3 years of medical school, receive training in all of the normal processes of the voice, speech, and language, their pathology, and re-educational techniques. They are, thus, not specialized solely for the deaf, and it is the choice and quality of their subsequent training which will better orient them toward education of the deaf.

It is unfortunate that training of teachers for young deaf people is the responsibility of one of the two ministries already mentioned. The promised university independence, theoretically now being practiced, should allow the multidisciplinary university training of professors for the deaf, modeled on the training program for orthophonists. This new high level training would certainly advance the quality and philosophy of re-education for the deaf child.

RESEARCH

Research projects in France are divided among a number of centers of audiophonology and university and hospital clinics of otorhinolaryngology.

Suzanne Borel-Maisonny of Paris, founder of orthophony in France, has developed a number of tests for determining the levels of children, and her studies on language are useful for both normal hearing and deaf children.

Gabriel Decroix and J. Dehaussy of Lille are studying stereophonic equipment.

Jean-Claude Lafon of Besancon has developed a phonetic test and a compensating frequency machine.

A. H. Morgon of Lyon is studying evoked potentials.

Guy Perdoncini of Nice, founder of the Medical Centers for Phoniatrie and Auditory Reeducation, has established a general method of education for the deaf child, has invented the analytic *cynétique* pulsatone, several audiometers for obtaining absolute and differential thresholds, and is currently working with a multidisciplinary team on modification of the oral message which would make it accessible to the profoundly deaf.

Michel Portmann and J. M. Aran of Bordeaux have invented and perfected the use of the *cochléogramme.*

This list of researchers is not exhaustive. All those mentioned are doing research without the intention of pecuniary gain.

Research on deafness itself can be divided into three parts: (1) A number of medications are being studied which would attempt to develop either the auditory function or the cortical function. The results seem irregular, and it seems that the best results obtained in deaf adults come largely from the improvement of the subject's general state, which has an effect on the sense organs of hearing. This has been verified by studies of H. Roddier on differential thresholds. (2) Surgical treatment of deafness by P. Pailoux of Paris is based on research done on surgery of the internal auditory passageway and on the cochlea. (3) In cases of presbyacousis in the adult, it is best to seek the best selective amplifier, capable of nontraumatic dynamic amplification at certain low frequencies of the message. The considerations for deaf children regarding this equipment for presbyacousis are also useful, but inadequate. Research is, thus, based on the modification of the message in such a way as to increase the quantity of information which can pass through that narrow door which is the deaf ear.

The laboratory of the Medical Center for Phoniatry and Auditory Reeducation at Nice is currently working on these two considerations: dynamic amplification and enrichment of the message.

ORGANIZATIONS AND ASSOCIATIONS RESPONSIBLE FOR HEARING HANDICAPPED

Professional Associations

1. Association Francaise des Enseignants spécialisés dans la Rééducation des Déficients du Langage et de l'Audition (AFERLA): 254, Rue Saint-Jacques–75005 Paris.
2. Association des Rééducateurs de la Parole et du Langage parlé et écrit (ARPLOE): 10, Rue de l'Arrivée–75005 Paris.
3. Syndicat National des Médecins spécialisés en Logopédie at Phoniatrie: 16, Rue des Ursulines–93200 Saint-Denis.
4. Syndicat des Orthophonistes (see ARPLOE).

Nonprofessional Associations

1. ANPEDA: Association nationale des parents d'enfants déficients auditifs.
2. BUCODES: Bureau de Coordination des devenus sourds.
3. CNSF: Confédération nationale des sourds de France.
4. "EPHETA": Association de sourds et d'entendants.
5. FNAPEDIDA: Fédération nationale des Associations de parents d'élèvès des instituts de déficients auditifs.
6. Ligue contre la Surdité.
7. UNISDA: Union national pour l'intégration sociale des déficients auditifs.

Because phoniatry is a very recent medical discipline situated between the orthophonists and the otorhinolaryngologists, the *Syndicat des Phoniatres* has been formed to establish its procedures.

The list of professional and parental organizations contains almost all of the interested groups. These organizations are very active in defending their professional and private rights.

Despite several laws, some even dating from the last century, French organization of activities on deafness is more a matter of habit than of any systematic law.

Nonetheless, a new legislative bill written a few weeks ago will soon be introduced for the approval of the Parliament.

PERIODICALS ON HEARING PUBLISHED IN FRANCE

1. Bulletin d'Information de la Société centrale d'Education et d'Assistance pour les Sourds-Muets en Fr ance: 254, Rue Saint-Jacques–Paris (5°).
2. Communiquer (Revue de l'ANPEDA): 63, Rue de Romilly–Mesnil-Le-Roi 78600.
3. La Revue de l'OUie: 57 Rue Caulaincourt–Paris (19°).
4. La Voix du Sourd (Revue de la CNSF): 20, Rue Thérèse–Paris (1°).
5. Rééducation Orthophonique (Revue de l'ARPLOE): 10, Rue de l'Arrivée–Paris (5°).
6. Revue générale de l'Enseignement des Déficients Auditifs (Revue de l'AFERLA): 166, Boulevard Voltaire–Paris (11°).

chapter 8

Communication for Hearing-handicapped People in Spain

Joseph Gisbert Alos, M.D.

Everyday we are more convinced that the last decade has been characterized by a wide interchange of experiences among professional audiologists in Spain. This interchange has served greatly to propagate new methods used in the habilitation of the deaf child. Some of the methods compete among themselves, but it could be safely stated that no one has superseded the results of the pure oral method of habilitation.

The oral method for deaf habilitation is the result of an auditory training that is aimed in the first place to establish proper audiophonatory circuits. These circuits have greater possibility of being created if the habilitation has an early start. However, in some particular cases of profound deafness or auditory agnosia, these audiophonatory circuits are rather difficult to establish. Anyway, whether they are difficult or not, at the beginning of the process of oral habilitation, there is always a linguistical structuralization that should be provided to the child. Structural linguistics has been demonstrated over the past few years to be more important to the habilitation process than the building of a simple vocabulary or than the purely phonetic approach. Today the importance of structural linguistics in the speech habilitation, rather than simply building a vocabulary, is universally accepted. It is embarrassing for a qualified professional to observe that still, in some circles in Spain, the need for structural linguistics is not recognized as yet; in these circles, the building of vocabulary and nucleus of interest for the deaf or the aphasic child is solely emphasized. However, building a vocabulary is not useful when structural linguistics is lacking.

Therefore, in our opinion, the effort of Dr. H. Oyer to bring up to date in a book the universal experience in the habilitative and rehabilitative audiology is a very commendable one and also a proof of the international concern to improve the methods and results in this field. Indeed nobody is entirely satisfied with the present status of habilitative and rehabilitative audiology. There is a strong need for research, especially in order to provide alalic children with acceptable speech. Hopefully, the new techniques of diagnosis, such as cortical audiometry, will help to pinpoint the respective etiology and, consequently, provide sufficient information for building a base for therapy in each case.

One problem, not solved as yet, is the one concerning the aphasic child, the one who has never spoken, who had "auditive permeability," but behaves nevertheless as a deaf child. The approach of habilitative audiology here should be completely different from the approached used for the peripherally deaf child.

Until recently, aphasic children were confounded with purely deaf children, and placed in six or seven vaguely defined categories. The findings of cortical pathology studies have brought things into better perspective. The aphasic children definitely produce pitch and melody after they acquire language, which excludes the possibility of a conductive loss. The auditive agnostic child, who even ignores his own name in spite of the fact *that he is able to listen to it*, presents even a more difficult task for the habilitative audiologist than the aphasic or simply the deaf child. A big problem for the aphasic child is how to acquire a linguistic structure. For these children, even the same phoneme has to be recognized every time it is discovered in a new word; they lack power of generalization.

The shift in the goals of rehabilitative therapy observed recently almost universally is indeed the by-product of the interchange of experiences and better communication of the professionals devoted to providing the nonoral child with language and voice communication. A few years ago the word "deaf-mute," and the social segregation implied by that label, was universally admitted. Today there exists an automatic repulsion toward the use of such a term and to that segregationistic implication. The prevalent concept today is habilitation and integration of the handicapped children into society. The chances of being successful with an habilitation procedure are directly proportional to the moment the program started: the earlier the better. There is now a consensus among professionals that integration of a classroom with, for example, one-third handicapped children and two-thirds normal children provides a benefit to both parties and society in general. This is the model in which any habilitative program should be based: integration. The author hopes that this chapter will contribute toward this goal.

DEFINITION OF AURAL REHABILITATION

To orally habilitate a deaf child consists of creating a language by using the residual hearing, exercising the discrimination potentials of the child, especially those concerning the most general parameters of sound and speech, namely, intensity, frequency, duration, and rhythm. This training must start as early as possible; emphasis on discrimination should be carried as far as it can be within the capabilities of each child. The author distinguishes *peripheral deafness*, in which the organ of corti is affected, and *central deafness*, in which the central areas are impaired. In this case the handicapped child is unable to recognize, associate, and integrate the perceived speech acoustic stimuli, or the praxic areas fail to coordinate properly the motor impulses. Result in both cases is an alalic aphasic child. Most often these children do not present cerebral lesions as detected by electroencephalograms. These infantile aphasias can be sensorial, motor, or mixed. In all instances, these handicapped children are unable to create their own speech and need professional help to develop a reasonable voice communication capability.

Both the peripherally and the centrally deaf children need to develop their auditive function; but while the peripherally deaf child must use amplification headsets in the classroom and hearing aid after school, the centrally deaf child does not need amplification. Headsets are used only for training on auditive discrimination, with little amplification.

The prognosis for the peripherally deaf child can be established with excellent accuracy when both the audiometric curve and the intelligence quotient coefficient are known. On the other hand, the prognosis for the centrally deaf child is difficult to establish and erratic. The "index of audiometric disjunction" that is discussed later in this chapter could give one an approximate idea concerning the probable evolution of the patient.

The creation of a true language involves not only good articulation and intelligibility but also the mastering of the linguistic structure of the language utilized in the habilitative process. The linguistic structure is either acquired during the first steps of the training or never. It is more important than the building of a vocabulary since it is possible in later stages to extend the initial vocabulary, but not the basic linguistic structure.

HISTORICAL REVIEW

This historical review is based on information from Sordomudez (Perello and Tortosa, 1968).

Pedro Ponce de Leon (1510–1584), a Benedictine monk, born in Sahagun de Campos, started in 1555 the education of a deaf child from a noble family, at the convent of San Salvador de Ona, near the city of Medina del Pomar, province of Burgos.

Manuel Ramirez de Carrion (1579–1652), born at Hellin, inspired by the teaching of Ponce, took over the education and habilitation of several deaf children from Castilian nobility. Ramirez de Carrion kept his method secret.

Juan Pablo Bonet (1579–1633) was born in Torres de Berellen, province of Zaragoza. In 1620 he published the first known book on education of the deaf-mute child. He emphasized articulation and did not use lipreading at all.

Bonet lacked the necessary experience since he only taught one student, already with speech, previously trained by Ramirez de Carrion. Actually Bonet limited himself to imitating Ramirez de Carrion. The merit of Bonet consisted of having the method used by that teacher of the deaf disseminated. The book by Bonet created a school of thinking and attracted widespread interest in the deaf. He contributed to the destruction of current superstitions about teaching deaf children that existed at that time. Proof that Bonet simply copied Ramirez de Carrion is deduced from some sentences from the book that Bonet wrote in 1620.

According to Bonet, the best age to start the habilitation of a deaf child is from 6–8 years of age. However, to let the child remain inactive up to a more mature age could cause atrophies and lack of flexibility of the structures of the vocal tract that could impair the whole process.

Bonet discarded lipreading as a means of perceiving speech. He recommended ideomimetic procedures and a manual alphabet. He stated that lipreading would detract from, rather than help, the process of habilitation.

The Abbot L'Epee, together with other Frenchmen, Sicard, his successor, and Clerc, a deaf man himself, started the teaching of deaf persons by grammatical means. That is, they classified words according to their grammatical function within sentences. Grammatical rules served as a base for construction of sentences. L'Epee was partial to the use of sign language. The sign alphabet he originated used both hands to express proper nouns. Verbs and most parts of the sentences were expressed with gestures. For instance, a soldier was expressed by the gesture of presenting arms; a cat by a gesture evoking his mustaches; bread by the gesture of cutting a slice; white color by showing the shirt; the past by moving the arm back toward the shoulder. L'Epee rationalized the use of gestures, arguing that they are natural, spontaneous, and descriptive. He proposed exercises of dictation to his students: they had to write in French what L'Epee "dictated" to them by these standard gestures, which included some of purely grammatical nature, to express genre, number, conjugations, etc. Of course, these rules rendered the process quite artificial, contrary to the claims brought by L'Epee. He did not realize this fact because he was convinced that grammar is the expression of reason and that everything within reason is natural. He did not appreciate oral habilitation, which put him a step back with respect to Pablo Bonet.

Heinicke, on the other hand, believed in the advantages of oral habilitation of the deaf, as well as in lipreading. These two different schools of thought kept the controversy going for a long time, up to 1879, the year that the Paris International Congress of Teachers of the Deaf adopted a resolution favoring oral habilitation rather than the sign language. The Congress of Milano reaffirmed this resolution.

Fray Diego Vidal Rodriguez (1675–1740), born in Tauste, taught the deaf persons of Zaragoza with a great deal of success, mainly because of his enthusiasm, faith, and dedication to his job. He emulated many foreign colleagues.

Don Manuel Godoy managed to promote the creation of the first official Institute for the Deaf, in Spain, August 29, 1795. This institute was part of the School of Lavapies (Collegium of San Fernando). The first director of this official institute was the Calasancian priest, Jose Fernandez Navarrete, educated in Italy by another priest of the same Order, Juan Bautista Octavio Assaroti.

In 1795, the Jesuit, Lorenzo Hervas Panduro (1735–1809), born in Horcajo de Santiago, province of Cuenca, published the book *Escuela Espanola de Sordomudos.*

Father Panduro was the first to use the word deaf-mute, as opposed to deaf, as previously used. The Municipality of Barcelona authorized Father Albert Marti on February 4, 1800 to teach the deaf, using a large room in the city hall.

In Madrid, the Royal School for the Deaf was founded on March 27, 1802. The first director was Antonio Josef Rouyer y Bethier. This school was sponsored by the Association Amigos del Pais. The headquarters were in the Plaza Mayor of Madrid, in the House of the Bakery.

Fray Manuel Estrada was appointed teacher of the deaf in Barcelona in 1815.

In the article 108 of the General Education Law of September 9, 1857, creation of special schools for the deaf was prescribed. These schools were to be organized within university districts.

In 1898 the Madrid School for the Deaf, at 71 La Gastellana Ave., was founded. During that year 300 students were enrolled. Dr. Vieta of Barcelona introduced, at the July 10, 1905 session of the Academy of Medicine, several trained deaf who were able to write and to utter several sentences and proper nouns.

Emilio Tortosa Orero founded in 1904, in Barcelona, the Catalan Institute for the Deaf, the first private institution in Spain devoted to the habilitation and rehabilitation of deaf persons.

In summary, the oral method was invented by Ponce de Leon; it was ignored by L'Epee, and then sponsored again by Heinicke. The Congress of Milano accepted this method internationally as the most proper for the habilitation of the deaf.

This method was reintroduced in Spain by the teacher of the deaf, Tortosa Orero, who imported it from Italy in 1904. Tortosa Orero used the oral method in his private institute, calling it "pure oral perceptive method," since it eliminated all gestures and emphasized lipreading.

The National Administration for the Deaf, Blind, and Mentally Retarded was organized in 1914, in Madrid. The headquarters of this administration were at the National School for the Deaf, 33 Granada St., Madrid, until the civil war. After the civil war was over, these headquarters were moved to San Mateo St., being inaugurated in July 1948.

Habilitation of the deaf was first oral in Spain. Then it was transformed in a mimic mode following the teachings of L'Epee, since this method proved to be easier and more immediate success was obtained through its usage. This approach is not completely satisfactory because of the fact that, if the deaf person does not speak, he or she cannot be considered habilitated; hence, a hybrid method has been adopted, especially in the U.S.A.

In 1880 the Congress of Milano imposed again the pure oral method, excluding mimics. This approach ignores the special psychological needs of the deaf.

In 1925 Herlin created the global method that includes special consideration of child psychology and development. It departs completely from the traditional approach and demands too much from the deaf to communicate spontaneously.

GENERAL DESCRIPTION OF PRESENT PROGRAMS OF AUDIOLOGICAL HABILITATION AND REHABILITATION IN SPAIN

The habilitation programs for deaf children include all the normal topics but emphasize the sensorial and linguistic aspects.

A few years ago the programs were very heterogeneous in Spain but, since the adoption of the general basic teaching, an improvement has been observed. Indeed, this progressive programing by areas, from a modern point of view which gives special consideration to the broader linguistic approach to language (rather than a grammatical one), allows the deaf child between 6 and 7 years of age to initiate the first level of general basic learning together with a normal child.

Naturally, this approach requires a greater effort for the special training of deaf because it is necessary to add auditory training, breathing exercises, gymnastics involved with the articulatory muscles, rhythm, and acquaintance with the different sounds and particularly the exercises of orthophonetic to the normal school work. These exercises take a lot of time and are indispensable for the deaf child if he is to acquire language with a solid foundation.

The flexibility that presently exists in the general basic teaching should be extended when it is applied to handicapped children, since some of the topics could be very difficult or impossible to teach in these circumstances. Imagine for instance a dictation within a classroom including all normal children and several deaf children. It is obvious that, even with the greatest possible help, i.e., sitting near the teacher, observing his or her excellent articulation, etc., the errors of orthography could be attributable to a deficit of reception rather than to actual lack of knowledge of correct spelling. If both the normal and the deaf children are treated with the same standard for grading, then the injustice is obvious. On the other hand, if the deaf child is encouraged to request repetition when he does not understand a given sentence, then injustice toward the normal children is also obvious here. The best way for these general programs to become effective depends on the clear enunciation of the goals considered for the habilitation of the deaf child.

If such deaf child must continue his professional training within a center for the deaf, the general learning should be obtained within that center; on the contrary, if the goal rather is to integrate him socially as soon as possible, he could initiate first grade in a normal school. Since classes in a normal school are held in Spain usually during half a day only, the remaining part of the day could be spent by the deaf child within a special center for the deaf.

This hybrid approach could be maintained from 1 to 3 years according to the degree of deafness and the adaptability of the deaf child, his intelligence, and personality characteristics.

Financing these programs is sometimes from governmental sources and sometimes from private sources. In addition, the Ministry of Science and Education sometimes grants scholarships to help pay for this very costly training. Additionally, the Ministry of Work grants 1,500 pesetas monthly to families with one or more handicapped members. There exists also Social Security help within different unions that can be granted to a member who has handicapped children.

Finally, it should be pointed out also that there are centers for habilitation for the handicapped which depend upon the provincial governments. Here, patients pay no fees for services or perhaps only a token fee. The church also provides some services of this type, supported by generous patrons.

We believe that the day will come in Spain when services to rehabilitate handicapped children will be available to everybody regardless of the family's economic status. Our hope is that the Social Security and Ministry of Work will one day arrange for some kind of agreement to make this possible as it is presently carried on in France and in some other countries.

DIAGNOSTIC PROCEDURES

Pediatric audiometry presents a great number of difficulties because of the limited intelligence and early age of the children involved who certainly cannot be considered like a small adult. Their reactions are qualitatively different from the adult reaction.

There is no purpose to review here all the procedures used by eminent audiologists to condition the deaf children to the different sounds in order to obtain from them responses that are above their thresholds. Rather it is of more interest to focus on a diagnostic problem that is usually ignored. This aspect concerns obtaining a general notion of the response of the child to sound. To this end, nothing is better than to play with him the game of uttering onomatopoeic, short words or any kind of vocalic or consonantal sounds; these utterances can provide the audiologist with an orientation concerning the timbre and melody of the deaf child's voice. This game is played without using headsets or audiometers that act as perturbing elements.

This is not an easy task, but should be diligently pursued, especially when, during the anamnesis, it is disclosed by the parents that the child spends time "lalling" although the utterances are unintelligible.

We start testing the child by using manipulative tests that amuse the child and make him feel at ease and become familiar with the clinician. These manipulative tests are very useful to determine the mental level of the child.

For these tests, we use noisy toys. We imitate the type of noise produced by the toy and attempt to elicit from the child the same noise. Other procedures consist of playing songs through a tape recorder that we present alternately to his ears and then to our ears. We hum along to stimulate an imitative articulation of the child.

Very often, when we have reached the point of giving up, the child starts emitting sounds spontaneously, reproducing some of the various noises to which he has been exposed previously. These utterances can provide a very good indication of the status of the child's audiophonatory circuit. For this reason, we label this part of the diagnostic procedure as "exploration of the audiophonatory circuit." If such a circuit does indeed exist, the child's acoustic emissions are melodic, modulated, and may be characterized by very well-defined timbre and rhythm.

In those cases in which all these assets are evident, and if the mental age of the child corresponds to his chronological age, we have a strong clue that the peripheral receptors are normal and, hence, that the acoustic stimuli actually reach the cortex. This situation clearly defines, then, an infantile aphasia rather than deafness.

Next we carry out conditioned audiometry within a sound isolated booth, first in a sound field, then by using a bone oscillator, and finally using headsets. This exploration allows detection of possible differences between the right and the left ear. During these tests we try to give to the child simple instructions as possible, in accordance with his mental age. We check the results of these tests by other means, i.e., by playing musical instruments behind the child at his left or right sides in order to observe whether or not he is able to perceive and localize the source. We check pertinent data from the anamnesis obtained through the parents.

If, after these steps, some doubt remains about the child's condition, we recall the child to perform evoked response audiometry. The technique of evoked response audioelectroencephalography, produced with the help of a computer, very often clarifies our doubts concerning aphasia, the behavioral symptoms of which are similar to those of deaf children. Clearly, in these cases, the patient has no impaired hearing structures up to the level of the cortex. There exists, however, a sensorial aphasia, namely, auditive agnosia.

Information given by the parents that should alert the clinician to suspect aphasia rather than deafness is an expression of doubt as to whether or not our child is really deaf because sometimes it looks like he can hear and other times he does not seem to hear even very loud noises.

On the other hand, the peripherally deaf child lacks spontaneous phonic emissions to express himself, and his voice lacks normal timbre. The period of spontaneous babbling is short, and the parents express no doubt about his deafness, except for very loud sounds or very low frequencies that he perceives as vibrations through the tactile receptors.

We have seen children with an obvious aphasia but with intact acoustic perception, including high frequencies, after some training sessions. In some of these cases, there were relatives or parents with impaired hearing caused by toxic, iatrogenic or noxious effects of some drugs (Streptomycin in particular). In most of these cases, the child patient has also received some ototoxic medication during the first months of his life; therefore, the question arises: can such ototoxic drugs affect not only the organ of corti but also the central pathways, the association circuits and the myelination process.

REHABILITATION PROCEDURES

Centers of Re-education for Deaf Children in Spain

We have surveyed each of these centers through the following questionnaire:

1. Name of the center
2. Director and title
3. Address
4. Sponsoring agency
5. Type of school: boarding school, semi-boarding school, day school
6. No. of students: Boys, girls, adults
7. Age of admittance: age of obligatory termination
8. Methods used
9. Class units
10. No. of classrooms which use amplification
11. No. of children that use hearing aids
12. Persons who are involved in diagnostic procedures:
    Audiologists___Phoniatrist___
    Psychologist___Pediatrician___
13. If diagnostics are not obtained in the center, where are they obtained?
14. Personnel involved in special pedagogy: Teachers___Psychologists___Others___
15. Auxiliary personnel
16. Professional training: yes___no___
17. If professional training is given; a type of trade taught, and maximum age at which the trainee should leave the school
18. Predominant communication method used: Audiophonatory___Lipreading___Sign language___
19. In case of sign language used: Alphabetic-symbolic___Motor idea expression___Others___
20. Parents counseling: yes___no___
21. Reports to parents: yes___no___ Frequency of reports______
22. Summary of the pedagogical experiences during the last 5 years
23. Present orientation
24. Other data of interest

This questionnaire was sent to 87 habilitation centers for deaf children, officially recognized by the Spanish Ministry of Education and Science. Only 24 centers replied, including the two directed by the author, but the 24 answers received were very representative of the totality of Spanish centers. The statistics derived, considering 100% the sum of figures from the 24 answers received, are as follows: official centers, 13 (54%); private centers, 7 (29%); private centers within the regimen of patronage, 2 (8%); centers belonging to the school board, 1 (4%); and centers sponsored by the church, 1 (4%).

Regarding Question 5, we obtained the following information: boarding schools, 39.8% (1,180 available places); semi-boarding schools, 31.58% (957 available places); day schools, 28.62% (870 available places); total, 3,007 available places.

Extrapolating these figures to the total number of centers in Spain, the figures become 4,368 (3,469 and 3,153, respectively), with a total of 10,990 available places. Statistics on the number of deaf children and adults that are not receiving training are not available. (Possibly these statistics may be obtained through the Ministry of Work and through the Minusval 74 Congress.)

Regarding Question 6, girls comprised 43% and boys comprised 57%. Regarding Question 9, the average of students per each class unit was 9.8% and the number of students for each teacher was 7. Regarding Question 10, 62% of the classrooms had auditory amplification.

These figures tell us that the auditory methods are expanding in spite of the fact that some of the classrooms with amplification are not used because of resistance of some of the teachers of the deaf. The averages of seven children for each teacher or the 9.8% children per class are also significant figures that indicate that Spain is within the international standards. It is important that these figures should be maintained in order to provide the necessary intensive care to meet needs of each deaf child.

FUNDAMENTAL ROLE OF AUDIOLOGIST, PHONIATRIST, AND PSYCHOLOGIST

Through these questionnaires it became apparent that the most important centers in the country have professionals on their staffs. Actually 50% of the centers have phoniatrists, 40% have audiologists and psychologists, and the remaining 10% of the centers also have pediatricians, psychiatrists, otorhinolaryngolists, dentists, and ophthalmologists.

HEARING AIDS USAGE

Of the 2,282 children within the 24 centers surveyed, only 845 (57%) habitually use hearing aids. In our opinion, this is too low a percentage considering the predominant status of the audiophonatory habilitation method. On the other hand, the hearing aid involves continuous and constant technical maintenance.

Sometimes one might think that the hearing aid is not too useful, but a close look may reveal that the problem is that the child has turned off his hearing aid or that the batteries are low, etc. Also, it should be noted that hearing aids are being improved through better design and testing which increase their potential for use. A feature very much in fashion lately is the usage of bilateral hearing aids, similar to the ocular correction. With this bilateral prosthesis not only does the child receive greater auditory amplification, but also he can also locate the source of sound more easily. This stereophonic audition is used presently within classrooms provided with amplification. Of course, this demands the existence of two microphones.

AGES OF ADMISSION AND TERMINATION

The minimum age of admission of the deaf child to these habilitation centers is at 3–4 years of age. This is true for 13 of the 24 centers surveyed. Percentage of children admitted at 3 years of age is 21% and at 4 years is 33%, making a total of 54% for this range of ages. This makes clear the tendency to begin the habilitation process as soon as possible. In two of the 24 centers surveyed, it was found that they admitted children 2 years old or younger. This training is given for 2.5 hours each morning and continues at home by the parents, under the guidance of the clinician.

It was found that 16.5% of the centers will not admit the child until he is 6 years old, and 8% of the centers surveyed establish the admission age of 7–8 years. In our opinion, these requirements are superseded by modern standards.

The obligatory age for termination of training depends fundamentally on the philosophy and the objectives of the habilitation program of each center. Approximately 46% of the centers surveyed in Spain have set this age at 18 years, whereas 12.5% have set it between 15 and 16 years. The author does not agree with this because, if the habilitation process has an early start, the child at age of 9 or 10 years should be integrated into a normal school where he can interact with normal hearing children.

This ideal objective seems too far and unreachable for many professionals in this field. Their limited objective is to provide the deaf child with a practical trade, in such a way he may become self-sufficient in spite of the fact that he must live a life segregated from the world of normal hearing people.

In the opinion of the author, this is the wrong approach. All habilitation programs should be aimed at obtaining the maximum social integration. In order to accomplish this, proper information should be given not only to the professionals but also to the handicapped people and to their families and to society in general, in order that everyone becomes aware of the handicapped and prepared to receive those who are habilitated into a normal life. It seems that the Congress of Minusval held in Spain in February 1974 will contribute toward this ideal goal.

METHODS UTILIZED

While the oral and lipreading methods are used with about 50% of the total deaf persons habilitated and rehabilitated, the other 50% are trained with a variety of methods other than the two already mentioned. However, the acoustic method is expanded and gaining support day by day, even with the most reluctant teachers of the deaf. The reason is that the results relative to the language structure and timbre of the voice are exceedingly superior to the results obtained by any other method. The usage of the audiophonatory circuit, even though meager, always improves the communication of the deaf person. In this context, one premise should be absolutely clear and fundamental to everyone: amplification, filtered or not, does not suffice. Training on discrimination and on the fundamental parameters of the auditory function is always necessary. Incidentally, the auditory function can be developed early in the deaf child through proper training. This goal should be the basic one irrespective of the type of methodology employed.

TRADE SCHOOLS FOR DEAF CHILDREN

Only 37.45% of the centers surveyed offer programs providing trade instruction for deaf children. The author considers these programs a valuable contribution; however, he adheres to the philosophy already discussed, namely, that of directing effort in the centers toward the goal of total integration of the deaf child into the normal world. With this in mind, the trade programs are not in keeping with this philosophy.

The different trades taught and the percentage of trainees involved are as follows: (1) woodworkers, 32.28%; (2) seamstress, 20.80%; (3) electricians, 16.64%; (4) needlepointing, 16.64%; (5) binding, mechanics, draft, tailoring, and cooking, 12.48%; (6) barbers, ceramics, shoemaking, 8.32%; (7) dental mechanics, watchmakers, photographers, plumbers, painters, locksmiths, printers, masonry, body-shop repairmen, 4.16%.

There are actually quite a variety of trades a deaf student can select according to his or her aptitude.

PREDOMINANT POSTHABILITATION LANGUAGE

Approximately 79% of the trainees use audiophonatory language, and 83.2% complement that language with lipreading. The sign language is currently used by 16.64% of the deaf people who rely on the alphabetic type and 4.16% on the ideomotor one.

We estimate that these statistics are tenuous, considering that the sign language is very much utilized by the deaf when they communicate among themselves, even though they use speech when they try to communicate with the normal listener.

Lately there is a trend to impose a universal gesture language that would allow all the deaf persons of the world to communicate among themselves very easily, a kind of esperanto for the deaf. It is the opinion of the writer that this segregational movement has a poor chance of succeeding.

Again, we reiterate that the goal of any program of habilitation for deaf children, whatever the method used, must be aimed toward the total integration in society at the most efficient level possible.

INTERPROFESSIONAL RELATIONSHIPS

Relationship between professionals of audiology and habilitation and rehabilitation of deaf persons ought to be very close and cordial, especially because of the great difficulties encountered in diagnosing deafness in children. The writer believes that presently only the most important centers in Spain have the potential for making truly accurate diagnoses through teamwork. The minimum staff for this task should be composed of an otorhinolaryngologist, a neuropediatrician, a phoniatrist, an audiologist, an electroencephalographer, and a psychologist. The logopedist and the teacher of the deaf not only need an accurate diagnosis but also should receive the candidate for training already fitted with the proper hearing aid. They need, as well, periodic checks of the effects of training. These checks should be provided by the audiologist, phoniatrist, and psychologist. Sometimes these checks may rectify a wrong diagnosis or prognosis. Any center of minimal status should include a psychologist and an audiophoniatric physician on its staff, who should be able to perform these periodic checks. However, sometimes a neuropediatrician or a neuropsychiatrist should be called as consultants to solve special problems.

During recent years, most professionals are becoming convinced of the need to interact more closely in order to increase the efficiency of the habilitation processes for the deaf and to avoid, as much as possible, errors of diagnosis. These errors or particular approaches when professionals work in isolation are very perturbing for the parents of the deaf child because they seem to believe that every professional who examines their child discovers a different impairment.

To summarize, the author believes strongly that the intensification of the interprofessional relationships among the professionals and social workers involved in the training of deaf persons will bring about a better human approach to the problem as well as a greater success.

PARTICIPATION OF THE DEAF PERSON'S FAMILY IN HIS/HER TREATMENT

Years ago the parents of a deaf child did not become involved with the training program or therapy. Presently parents are counseled as early as possible in order that they can become efficient collaborators in the process of habilitation of their child. And so, immediately after the diagnosis of deafness is established in a child several months old, parents are instructed by a phoniatrist or audiologist as to how to produce a series of auditory training exercises in order to help stimulate the residual hearing of the child. When this child reaches the age of 3 years, he then can be referred to a specialized center to continue with a more technical program.

This period of pretraining by the parents serves also to convey to them and to have them understand the magnitude and difficulties of the problem. Parents should be informed of the progress attained through the exercises they give to their child; in this way they are rewarded and their interest does not wane. Communication with the parents must be maintained continuously, providing them with complete reports on the results of the habilitation program and on how to improve communication with the child, etc. Vacation periods, like Christmas or Holy Week, when the child is taken home, are most appropriate for the parents to put into practice what they have learned about communication with the deaf child. Weekends in Spain are the best days for the clinician to counsel the parents.

Summer vacation should not interfere with the continuity of the habilitative program. Parents should continue at home putting into practice the "real life" communication with the infant, even if he is being tutored by a third party. Parents should understand the value of "spontaneous communication" for ultimate success of habilitation of deaf children. These notions must be emphasized at all times to the parents, to avoid their withdrawal from this duty because of different excuses, such as "too much pressure," "no time because of profession or work," etc.

Since January 1974, a monthly magazine, *PROAS*, published by The Fundacion General Mediterranea (Institute for Assistance to the Deaf), has appeared with the goal of providing the parents of deaf children with this type of knowledge and understanding of the problem. This journal serves also as a means of disseminating information on what the deaf can give to society in general. The image of the deaf person in Spain may improve through the positive action of *PROAS*. Some congresses invite parents of deaf children to participate in their sessions, for example, the First Symposium of Auditory Reeducation held in Barcelona, November 23–26, 1972. This participation may be encouraged; however, there is a danger of creating too great an involvement with parents who may exert pressures on the habilitative programs, in the belief that their recommendations are the right ones. This should not occur since parents are not experts in audiology. Being at the same time the judge and the defendant may lead to recommendations of new and miraculous procedures, not sufficiently tested, and, thus, make a guinea pig of the deaf child. This danger should be avoided, although the dialogue of clinician with parents should always be encouraged.

The relatives of an adult who became deaf also can participate in his/her rehabilitation. They should be taught how to communicate with the deaf relative, i.e., to speak slowly, loudly, with excellent articulation and facing the patient, in order that he can lipread with a minimum of difficulty. Relatives should be shown, in a dramatic way, the problems of the adult deaf, for example by providing for them various experiences that the deaf must endure.

TRAINING OF PROFESSIONALS IN THE FIELD OF HABILITATIVE AND REHABILITATIVE AUDIOLOGY

The audiologist as an independent professional does not exist in Spain. Audiology is a specialty within otorhinolaryngology. Pediatric audiology, as opposed to adult audiology, demands the exclusive dedication of some former otorhinolaryngologist. On the other hand, the physician phoniatrist, who does not receive formal training within the Spanish universities, always is an autodidact, like the Spanish pioneer in this field, Dr. Jorge Perello, who has been responsible for the development of this discipline in Spain. The assistants of the phoniatrists, the logopedists, have no available formal training programs here either. If they are teachers, they may pursue some special courses offered by the Ministry of Education and Sciences. After completion, they receive a diploma of Teacher for the Handicapped. Some informal training sessions on logopedics are offered also by the

Social Security Office. On the other hand, there exist in Spain the teachers of the deaf who obtain their certification by completing brief courses dealing with habilitative pedagogy for deaf children.

Graduates from the Faculty of Philosophy may specialize in special pedagogy by taking some courses offered by the Faculty of Medicine. They are, for all practical purposes, in a worse professional situation than those teachers with a degree in pedagogy for the handicapped.

From this information the reader may conclude that it is imperative that Spanish universities offer formal programs for both the phoniatrist and the logopedist. If this happens in the future, a grandfather clause should be established to protect the present practitioners who did not receive formal training.

RESEARCH

Research in audiology and speech sciences has not received official attention in Spain. Therefore, the only research done in this field is on a private basis exclusively.

One of the private institutions, concerned with research in the field of the habilitative audiology, was ARANS, organized from November 23–26, 1972, in Barcelona, the First International Symposium of Auditory Reeducation. This symposium was focused upon research and provided for useful interchange of experiences among persons engaged in research.

In spite of the lack of formal research programs, the author believes that the practice of habilitative audiology in Spain is comparable to that existing in some other countries. Some Spanish studies are appreciated abroad, although most of the audiological knowledge in Spain is imported.

Universities in Spain have the responsibility and the duty to promote and encourage research in our field, in order to produce men of the stature of Thomas Navarro, whose contributions to phonetics have transcended our national borders. Linguistic research could have a two-fold purpose in Spain: (1) to find the proper structures to habilitate linguistically the language impaired child, and (2) to teach Spanish properly to foreigners. These certainly are not easy tasks, but they should be undertaken in the future.

ASSOCIATIONS CONCERNED WITH DEAF AND HYPOACUSIC PERSONS

We have already discussed the existence of Associations of Parents of Deaf Children in Spain and the publication of the magazine *PROAS*, edited by the Fundacion General Mediterranea, the purpose of which is to inform and to create groups of parents. There is presently a tendency to create similar associations in many Spanish provinces.

The author would like to discuss, in this last section, the Associations of Deaf Adults that exist in many provinces. Goals of these nonprofessional associations are many, but all converge to improve the lives of their handicapped members. Some areas covered by these associations are as follows:

1. Religious. A deaf priest or one specially trained in sign language is in charge of the religious needs of the members.
2. Cultural. These associations maintain a library and offer courses in speech, written language, and arithmetic to the members.
3. Sports. Many sports and games are offered to the members, like football, swimming, baseball, gymnastics, ping-pong, and chess. Many of these associations participate in an annual contest organized by the Committee on Silent Sports.
4. Recreational. Mime theater, special films, cultural tours, and excursions are currently offered to the members.

All of these activities are facilitated and centralized through their association headquarters. Some of these associations possess excellent and functional buildings, as the Association of Gijon, erected in 1950 with funds from the Spanish Development III Plan. Other associations are housed in more humble headquarters, provided often by the local municipality, as in the case of the Association of Sabadell.

All of these associations are members of the National Federation of Spanish Associations of Deaf-Mutes with headquarters in Madrid. There are 45 associations for the deaf-mute in Spain, with 4,000–5,000 members totally. Approximately 55% of the members are male and 45% are female. The oldest association is the one in Zaragoza, founded in 1932. It is interesting to point out that members come from different social classes, but all of them interact on equal bases within their associations.

Funds to sustain these associations are always scarce. The sources of income are the social dues and donations of patrons. Even with meager funds, all these associations are able to fulfill their goals effectively and with great enthusiasm.

These associations are very meritorious indeed; however, the author sees a potential danger that deaf people may become segregated from society in general. These clubs could eventually become a "ghetto" by grouping together only handicapped people.

The Congress Minusval 74 recommended against this type of segregation. In keeping with this notion, it is interesting to point out the presentation of Professor Hellbrügge of Munich at the First Spanish-German Symposium for the Rehabilitation of the Child with Psychomotor Deficit, held in Valencia in May 1974. Professor Hellbrügge reported that all centers in Munich for habilitation of deaf children related to the local university have their pupils interacting a couple of hours each day with other handicapped children (cerebral palsied, retarded, etc.) and with nonhandicapped children in the proportion of one-third handicapped and two-thirds nonhandicapped. After 3 years of experience with this program, Professor Hellbrügge reported that the parents of the nonhandicapped children were most enthusiastic about the exposure their sons and daughters were able to have with handicapped children. They felt that this opportunity provided their children with a unique and important social learning experience. It is felt by the author that this early interaction may help to destroy the roots of segregation that, if allowed to grow, poison the entire society.

ACKNOWLEDGMENTS

The writer acknowledges the Associations of the Deaf of Cordoba, Gijon, Leon, Las Palmas de Gran Canaria, Sabadell, and Zaragoza, who helped to provide the data for this chapter.

SCHOOLS FOR DEAF CHILDREN THAT EXIST IN SPAIN

1. Centro de Educacion Especial, Merida (Badajoz).
2. Colegio de Sordomudos, Salas, 46, Palma de Mallorca (Baleares).
3. Instituto Educativo de Sordomudos y Ciegos de "La Purisima" Pase General Mola, 8, Barcelona.
4. Centro de Reeducacion diferencial "San Guillermo" Tolra, 23, (Horta) Barcelona.
5. Centro Piloto de Reeducacion Auditiva, Verdi, 254 (Torre) Barcelona.
6. Instituto Catalan de Sordomudos, San Fructuoso, 71, Barcelona.
7. Centro de Audicion y Lenguaje, Descartes, 6, Barcelona.
8. Colegio de Sordomudos, Madrid, 45, Burgos.
9. Instituto Psicopedagogico "Cruz Roja-Afanas," Beata M[a] Soledad, 9, Cadiz.
10. Hogar Provincial "San Vicente," Plaza Fradell, 3, Castellon.
11. Escuela Especial de Sordomudos, Isabel Cabral, 9, Ceuta.
12. Colegio Provincial de Sordomudos. "Ponce de Leon," Doña Berenguela, 4, Cordoba.
13. Instituto de Lenguaje, Almendro, 6, Cordoba.
14. Colegio de Sordomudos, Marques de Amboague, 1, La Coruña.
15. Colegio Regional de Sordomudos, San Cayetano, s/n., Santiago de Compostela (La Coruña).
16. Escuela para Sordomudos, Colon, 2, Cuenca.

17. Centro de Reeducacion del Lenguaje e Hipoacusia, Martinez Campos, 20-2°-izqda, Granada.
18. Colegio Especial "Sagrada Familia," Carretera de la Sierra, 1, Granada.
19. Asociacion de Reeducacion Auditiva "Arans-Gui" Alto de San Bartolome, San Sebastian (Guipuzcoa).
20. Escuelas del Patronato "San Miguel," Eibar (Guipuzcoa).
21. Centro de Educacion Especial para Deficientes del Lenguaje, Ceron, 21, Jaen.
22. Colegio de Sordomudos, Hospicio, 4, Astorga (Leon).
23. Hogar "San Jose," Plaza San Jose, s/n., Lerida.
24. Hogar Provincial, Marques de Murrieta, 80, Logroño.
25. Colegio Provincial "Santa Maria," Primo de Rivera, Lugo.
26. Colegio Nacional de Sordomudos, San Mateo, 5, Madrid.
27. Instituto Nacional de Pedagogia Terapeutica, General Oraa, 49, Madrid.
28. Instituto Municipal de Educacion, Mejia Lequerica, 21, Madrid.
29. Colegio Nacional "Claudio Moyano," cea Bermudez, Madrid.
30. Dispensario Central de Rehabilitation, Maudes, 32, Madrid.
31. Colegio "San Gabriel," Arturo Soria, 165, Madrid.
32. Colegio de la Purisima, Alcala, 215, Madrid.
33. Colegio de la Purisima, Ricardo Ortiz, Madrid.
34. Instituto Hispano Americano de la Palabra, Carril del Conde, 51, Madrid.
35. Instituto de Sordomudos "Ponce de Leon," Cardenal Cisneros, 61, Madrid.
36. Instituto de Sordomudos "Ponce de Leon," Los Negrales, Madrid.
37. Foniatria y Logopedia, Alfonso XIII, 164, Madrid.
38. Instituto de Ortofonia, Encinar, 12, Madrid.
39. Colegio de la Purisma, Morales Villarubia, Gamarra, Malaga.
40. Instituto Psicopedagogico "Dulce Nombre de Maria," Amador de los Rios, Malaga.
41. Casa Jose Antonio (Hogar Provincial del Niño) Acisclo Diaz, 8, Murcia.
42. Colegio Nacional Hermanos San Isidoro y Santa Florentina (Clases Especiales), Cartagena (Murcia).
43. Instituto Canossiano, Colegio de Sordomudos, Ezcaba, s/n., Chantrea, Pamplona (Navarra).
44. Instituto Pedagogico para Niños Anormales y Sordomudos, Magdelena, s/n., Junto al Portal de Francia, Pamplona (Navarra).
45. Colegio Fundacion Vinjoy de la "Sagrada Familia," Carretera del Cristo de las Cadenas, s/n., Oviedo (Asturias).
46. Centro de Educacion Especial "Jovellanos" Plaza Generalisimo, 8.2^{o}, Gijon (Asturias).
47. Sanatorio Martimo "San Bernardo y San Hermenegilgo" Colonia de Piles, Gijon (Asturias).
48. Colegio de Sordomudos, Granadera Canaria, Las Palmas de Gran Canaria (Las Palmas).
49. Colegio de Sordomudos, Palencia.

50. Colegio Provincial de Sordomudos, La Lanzada, El Grove, Pontevedra.
51. Residencia Provincial de Niños "San Jose," Vergara, 26, Salamanca.
52. Colegio del Corazon de Maria, Perez Galdos, 15, Santa Cruz de Tenerife (Tenerife).
53. Instituto "Padre Apolinar," Avenida Maura, 1, Santander.
54. Instituto Padre Apolinar, Paseo General Davila, 9, Santander.
55. Centro de Rehabilitacion y Educacion "Jesus del Gran Poder" Avenida Eduardo Dato, 30, Sevilla.
56. Residencia Escuela "San Luis" Colegio Provincial de Sordomudos, San Luis, 29-35, Sevilla.
57. Instituto de Orientacion Pedagogica "San Rafael" Carretera de Valls, 54, Tarragona.
58. Instituto Medico Pedagogico "Padre Manjon" Virgen de Olivar, 40, Torrente (Valencia).
59. Escuela Unitaria de Sordomudos, Pintor Fillol, 10, Valencia.
60. Asilo Hospital "San Juan de Dios," Senda de la Capelleta, 43, Valencia.
61. Colegio "San Jose," Sr, Sumsi, 3, Valencia.
62. Unidad de Educacion Especial, Na Jordana, 45, Valencia.
63. Instituto Valenciano de Sordomudos, Gaspar Torrela, 27, Valencia.
64. Centro de Ortofonia "Traspalvox," Sumacarcel (Valencia).
65. Centro Auditivo Montcabrer, Madre Carlota de Santa Teresa, s/n., Godella (Valencia).
66. Instituto Medico Pedagogico "San Juan de Dios" Carretera de Madrid, Km, 186, Valladolid.
67. Obra Social del Santuario Nacional, Jose Mª Lacort 9, Valladolid.
68. Centro de Educacion Especial, Basauri (Vizcaya).
69. Colegio de Niños Subnormales "La Casilla," Plaza Calvo Sotelo, Bilbao (Vizcaya).
70. Colegio de Sordomudos de Vizcaya, Avenida Madariaga, 72, Deusto (Vizcaya).
71. Escuelas de Educacion Especial "General Varela" Durango (Vizcaya).
72. Centro de Educacion Especial "Angel Iturricha" San Juan de la Cruz, 57, Bilbao (Vizcaya).
73. Colegio de al Purisima, Corona de Aragon, 54, Zaragoza.
74. Colegio de la Consolacion (Para Sordomudos) Castellon de la Plana.
75. Colegio Provincial de Sordomudos (Diputacion Provincial) Calle de Sevilla, 13, Cordoba.
76. Sanatorio Infantil de "Santa Angel," Cordoba.
77. Colegio Regional de Sordomudos (Diputacion Provincial), Santiago de Compostela.
78. Colegio de Sordomudos de Santa Cruz de Tenerife, Tenerife.
79. Colegio de Sordomudos, Caballeros, 19, Castellon de la Plana.
80. Colegio de Sordomudos (Casa Beneficencia Patronato) Sor Valentina Elola, Cuenca.
81. Escuela Municipal de Sordomudos, de Gijon, Gijon.
82. Colegio de Sordomudos de Rr. Franciscanas, Camino de son Rapina, s/n., Palma de Mallorca.

83. Colegio de las RRTT Franciscanas, Arzobispo Mayoral, 4, Valencia.
84. Centro de Reeducacion Auditiva de Sabadell, Parque Tauli, Samuntada, Sabadell.
85. Centro Municipal Fonoaudiologico "Jose M[a] de Porcioles" Parque de Montjuich, Barcelona-4.
86. Instituto Nacional de Pedagogia de Sordos, Carretera de Vicalvaro, Km. 2,3, (Gran San Blas) Madrid, 32.
87. Colegio Provincial de Sordomudos, Paseo de Campoamor, 6, Alicante.

SOCIETIES FOR THE DEAF THAT EXIST IN SPAIN

1. Accion Catolica de Sordumudos de Madrid, Cardenal Cisneros, 61, Madrid-10.
2. Accion Catolica de Sordumudos de Baleares, Jeronimo Rossello, 75-A, Palma de Mallorca.
3. Accion Catolica de Sordumudos, Valencia, 358-principal-1[a], Barcelona-9.
4. Agrupacion de Sordumudos de la Comarca del Llobregat, Buenos Aires,27, Hospitalet de Llobregat.
5. Casa del Sordomudo de Barcelona, Neuva de D. Francisco, 9-principal-1[a], Barcelona.
6. Casa del Sordomudo de Manresa Y Comarca, Sobrerroca, 28, Manresa.
7. Centro de Altatorre, San Marcelo, 5, Madrid-17.
8. Sociedad Federada de Sordomudos, Marques de Moya, 1, Malaga.
9. Agrupacion de Sordomudos de Zaragoza, Arzobispo Soldevilla, 2, Zaragoza.
10. Asociacion de Sordomudos de Oviedo, Campomanes, 17-bajos, Oviedo (Asturias).
11. Asociacion Provincial de Sordomudos, San Miguel, 8-bajos, Cadiz.
12. Asociacion de Sordomudos de Gijon, Dindura, 33-1[o]-A, Gijon.
14. Hogar del Sordomudos de Lerida, Avenida Garrigas, 15-1[o]-1[a], Lerida.
15. Asociacion de Sordomudose de Tenerife, Viera Y Clavijo, 32, Santa Cruz de Tenerife (Canarias).
16. Agrupacion de Sordomudos de Granada, Recogidas, 13-1[a], Granada.
17. Asociacion de Sordomudos de Elche, Comisario, 2, Elche (Alicante).
18. Asociacion de Sordomudos de Toledo, Circo Ramano, 16, Toledo.
19. Federacion Nacional de Sordomudos, Beneficencia, 18, Madrid-4.
20. Asociacion de Sordomudos de Jerez de la Frontera, Angel Mayo, 21-2[o], Jerez de la Frontera.
21. Asociacion Valenciana de Sordomudos, Llano de la Zaidia, 18, Valencia-9.
22. Asociacion de Sordomudos de Sevilla, Conde de Ibarra, 10, Sevilla.
23. Union de Sordomudos de Guipuzcoa, San Juan, 14, San Sebastian.
24. Accion Catolica de Sordomudos, Viciana, 8, Valencia.
25. Agrupacion de Sordomudos de Vich, Riera, 31-bajos, Vich (Barcelona).
26. Asociacion de Sordomudos de Vigo, Callejon del Estrecho, 22, Vigo (Pontevedra).

27. Sociedad de Socorros Mutuos entre Los Sordomudos, San Fructuoso, 71, Barcelona-4.
28. Comite de Deportes de la F.N. S.S.E., Beneficencia, 18-bis, Madrid-4.
29. Asociacion de Sordomudos de Vizcaya, Zabalburu, 3-bajos-derecha, Bilbao-12.
30. Asociacion de Sordomudos de Bilbao, Santo Domingo de Guzman, 11, Bilbao.
31. Asociacion de Sordomudos de Vallodolid, 18 de Julio, 42-bajos, Valladolid.
32. Asociacion Provincial de Sordomudos de Cordoba, San Fernando, 20, Cordoba.
33. Asociacion de Sordomudos de Sabadell, Perez Galdos, 110, Sabadell (Barcelona).
34. Asociacion de Sordomudos de Caceres, Medina, 1, Plasencia (Caceres).
35. Asociacion de Sordomudos de Pamplona, Magdalena, 8-1º-derecha, Pamplona (Navarra).
36. Asociacion de Sordomudos de Santander, Los Escalantes, 5, Santander.
37. Agrupacion Salmantina de Sordomudos, Avenida de Mirat, 12, Salamanca.
38. Asociacion de Sordomudos "Fray Ponce de Leon," Paseo de la Quinta, 13, Burgos.
39. Asociacion de Sordomudos de Langreo, Gregorio Aurre, 7, La Felguera (asturias).
40. Asociacion de Sordomudos de Alcoy, Poeta Arolas, 3, Alcoy (Alicante).
41. Asociacion de Sordomudos de Leon, Avenida Fose Maria Fernandez, 3, Leon.
42. Centro de Sordomudos de Alava, Beato Tomas de Zumarraga, 30, Vitoria.
43. Asociacion de Sordomudos de las Palmas de Gran Canaria, Agustina de Argon, 13, Las Palmas de Gran Canaria.
44. Agrupacion de Sordomudos de la Coruña, Barrio de Las Flores, Bloque, 34, commercial, 76, La Coruña.

LITERATURE CITED

Perello, J., and F. Tortosa. 1968. Sordomudez Ed. Cientifico-Medica, Barcelona.

chapter 9

Communication for Hearing-handicapped People in Sweden

Tore Lundborg, M.D.

Impaired communication related to hearing disorders of any type has profound sociological effects, which are particularly apparent and for a long time recognized in children, but, when acquired in adults, also cause grave social consequences. However, the latter group constitutes the larger number of the patients and will be stressed in this chapter.

PHILOSOPHICAL POSITION OF WRITER IN RELATION TO CLINICAL PERFORMANCE OF AUDIOLOGICAL ACTIVITIES

The size of the problem is not readily apparent and can only be estimated for the population. Although exact statistics on the matter are not available, the experience from several western countries indicates that the number of the total population needing audiological service of any kind, i.e., with socially significant hearing loss, is approximately 4%, whereas profound prelingual deafness in children is thought to be on the order of 1–2/1,000 live births. The latter patient group, although from every point of view important, constitutes statistically only a relatively small minority of the case material with hearing and communication problems. The preschool children with profound deafness have been taken care of rather adequately in most countries through different types of organizations and, as a rule also, long before there have been available corresponding audiological activities for all other patient groups needing audiological attention.

It is difficult and also somewhat confusing to try to compare the institutional structures, staffs, and programs of different audiological units, hospital based or not, since case materials, goals, and scientific or training interests, etc., in many respects, are vastly different. When observing these units, it is obvious that, for these reasons, any evaluation on a scale of efficiency or suitability never would be meaningful.

On the other hand, in the framework of an international perspective, it seems meaningful to present experiences gained from a hospital-based audiological unit with activities, institutional capacity, and structure of staff well defined. Such an organization is based on the thinking that an organization which is thought to be relevant to the management of hearing loss patients, including staff training and research aspects, can only be based on the problems as they exist in the field.

The following report is aimed to reflect how audiological clinical programs are utilized by the patient groups needing them with reference to the otolaryngologists referring the patients to the audiological unit of the Department of Audiology, Sodersjukhuset, Stockholm, which in this case is serving an urban area of approximately three-quarters of a million. In many respects, the following description reflects the present status of a Swedish hospital-based audiological unit and its care of hearing-handicapped patients who sustain communication problems.

DEFINITION OF AURAL REHABILITATION

It must be stressed again that the hospital-based audiological organization in Sweden is supposed to take care of hearing-handicapped patients of any age and with any problems that are not handled within a traditional otolaryngological department. Thus, these patients are for the most part referred by otologists and, to some extent also, by neurologists, pediatricians, etc. At the risk of oversimplification, it might perhaps be said that hospital-based audiology is a consequence of recent remodeling of otology, from which it is functionally derived. This holds at least in the sense that the doctors starting the above-mentioned audiological activities within the hospital units, using a multidisciplinary staff, were trained otologists, who also, after having acquired experience, became self-made audiologists. The program of activities, as mentioned, is medically based, and the task is diagnosis, therapy, and prophylaxis of the hearing loss and communication problems in the patient groups concerned. These activities, on the other hand, do not cover the educational activities necessary to take care of hearing-handicapped children nor the vocational needs for young and adult hearing handicapped. These particular programs are handled by school or vocational authorities and are performed outside the hospital.

HISTORICAL OVERVIEW AND GENERAL DESCRIPTION OF PRESENT PROGRAMS

Faced with foreign achievements in the field of hearing rehabilitation and electronics and with the results of rapidly developing modern otosurgery, the Swedish government in 1954 passed an act authorizing audiological service to be developed by the setting up of audiological departments, connected to otolaryngological departments, and run by medical authorities. In practice, these institutions were to be structured on the basis of medical, technical, pedagogic, and social teamwork under medical guidance.

Supplementary medicolegal decisions have regulated the prescription of hearing aids as well as of special technical devices in addition to hearing aids and further the aural rehabilitation required (often referred to as *audiopedic measures*), i.e., instructional courses in the use and handling of the hearing aid as well as the functional rehabilitation in the form of auditory training, speech correction, sign language, etc.

Specialists with training in these audiopedic activities (referring to therapeutic measures with the hearing-handicapped patients, excluding educational and vocational activities) have successively completed the staffs of the audiological departments.

Audiological Departments: Structure and Staff

In Sweden, clinical audiology is a medical specialty. The activities of an audiological department, as mentioned above, are based on the joint efforts by staff members from the fields of medicine, technology, psychology, and pedagogics, as well as social work.

This system was adapted in Sweden during the 1950's from Danish models and was remodeled in certain respects. Several activities followed other directions of development. Both institutional structure and programs show many local variations.

It differs considerably from the pattern of U.S. centers, where the staff usually has several members holding university degrees in nonmedical disciplines and the head frequently is a Ph.D. In Swedish audiological institutions, *the medical members* are ear, nose, and throat (ENT) specialists with complementary training in audiology. They handle much of the diagnostic work with both conductive and sensorineural hearing loss patients. In some institutions they also participate in otosurgery and, furthermore, they take part in training programs, administration, etc.

An important member of the doctor's staff is the *audiological assistant,* who performs audiometry of various kinds, as well as hearing aid fitting, etc. The assistant is not university educated, but has a basic training period of 1 year, and functions in much the same manner as the laboratory assistant in radiological or chemical laboratories.

The engineers, mostly electronic engineers of the M.A. or B.A. level, are in charge of the electronic and electroacoustic equipments used in diagnostic and therapeutic purposes. They perform part of the diagnostic work and also participate as technical instructors and advisers.

Service technicians handle the control and repair of hearing aids, installation and control of special devices, earmold preparation, etc.

The hearing aid dealers serve mainly as importers and distributors of hearing aids. The direct distribution of hearing aids to the audiological departments and hearing centers is mostly handled by the Purchasing Center of the Swedish County Councils, which is a nonhospital organization for distribution, service, repair, etc. of various types of hospital equipment. The organization also has service units in connection with hospitals or within the hospital localities throughout Sweden for repair of hearing aids, installation of special devices for hearing handicapped, etc.

The *hearing pedagogues-"audiopedes"* perform the therapeutic work and give instruction courses concerning the communication instruments recommended and functional training to compensate for impaired communication, i.e., auditory training, speech reading, etc.

Social workers and, if available, *psychologists* handle the psychosocial measures necessary to compensate the hearing handicap.

In Sweden, with a population of approximately 8 million, there are 11 fully staffed audiological departments with the 11 largest otolaryngological (ENT) departments. There are, furthermore, 38 hearing centers, connected to the same departments of the county hospital, staffed with part of the above mentioned specialist team (Figure 1).

Activities of Audiological Institutions Connected to Hospitals

As previously mentioned, the Department of Audiology, Sodersjukhuset, differs from many other audiological units because of the medical structure chosen, i.e., combining clinical diagnostic work, partly otological, with hearing aid fitting and aural rehabilitation. The experiences reported, of course, are reflecting the structure chosen.

With sufficient institutional capacity available, patients with any hearing problem suspected or manifested at any age may be referred to the audiological department. This implies principally all well known diagnostic, therapeutic, and prophylactic audiological measures, based on medical admissions, but, as mentioned earlier, excluding educational and vocational tasks.

While in the past concerned primarily with diagnostic work-ups and hearing aid fitting of patients with both conductive and sensorineural hearing loss, at the present time more and more of the activities outlined above have been realized, but with many local variations. It is to be hoped

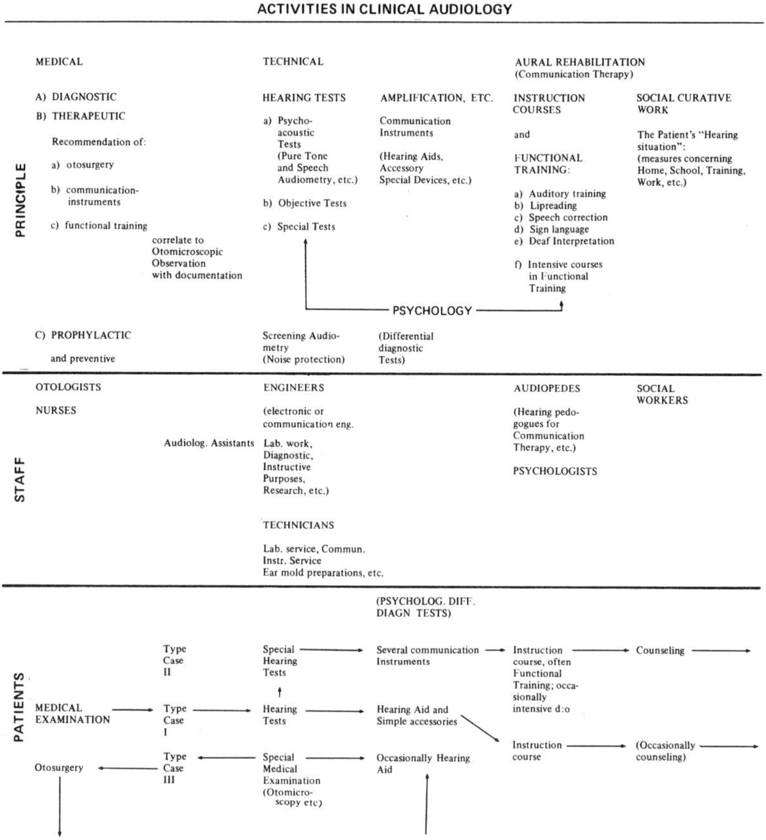

Figure 1. Sketch of audiological activities. Working principles, staff members concerned, and therapeutic measures in various types of cases.

that within a period of 10 years all the needed audiological activities can be taken care of by adequately trained and experienced audiological staff members.

Staff and Case Material

The caseload taken care of and the size of staff performing the service may give an idea of the activities.

There are approximately 40 full-time staff members and part-time consultants working within the unit and additionally 10–15 technicians for hearing aid service, installation of special devices, and ear mold preparations.

Clinical Investigations

In 1973, there were 714 patients referred for preoperative evaluation of *transmission hearing loss* with operative performance in either of the otolaryngological departments of Sodersjukhuset and Sabbatsberg.

In 1973, 549 patients were referred for diagnosis of *sensorineural hearing loss* with further clinical care, if necessary, in the otolaryngological departments or occasionally within the neurological clinics.

Both of these groups of patients are handled within the clinical diagnostic section of the department of audiology by otologists, nurses, electronic engineers, and audiological assistants.

For clinical and didactic reasons, the communication between the audiological and otolaryngological departments is arranged as weekly staff meetings in each of the latter units, and all cases of particular interest are demonstrated in slides with documentation of essential facts, including color photos of every middle ear lesion. This work is rather time consuming but is found to be necessary for optimal otoaudiological cooperation.

A practical and economical consequence of these arrangements is that very few clinical evaluations, approximately 10 out of 1,000 admissions, have to be performed with the patient hospitalized.

Hearing Aid Fitting

Patients admitted for hearing aid fitting, for other communication instruments, and for functional and rehabilitative training constitute the largest group. In 1973, 3,705 patients were fitted with hearing aids. Of these, 3,500 patients were fitted with 10,500 special devices in addition to the hearing aids. The hearing-aid-fitting procedures are performed by audiological assistants within the hearing center; the other services mentioned are taken care of within the audiopedic section by either hearing pedagogues (audiopedes) or electronic engineers (Figure 1).

Other Patient Groups

School children service is based mainly on admissions as a result of regular screening procedures within the schools. Each pupil is screened during his 1st, 4th, and 7th year. During 1973 there were 451 visits.

Preschool children service is given to admissions from the pediatric care service, particularly in connection with the control program of all 4-year-old children within Stockholm. During 1973 there were 425 visits.

Patients with noise-induced hearing loss, whose admissions are based on a recently passed insurance act aiming to benefit patients with severe communication problems of this type, are also seen.

An ambulant audiological service to screen (and take care of) all noise-exposed industrial employees has been planned and discussed for many years, but so far nothing of the service is realized.

DIAGNOSTIC PROCEDURES

The diagnostic procedures in a hospital-based audiological unit of the type described cover a wide range of lesions. For obvious reasons, the performance of tests and the interpretation of test results require cooperation from several medical, as well as nonmedical, staff members.

The audiological examination constitutes one part of a broad medical examination also including such contributions as otoneurological, neurological, and roentgenological.

The task of the diagnostic procedures is to assess the type of hearing loss according to pure-tone-audiogram/hearing threshold level (HTL) and discomfort level (DCL) as a function of frequency/and speech-audiogram/ speech reception threshold (SRT) and discrimination score, considering also the relation between pure tone and speech audiogram. Is the hearing loss of organic or functional type? In organic hearing loss, where is the site of lesion (conductive, cochlear, retrocochlear, or situated within the central nervous system)? With conductive lesions, there is assessment of reduced sound collection because of drum perforation, reduced sound conduction because of rigidity or interruption of chain, and further reduced sound protection in patients with large drum perforation and exposed labyrinth windows, i.e., "window hearing" cases, etc.

With sensorineural lesions, do the findings suggest a cochlear test pattern, a retrocochlear test pattern, or a central hearing loss type? In functional hearing loss, is the psychogenic HL aggravation or malingering?

An additional sociomedical evaluation has to consider the social handicap of the patient's hearing loss (in relation to home, school, training, work, etc.).

Assessment of Hearing Loss

In the great majority of adult and young hard-of-hearing patients, the type and severity of hearing loss can be evaluated using customary psychoacoustic tests (pure tone and speech and audiometry, etc.). Objective methods, for instance, impedance tests, are used together with the psychoacoustic tests as an additional part of the test battery. Certain patients who are not cooperating for various reasons require some form of objective audiometry, i.e., ERA. Preschool children (newborn children and, occasionally, fetuses) require special methods (play audiometry, registration of palpebral reflex, change of heart rate during sound stimulation, etc.).

The diagnostic procedures performed in routine clinical praxis will be briefly described and commented upon in connection with Figure 2. In the great majority of cases, these procedures constitute a sufficient basis for therapeutic prescription, i.e.: (1) otosurgical or other medical treatment, (2) hearing aids or other communication instruments, and further (3) audiopedic measures, i.e., instruction and aural rehabilitative measures, occasionally also social counseling. In many cases, there is a need for more than one of these procedures in the same individual. This fact, as experienced over many years in a considerable part of the total patient material handled within the Department of Audiology, Sodersjukhuset, is one main reason for performing the whole diagnostic and therapeutic program within the same clinical framework.

Considering Middle Ear Lesions Otoscopy and conventional pure tone and speech audiometry generally give a clue to the following classification: (1) hearing loss of conductive type and intact drum (CL); (2) hearing loss of conductive type and drum perforation (CL); and (3) hearing loss of sensorineural type (SNL).

It is unnecessary to be reminded of the rather often concomitant presence of both conductive and sensorineural type of hearing loss, occasionally requiring investigation of both these components.

The aim of the procedures is to suggest whether or not a surgical performance is indicated and, if possible, also to suggest the type of operation as described by Lundborg and Linzander (1970).

Some of the most common middle ear lesions with transmission hearing loss encountered in the unit's diagnostic work are briefly commented upon with reference to the otosurgical measures. There were 714 patients in 1973. The evaluation of transmission hearing loss cases attempts to state which of the types of lesions were encountered.

With one single localization of the lesion, either tympanic membrane, stapes or long incudar process, the otosurgical procedure and the expected postoperative result are more favorable than if there is more than one site of lesion. The cochlear function, as well as the tubar function, of course, are also considered as well as the question of whether an operation or a hearing aid is indicated.

Conductive hearing loss with *intact tympanic membrane* has to be evaluated indirectly by otomicroscopy and impedance tests, including the Gelle tests. A test tone in the outer auditory meatus is partly reflected by the tympanic membrane and is partly transmitted through the middle ear,

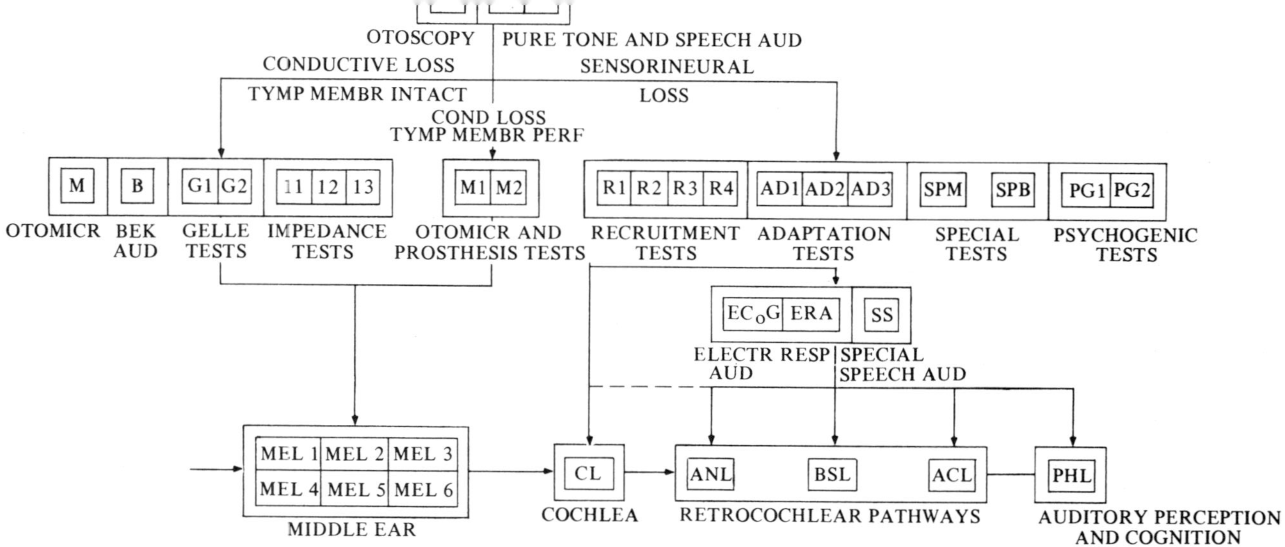

Figure 2. Sketch of the audiological test battery utilized in various types of hearing loss. The procedures: *O*, otoscopy; *A1*, pure tone audiometry (air and bone conduction, etc.); *A2*, speech audiometry (speech reception threshold and speech discrimination). *M*, otomicroscopy; *B*, Bekesy audiometry (continuous and interrupted tone tracing); *G*, Gelle tests (air conduction and bone conduction); *I1*, tympanometry (impedance, absolute value); *I2*, tympanometry (admittance–conductance and susceptance values); *I3*, stapedius reflex registration. *M1*, otomicroscopy and microphotography; *M2*, prosthesis test. *R1*, Bekesy audiometry; *R2*, Fowler test; *R3*, SiSi test; *R4*, other tests. *AD1*, Bekesy audiometry; *AD2*, tone decay test; *AD3*, reflex decay test. *SMP*, monaural difference limen tests; *SPB*, binaural difference limen tests, including auditory localization tests; tests for preschool children. *PG1*, Bekesy audiometry; *PG2*, Lombard, Steger, etc. *ECoG*, electrocochleography (near field or far field); *ERA*, electrical (evoked) response audiometry, especially late response. *SS*, special speech audiometry (speech in noise, distorted speech audiometry, etc.). The Lesions–Middle Ear Lesion: *MEL1*, otosclerosis; *MEL2*, tympanosclerosis, e.g., fixed malleus syndrome, residuae, etc., tympanic membrane intact; *MEL3*, ossicular chain defect tympanic membrane intact; *MEL4*, tympanic membrane perforation (ossicular chain intact); *MEL5*, tympanic membrane perforation and tympanosclerosis; *MEL6*, tympanic membrane perforation and ossicular chain defect. *CL*, cochlear lesion. *ANL*, acoustic nerve lesion; *BSL*, brain stem lesion; *ACL*, auditory cortex lesion. *PHL*, psychogenic hearing loss.

and the latter portion may be perceived by the test subject. In impedance test procedures, the middle ear is evaluated by means of the reflected part of the stimulus; in the Gelle procedure, on the other hand, the transmitted portion of the test stimulus, utilizing fixed frequency Bekesy tracing, is evaluated during pressure variations of the outer meatus. This type of lesion is mostly comprised of: (1) otosclerosis, i.e., fixation of the stapedial footplate in the oval window niche, i.e., MEL (middle ear lesion *A*) in Figure 3. Stapes surgery consists of removal of the fixed stapes, replacing it by a prosthesis, vein and wire or polyethylene tube; in more than nine out of 10 operated cases, these procedures are successful, resulting in normal sound transmission to the inner ear via the "corrected" middle ear; (2) tympanosclerosis, e.g., fixed-malleus syndrome, e.g., fixation of the ossicular chain by formation of tympanosclerotic tissue in the middle ear, for instance, around the malleoincudal articulation, in the oval window niche, etc. (MEL *B* in the legend). Reconstructive middle ear surgery comprises "lysis" and removal of adhesions, etc., occasionally resulting in mobility of the ossicular chain.

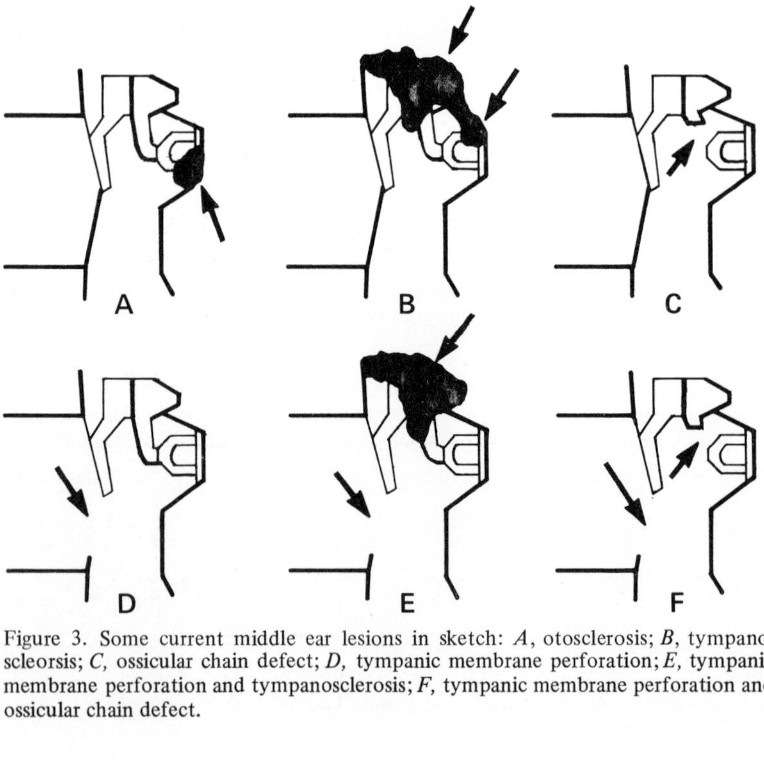

Figure 3. Some current middle ear lesions in sketch: *A*, otosclerosis; *B*, tympanoscleorsis; *C*, ossicular chain defect; *D*, tympanic membrane perforation; *E*, tympanic membrane perforation and tympanosclerosis; *F*, tympanic membrane perforation and ossicular chain defect.

Conductive hearing loss with *perforation of tympanic membrane* is examined by otomicroscopy directly or indirectly by using a small mirror in middle ear position, thorough investigation of the ossicular chain and other parts of the middle ear, including palpation by silver probe to demonstrate the anatomical mobility. Certain *functional tests* (covering prosthesis, stapes-contact prosthesis, etc.) considering the physiological mobility of chain and labyrinth windows also have to be performed as, for instance, described by Lundborg and Linzander (1970).

Sequelae after middle ear infection with *tympanic membrane perforation with the ossicular chain intact* is the most common condition encountered (MEL *D* in the legend) among conductive hearing loss patients. The perforation of the tympanic membrane is often repaired with a temporal fascia and this also, as a rule, results in an anatomically and functionally normal middle ear.

Sequelae of chronic otitis with defects in *tympanic membrane* and with *formation of tympanosclerotic tissue around the ossicular chain* reduce its mobility (MEL *E* in the legend). Reconstructive surgery has to include both removal of pathological formations, as in MEL *B,* and repair of the perforation, as in MEL *D.*

Tympanic membrane perforation and *ossicular chain defect,* the final state of chronic otitis, as in MEL *F,* reveals lesions both in drum and chain and, thus, requires reconstruction of tympanic membrane as in MEL *D* and Columella operation as in MEL *C.* As mentioned above, a reconstruction of more than *one* site of lesion within the middle ear cannot be expected to give as favorable (anatomical and functional) results as within conditions with only one site of lesion.

Considering Sensorineural Hearing Loss In sensorineural hearing loss, particularly if unilateral, the question is whether the lesion is of the cochlear or of the retrocochlear type. With a certain simplification, it may be said that the test battery used in cochlear lesions reveals recruitment signs but normal adaptation, i.e., a consistent cochlear test pattern. On the other hand, adaptation without recruitment signs reveals a consistent retrocochlear test pattern. Figure 2 shows the test battery utilized which empirically has been found to be useful. The number of tests has to be restricted to permit sufficient experience in performance and evaluation. It is assumed that no single test is pathognomic: typical cochlear or retrocochlear test pattern, according to experience, is expected to be revealed in the great majority of the cases encountered. In inconsistent test patterns, the audiological tests are not considered to constitute a sufficient diagnostic basis and, thus, according to Lundborg (1971), complementary investigations (neurological, radiological, etc.) have to be performed.

Cochlear type of hearing loss refers to lesions not only in the cochlea but also in the ganglion spirale. Electrocochleography (ECoG) may contribute to differential diagnosis between cochlear lesion with no cochlear microphonic (CM) or nerve action potential (AP) and nerve lesion (with CM but no AP).

Retrocochlear lesions refer to site of lesions between ganglion spirale, i.e., nuclear cochleares, central auditory pathways, and auditory cortex bilaterally. Level of lesions within the central nervous system may further be established by means of: (1) *distorted speech audiometry* as described by Korsan-Bengtsen (1973), a subjective method, and (2) auditory evoked response audiometry (ERA), an objective method. Site of lesions within the auditory pathways can also be established by means of *special binaural methods*, assessing a patient's ability to estimate the direction of a sound source, an ability which is corresponding to his ability to detect interaural differences in time and intensity as described by Nordlund (1963). There are also some tests (Lombard, Stenger, etc.) used to establish psychogenic hearing loss or malingering. These conventional methods can be complemented by ERA.

Evaluation of Hearing Loss in Preschool Children Infants, newborn babies, and, occasionally, fetuses, require special test procedures utilizing some form of infant audiology systems.

Children under the age of 4 years are tested, for instance, with the utilization of an *infant-audiology system*, which is based on conditioned orientation reflex (COR). The child patient may be seated between two cabinets with facilities for acoustical stimuli from a loudspeaker combined with screens for peep show. When the child is correctly reacting to an acoustic stimulus, he is rewarded by the appearance of a color picture on a screen or of, for example, a doll in a niche.

Infants under the age of 2 years are primarily tested by ERA and newborns by ERA, palpebral reflex elicitation, and, occasionally, registration of sound-induced heart rate changes.

Mentally retarded children have to be examined by these procedures regardless of age.

Anechoic Chamber There are several tasks within a stratified audiological department requiring an anechoic chamber (Figure 4):

1. Diagnostic procedures in free field with well-defined stimuli without additional reverberation sound energy as in electrocochleography (ECoG) and evoked response audiometry (ERA), determination of auditive directional hearing, and special psychoacoustic tests concerning binaural versus monaural signal detection, etc.

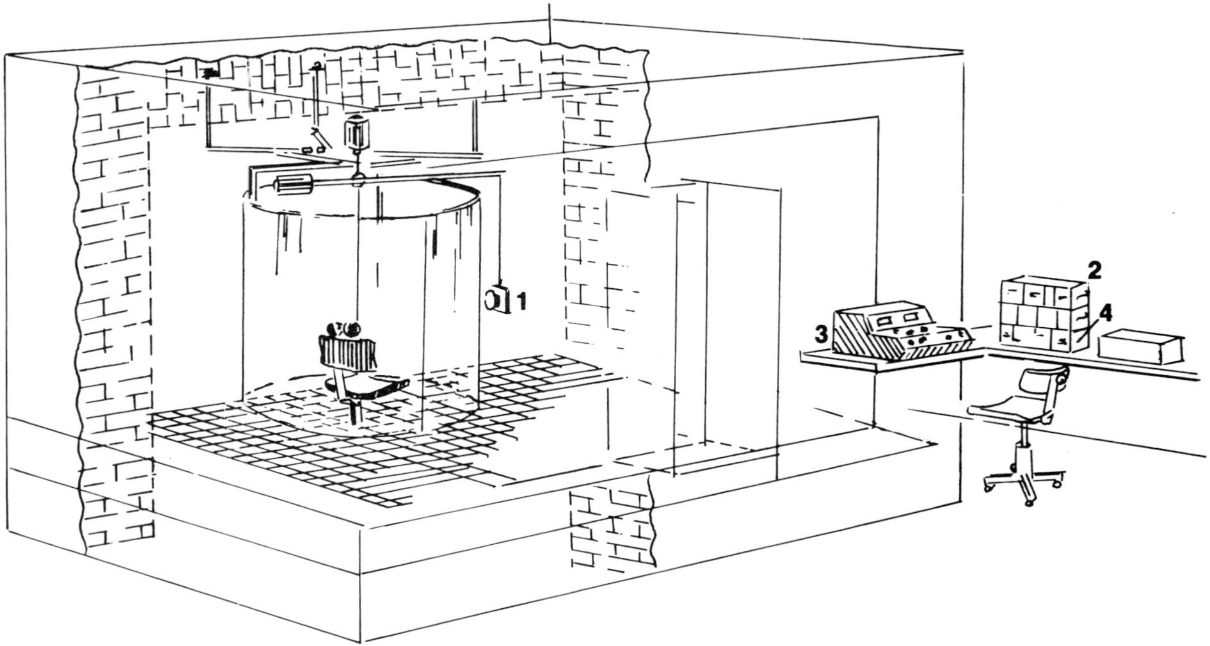

Figure 4. Anechoic chamber: outer size is 5 × 7 meters = 35 meters² (ca. 315 sq. feet); inner size is 4 × 6 meters = 24 meters² (ca. 216 sq. feet). Acoustic isolation: glass fiber material according to "Wurfelsystem BP" (3 layers), lower frequency bound–150 Hz.

2. Arrangements of controlled acoustic milieus to simulate, for instance, a hearing aid patient's various everyday situations.
3. Investigations on hearing aid patients in free field situations to evaluate the function hearing loss patient-hearing aid, for instance, determination of the ability of speech discrimination in noise (as in 2), determination of improved directional hearing with (binaural) hearing aid or with specially designed hearing aid with the purpose to improve the auditive localization ability.

An adequate utilization of the anechoic chamber requires a close cooperation with technical institutions which is currently developing at the Department of Audiology, Sodersjukhuset.

The movable loudspeaker (motor operated–special arrangement) functions to evaluate directional hearing for diagnostic purposes. The amplifier delay gate system, etc., have as their function sound stimulation. The audiometer has as its function sound stimulation. The control unit (special arrangement) has as its function positioning control and positioning the indication of movable loudspeaker.

REHABILITATIVE PROCEDURES

Hearing Aid Fitting

When choosing between different equipments in suitable cases of hearing loss, the prescription or recommendation of an electroacoustic amplifier, from the medical point of view, offers the same problem as selecting a pharmaceutical compound from among all available remedies as described by Lundborg et al. (1973).

There is still a lack of specific standards in the hearing-aid-fitting procedures and, thus, it is still necessary to use simple clinical routines and evaluate them empirically to fit the majority of hearing aid patients. There are three main factors to be evaluated in these procedures: *the hearing aid*, the physical characteristics of which can be described rather well by a number of tests, *the hearing loss* patient, who by means of pure tone and speech audiometry procedures, etc. can at least be partly evaluated, and, finally, the combination *hearing loss patient-hearing aid*, which still yields the essential problem both for clinical assessment and research. The relations between certain physical parameters and corresponding variables of subjective experience have to be thoroughly investigated and this requires extensive human-technological cooperation and research.

The overall performance of the hearing aid, i.e., the frequency response curve, the maximum acoustic gain, and the maximum output, are still much used for classification of the hearing aid assortment available.

The operational procedures of the hearing aid fitting will not be discussed in this connection, but the writer shall merely point out how the hearing aid characteristics are considered as guidance during the hearing aid fitting to demonstrate some typical clinical and rehabilitative situations.

The basic information from the hearing loss patient comes from pure tone measurements: hearing threshold, discomfort level, and also an estimation of the most comfortable level (MCL).

Most hearing loss patients are candidates either for a low output or a moderate output hearing aid. The high output aids should be restricted to the relatively few severely hearing-impaired patients who need particularly rehabilitative resources. Headworn hearing aids are mostly recommended to slight and moderate hearing loss cases and these aids also require more mechanical skill on the part of the patients. This is also true for hear-glasses, where cosmetic wants and considerations often are important.

During the preselection procedures mentioned above, hearing aid type and degree of output can be determined, and these steps may be followed by a comparison among a group of hearing aids which are identical on some basic parameters but have different frequency response characteristics, i.e., bandwidths corresponding to the patients' subjectively different estimation of "sound" when they are listening to standardized speech.

During this test situation, when the patient experiences the sound level and quality as comfortable, it is of practical interest to measure the hearing aid amplification of these comfortably perceived sounds.

The following examples from three hearing loss situations (Figure 5, *a*, *b*, and *c*) may illustrate the relations between degree of hearing loss and type of hearing aid selection, as well as the amplification practically utilized.

The case examples may demonstrate the action and function of the chosen hearing aids with reference to speech perception at the most comfortable level. The hearing ability has not changed, but, by utilization of an adequate hearing aid amplification (note in all cases, this is considerably below the maximal acoustic gain of the hearing aid chosen), the position of the speech elements has been changed in relation to the hearing loss patient's most comfortable level so that they can be adequately perceived.

Special Devices Recommendation of special devices, according to Lundborg et al. (1972), aims to reduce various communication problems involving the use of telephone, radio and television, the inability to detect

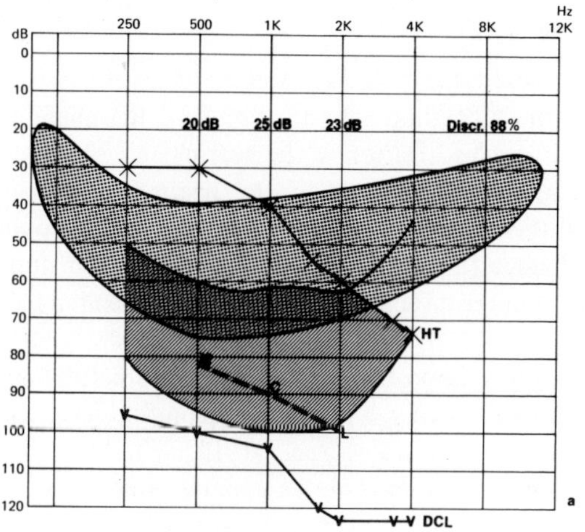

Figure 5a

Figure 5. *a*: Case 1. Moderate hearing loss in left ear. Approximate levels in dB: *HT*, 40, *DCL*, 110, *MCL*, 90. Amplification in dB: 20 (500 Hz), 25 (1 kHz), 28 (2 kHz). *Shadowed area* in *a*, *b*, and *c* represents a normal hearing listener's conversational speech area at 1 meter listening to comfortable speech sounds. Speech elements one HT-line not perceived. *Lined area* in the *a*, *b*, and *c* represents position of the area for amplified speech according to the calculated amplification as indicated in the record, i.e., approximately 25 dB. In case 1, moderate hearing loss in left ear at the 40-dB level, *MCL*, situated within the amplified speech area, demonstrates an adequate hearing aid fitting. Hearing aid selected–headworn, low output. *b:* Case 2. Represents a more pronounced sensorineural hearing loss in left ear. Approximate levels in dB: *HT*, 65, *DCL*, 110, *MCL*, 97. Amplification in dB: 18 (500 Hz), 41 (1 kHz), 39 (2 kHz). Pronounced hearing loss at the 65-dB level. Speech elements one HT-line, i.e., ca. 80%, not perceived by unaided ear. The position of amplified speech area with MCL level adequately between HT and DCL indicates a suitable HA-fitting. Hearing aid selected–headworn, high output. *c*: Case 3. Represents a severe sensorineural hearing loss on right ear. Approximate levels in dB: *HT*, 82, *DCL*, 120, *MCL*, 107. Amplification in dB: 30 (500 Hz), 41 (1 kHz), 45 (2 kHz). Severe hearing loss at the 80-dB level. Nothing of the speech sounds from a 1-meter distant speaker can be perceived by unaided ear. Position of aided ear's speech area adequately situated in relation to MCL. Hearing aid selected–body worn, high output.

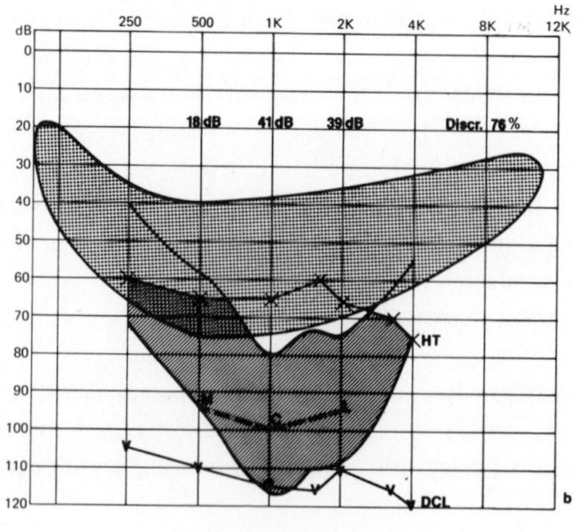

Figure 5b

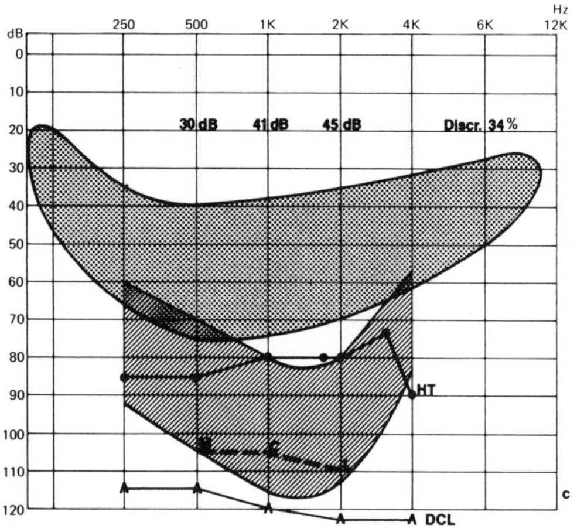

Figure 5c

signals from door chime, telephone bell, alarm clock, etc. Eleven of these communication facilities are simultaneously sketched in Figure 6. The following examples from typical patients' situations may illustrate the use and function of these devices:

1. Moderate degree hearing-handicapped patients, often not using a hearing aid, are utilizing: acoustical signals by particular pitch or extra strength for detection of door and telephone signals, a telephone handset with amplifier and thumb-operated volume-control for amplification of incoming telephone message, and a telephone headset for connection to television loudspeaker extra output for amplification of television sound. Another alternative is the television aid equipped with earpiece and volume control for connection to television loudspeaker extra output.
2. Patients with somewhat higher degree of hearing loss, using hearing aids besides signals for door and telephone and telephone amplifier, also use special devices for radio and television listening in the form of a small induction loop, connected to television loudspeaker extra output. When wanted, the hearing aid and induction coil can be substituted with a telephone headset for connection to television loudspeaker extra output for a television aid.
3. Pronounced hearing loss patients often use an auxiliary system of several devices serving all communicative possibilities.

The door signal can be detected either acoustically or by optical indication from flashing lampgroup with slow sequence. Telephone signal is detected in a similar way (acoustically or optically), with rapid sequence

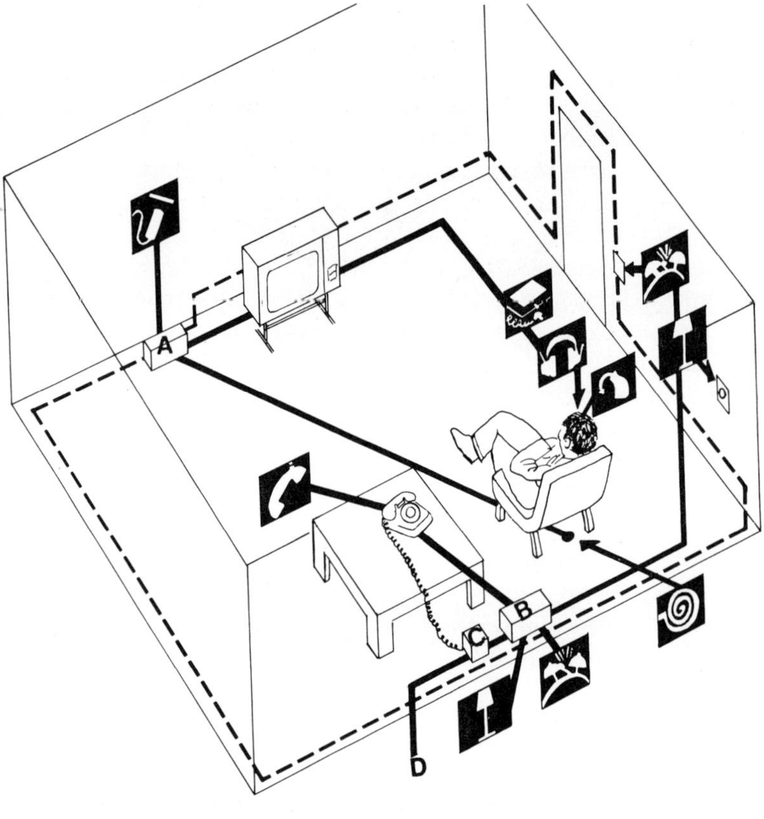

LEGEND OF FUNCTION OF DEVICES.

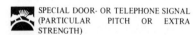

SPECIAL DOOR- OR TELEPHONE SIGNAL (PARTICULAR PITCH OR EXTRA STRENGTH)

AUXILIARY SIGNAL CONTROL ACTIVATING FLASHING-LAMPGROUP INDICATING DOOR OR TELEPHONE RINGING

TELEPHONE HANDSET WITH AMPLIFIER AND VOLUME CONTROL

TELEPHONE HEADSET FOR CONNECTION TO TV LOUDSPEAKER EXTRA OUTPUT

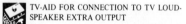

TV-AID FOR CONNECTION TO TV LOUDSPEAKER EXTRA OUTPUT

HEADWORN HEARING AID WITH INDUCTION COIL

SMALL INDUCTION LOOP FOR CONNECTION TO TV LOUDSPEAKER EXTRA OUTPUT

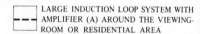

LARGE INDUCTION LOOP SYSTEM WITH AMPLIFIER (A) AROUND THE VIEWING-ROOM OR RESIDENTIAL AREA

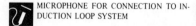

MICROPHONE FOR CONNECTION TO INDUCTION LOOP SYSTEM

Figure 6. Chamber for instruction and assessment of need for communication instruments. Eleven various communication facilities in sketch.

by means of two relay devices (*B* and *C* in Figure 6) connected to the telephone. Incoming telephone messages are detected as in A.

The television listener is using hearing aid with either a small induction loop plate in the chair position or by utilizing a large induction loop system requiring an amplifier (*A*) around the viewing room.

At choice, the hearing aid and magnetic coil can be substituted by a telephone headset for connection to loudspeaker extra output. A microphone can be coupled to the inductive loop system in residential areas for hearing-impaired school children and students (Figure 6).

4. Severely handicapped patients (with hearing rests or deaf) also need special devices for automatic alarm indication. An automatic alarm clock with an amplifier and relay can, at a preset time, activate a vibrating buzzer in position under the pillow to awaken the hearing-handicapped patient (Figure 7).

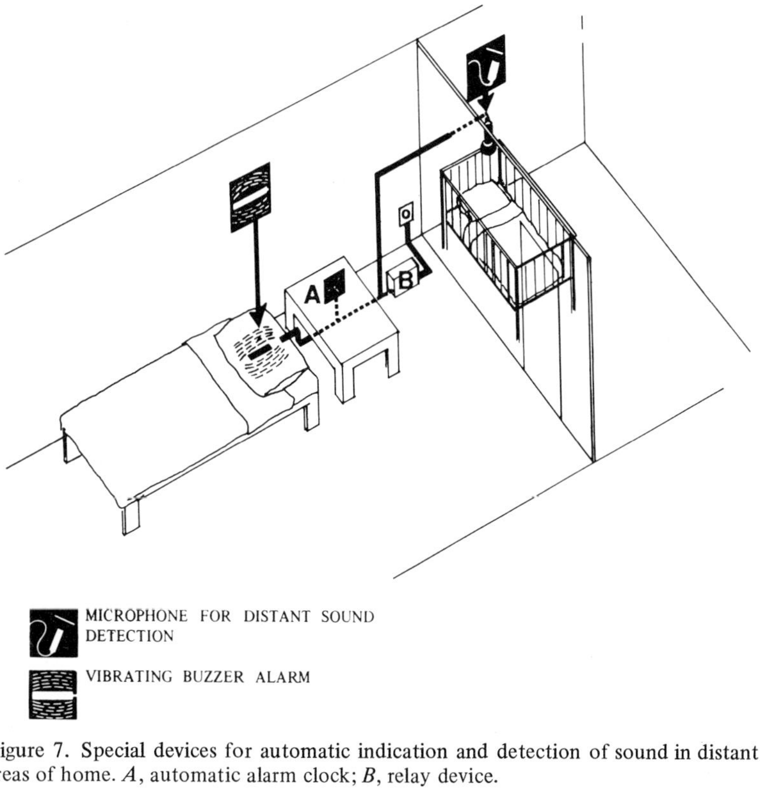

Figure 7. Special devices for automatic indication and detection of sound in distant areas of home. *A*, automatic alarm clock; *B*, relay device.

The detection of sound from other home areas, for instance, a crying baby in a room beside a deafened mother's room, is picked up by a microphone with an amplifier and, provided the sounds are strong and enduring enough, via the relay activating the buzzer signal system.

Recommendation of Instruction and Audiopedic Functional Training The great majority of patients taken care of within the audiopedic section are those being fitted with hearing aids.

For 3,705 hearing aid patients fitted in 1973, 6-hour instruction in the use of the hearing aid, etc. was recommended to 2,532 patients arranged in 393 groups. This means, as a rule, six to seven patients in each group and it also means that almost every new hearing aid patient participated in this service.

During the instruction courses, the patients are evaluated as to their need of special devices in addition to the hearing aid for particular communication purposes. The new hearing aid patients, together with patients previously fitted but returning because of additional communication needs, had a total of 10,500 special communication devices recommended.

The need for functional training is also assessed during the instruction courses with the result that 593 patients, approximately half of them new hearing aid users, i.e., about 10% of the total group having functional training, comprising, as a rule, 30 training situations. The other part of the group needed additional functional training.

Functional Training Programs Auditory training programs are arranged with six or seven severely hard-of-hearing patients or patients having moderate hearing loss but with pronounced loudness problems because of recruitment.

During the training, either the individual hearing aid or a group amplifier is utilized. The aim of this program is either an auditive reactivation or improvement of the patients' tolerance to amplitude variations in speech. Speech material consists of everyday speech either presented by the instructor (audiopede) or utilizing tape recorder. Internal television (ITV) is also used during combined audiovisual training. The training procedures vary in degrees of difficulty because of differences in speech material, change of speech, or speech material mixed with noise of different characteristics at different signal-to-noise ratios.

Speechreading A group amplifier is utilized only exceptionally, i.e., when the patients are informed about arrangements for the training program. The aim of the procedure is to improve the patients' visual communication when a hearing aid either cannot be used or improves the speech discrimination only insufficiently. Utilizing different speech material, either presented directly by the instructor or via film or television, the speech movements, mimics, and attitudes of the speaker are viewed. On the other hand, the patients are only occasionally watching static pictures of single speech sounds.

Radio-Emitted Speech This functional training system is offered, for instance, to the severely hearing impaired (most university or high school students) to make study possible for these patients (for communication during lectures, staff meetings, seminars, etc.) in situations when they are together with nonhearing-impaired individuals.

Comment Restricted experience is collected concerning the recommendation and use of radio emitters to severely hearing-impaired university students. Within the inner city area (about three-fourths of a million people), there are at the moment about 30 radio emitters used in these particular situations. This figure may be compared with some other relevant statistics. Wtihin the same area, there are approximately 75,000 school children of the age of 7–18 years. Of these pupils, about 200 are taken care of by special audiological arrangements. The majority of the children are in special *hearing classes,* the others are in ordinary classes.

The great majority of this patient group of children is equipped with an euxiliary communicative system serving all possibilities, including a microphone coupled to the inductive loop in the pupils' residence permitting a communication between the hearing impaired and visitors, etc. (Figure 6).

Sign Language Relatives of deaf patients, i.e., those who are not communicating in an auditive way and staff members handling these deaf patients in various professional situations, often need to perform the communication required in a nonauditive way, i.e., via sign language.

For this purpose, training programs for sign language have been arranged. During 1973, there were 144 groups with 930 persons participating. This rather high frequency may also reflect an accumulated need for this type of service. At present, a rapid development is characterizing the Swedish sign language system with the intention to adapt it to *speech language* and also, as far as possible, adapt the Swedish system to Scandinavian and international systems. There is, therefore, need for frequent remodeling of both teaching technique and material.

Sign Language Interpretation Service The various communication therapeutic services given since 1968, when the department of audiology was completed with a particular audiopedic section, have created new demands and have also developed further in various directions. This implies new sociomedical facilities on a medical basis. An example of this latter type of activity is *interpretation service* given to the approximately

TYPE AND LEVEL OF HEARING LOSS	COMMUNICATION INSTRUMENTS HEARING AID	SPECIAL DEVICES	AUDIOPEDIC MEASURES (INSTRUCTION AND REHABILITATION)	COMMENT
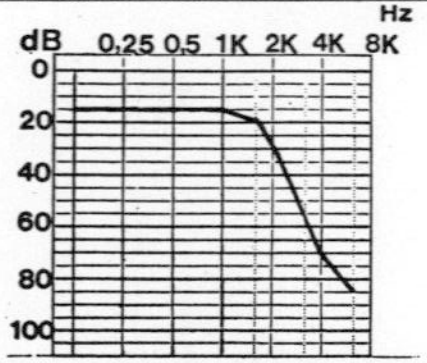 20–40 dB	0	1 DOOR AND TELEPHONE **Acoustical signals** Optical signals 2 TELEPHONE AMPLIFIER 3 DEVICES FOR TV AND RADIO **"TV-aid"** Acoustic cushion Telemagnetic loop Telephone Headset	INSTRUCTION COURSE in the use of a hearing aid. **Demonstration of special devices**	Additional case material ca 400 pts/year
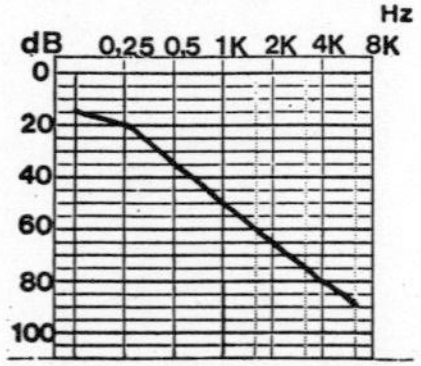 40–60 dB	Earworn hearing aid (hearglasses) 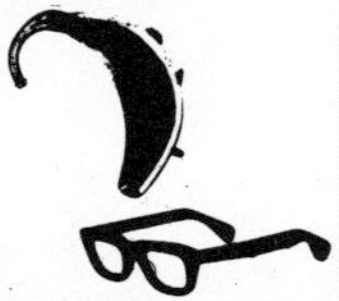	1 DOOR AND TELEPHONE **Acoustical signals** Optical signals **2 TELEPHONE AMPLIFIER** 3 DEVICES FOR TV AND RADIO "TV-aid" **Acoustic cushion** Telemagnetic loop Telephone Headset 4 ALARM DEVICES	**INSTRUCTION AND REHABILITATIVE TRAINING PROGRAMS** 1 Instruction in the use of a hearing aid 2 Demonstration of Special Devices 3 Assessment of need for Functional Training FUNCTIONAL TRAINING 1 Auditory training 2 Lipreading	ca 50% of case material (3850 pts) ← occassionally
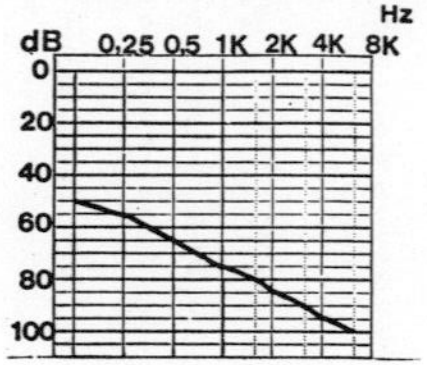 60–80 dB	Bodyworn or earworn hearing aids 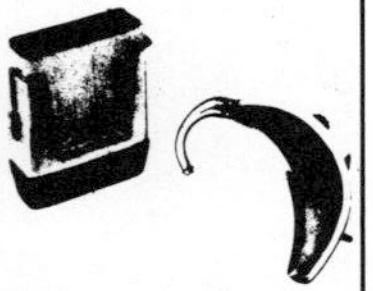	1 DOOR AND TELEPHONE Acoustical signals **Optical signals** **2 TELEPHONE AMPLIFIER** 3 DEVICES FOR TV AND RADIO "TV-aid" Acoustic cushion **Telemagnetic loop** Telephone Headset **4 ALARM DEVICES**	**INSTRUCTION AND REHABILITATIVE TRAINING PROGRAMS** 1 Instruction in the use of a hearing aid 2 Demonstration of Special Devices 3 Assessment of need for Functional Training FUNCTIONAL TRAINING **1 Auditory training** **2 Lipreading** 3 Speech correction 4 Sign Language	ca 40% of case material (3850 pts) ← ca 10%
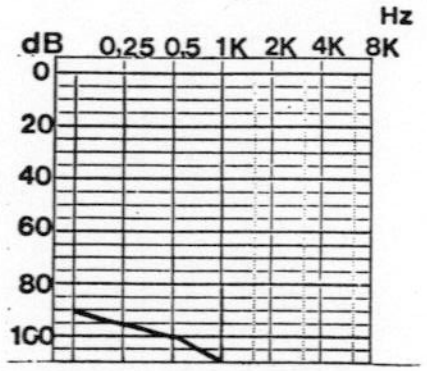 80 dB →	Bodyworn hearing aid 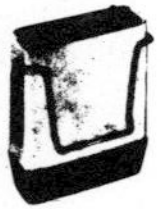	1 DOOR AND TELEPHONE Acoustical signals **Optical signals** 2 TELEPHONE AMPLIFIER 3 DEVICES FOR TV AND RADIO "TV-aid" Acoustic cushion **Telemagnetic loop** Telephone Headset **4 ALARM DEVICES**	**INSTRUCTION AND REHABILITATIVE TRAINING PROGRAMS** 1 Instruction in the use of a hearing aid 2 Demonstration of Special Devices 3 Assessment of need for Functional Training **FUNCTIONAL TRAINING** 1 Auditory training 2 Lipreading 3 Speech correction 4 Sign Language	ca 10% of case material (3850 pts) ← ca 40%

800 nonauditively communicating severely hearing impaired within the Stockholm region (population: 1.5 million people). Such service may be required during the patients' medical or dental visits and during visits to different kinds of authorities, social institutions, etc.

During 1973, the Department of Audiology performed 1,008 sign language interpretation measures.

A summary of the therapeutic recommendations and aural rehabilitative measures is outlined and surveyed in Figure 8.

Summary A survey is presented by Lundborg et al. (1973) of the therapeutic prescriptions, i.e., hearing aids, special devices, and audiopedic measures to 3,850 hearing loss patients in 1971. The patients with slight hearing loss referred by otologists for hearing aid fitting mostly did not need hearing aids, but could often benefit from particular acoustic signals for door and telephone and sometimes a television aid.

For the patients with PTA between 40 and 60 dB, about 50% of the case material is recommended: (1) hearing aids of the earworn type (or hearing glasses); and often (2) special devices of the acoustical type for telephone and door, telephone amplifier, and "acoustic cushion" for television listening; and (3) instruction courses in the use of a hearing aid with demonstrations of special devices and assessment of the need of functional training (required only occasionally).

For patients with PTA between 60 and 80 dB, about 40% of the case material is recommended: (1) body-worn hearing aids; (2) optical signals for telephone and door, telephone amplifiers, telemagnetic loops, and sometimes alarm devices; and (3) the instructional program and additional functional training (which are given to those who are able to utilize the therapeutic activities offered (10%)).

For patients with PTA above the 80 dB level, i.e., patients with only residual hearing or totally deaf patients (comprising about 10% of the case material) the following are recommended: (1) bodyworn hearing aids; (2) optical signals for telephone and door, telemagnetic loops, and sometimes alarm devices; (3) a full rehabilitative program (needed by every patient, but only 40% can utilize the therapy which is offered).

INTERPROFESSIONAL RELATIONSHIPS

The British Departmental Enquiry (1973) is a very thorough and comprehensive survey and analysis of the problems of hearing-handicapped patients and includes suggestions as to how to arrange for clinical and scientific progress in the field. It reflects many of the hearing-loss patients' difficulties and the handling of the corresponding training and scientific problems. It is generally agreed that a multidisciplinary approach is required involving staff members from many different disciplines in the care and treatment of hearing-loss patients. The constitution of an audiological team is very different depending on the type of organization (whether medical or nonmedical), the type of task chosen (clinical, scientific, or staff training work, etc.) among other things. The audiological activities described above are based on the thinking that the type of organization shall reflect a staff adequately structured to handle the communication problems of the hearing-loss patients as they exist in the field. With this premise, the framework of the above mentioned hospital-based audiological unit seems suitable. It may also be said that it has proved to function within its clinical framework, i.e., together with the otolaryngological and other medical departments, which are admitting the patients. Since it is a medical unit, the doctors, for obvious reasons, have a particular responsibility in this type of work. On the other hand, it seems quite clear that the medical and nonmedical (technical, psychopedagogical, etc.) contributions for the benefit of the hearing-handicapped patients have to be considered as quite equal parts in this multidisciplinary team. From the practical point, it seems meaningful and even necessary to have the departments of audiology and otology in close cooperation with the otologists handling the primary selection of patients for admission to audiological service for different kinds of diagnostic, therapeutic, and rehabilitative work when they find it useful.

With an adequate staff and equipment, it also seems important to structure an audiological unit in such a way that both *diagnostic procedures* (concerning transmission as well as sensorineural hearing loss), *therapeutic procedures* (recommendation of otosurgery, hearing aids, special devices in addition to hearing aid), as well as *audiopedic rehabilitative procedures* (instruction and functional training) are considered at the same time.

Figure 1 presents a framework of a hospital-based department of audiology and its clinical activities, displaying principles, staffing people, and patients' groups. The sketch may also show that this medical task, i.e., handling diagnostic and therapeutic procedures with hearing- and communication-handicapped patients, may be performed only to a lesser degree by conventional medical staff members (doctors, nurses, etc.), but to a greater degree by nonmedical staff members with either technical training (audiological assistants, electronic or communication engineers) or psychopedagogical backgrounds (audiopedes, i.e., hearing pedagogues for instructional and functional training, social workers, or psychologists). Basically, however, all the work performed is medical or, if put in administrative terms, it constitutes a medical production.

It is to be recalled that such broad teamwork with many disciplines involved probably never can be established without meeting and solving many problems concerning definition of spheres of interest. There are also occasional conflicts between various groups of staff. These attitudes may concern doctors with or without surgical training and interest, doctors with stress on diagnostic or rehabilitative work (including every type of patient or mainly paedoaudiological activities, etc.). They may also concern administrative groups of pressure groups, who may see a conflict between adult and preschool audiological work at a possible cost of the care of the latter group in units with a "total" aim concerning different patient groups and medical tasks, etc. They may further concern hearing pedagogues favoring either the oral or the visual method in speech training, including the question as to whether or not therapeutic work utilizing pedagogic methods should be performed within a hospital-based institution or if it only should be performed outside the hospital.

Should hearing aid fitting be performed in a hospital-based unit or should it be *reserved* for noninstitutional activities?

All these attitudes more or less have probably been manifested with some local variations wherever some people have tried to establish this type of cooperation. From the psychological point of view, this is certainly not difficult to understand.

When realizing these negative attitudes, one is also pointing to some of the dilemmas in the audiological activities. From the medical point of view, it could never be justified to favor one audiological area, for instance, one patient group or one type of activity (be it surgical, technical, or rehabilitative) at the expense of any other section of work. Recalling that many activities have started just because of some particular interest and assumption present (institutional, personal, administrative, economic, etc.), it seems easier to understand why there still are so many different patterns of activities. Assuming that all these different models have contributed to the mutual promotion of audiological activities, it seems also to become possible in the near future to create a rational pattern of institutional activities with all different specialists contributing on the same level. It is, on the other hand, as already has been mentioned, mainly a practical question that, within a medical organization, for obvious reasons, the medical staff member has a particular responsibility.

It is easy to say, but not that easy to realize, that all these nonadequate attitudes and matters of misunderstanding and occasional conflicts of interest have to disappear. With mutual understanding and interdisciplinary respect, based on experience, all the isolated specialist activities may be converted into a true medical program where such questions never should arise.

TRAINING PROGRAM FOR PROFESSIONALS

No official training programs for all the professional groups active within the Swedish departments of audiology have yet been outlined. This fact reflects one of the main problems still existing. It is hoped that these professional needs will be fulfilled within a few years. Some of the current training programs will be briefly sketched.

Medical Audiologists

The *basic* medical training starts after baccalaureate (with 19-year-old students as a rule) and consists of 5½ years of medical studies and 21 months of additional training and results in the licensed physician's degree (M.D. refers to the medical doctor's degree, requiring a particular dissertation, as a rule, and 3 years' further work).

The *complementary* training to become a specialist within medical audiology consists of 2 years of training within a department of audiology and 2 years of training in otorhinolaryngology. Half a year of the latter part may be substituted by training in medical phoniatrics. The *additional* training period of half a year may be performed within either the neurological block (neurosurgery, neurology, or neurophysiology) or the psychiatric block (psychiatry or juvenile psychiatry).

Audiological Assistants

The basic requirement is the grammer school (9 years) which may entitle a student to the 1-year training course within one particular medical vocational school to become an audiological assistant. The training period comprises 4 months of theory and 6 months of practice within some large and stratified department of audiology.

Both the responsible M.D.s, as well as the audiological assistants themselves, want a longer basic training period (at least 2 years) for the audiological assistants. So far, this is a wish that may possibly later be fulfilled.

Hearing Pedagogues (audiopedes)

These specialists are recruited from grammar school teachers, who, after 3 years of practice, may attend a 1½-year training period at the Teacher's Training College (special line for hearing-handicapped children). This training prepares them to become a hearing pedagogue within the special classes for hearing handicapped. An additional half-year training period permits them to teach totally deaf children.

So far, there are no special official training arrangements for the hearing pedagogues, who are performing the instruction and training programs within the departments of audiology. These specialists (fulfilling a medical task, but utilizing pedagogic methods) are often nominated *audiopedes* as a parallel with the logopedes within the phoniatric departments. The audiopedes have to be trained within the departments of audiology, but, there are in Sweden so far no special arrangements for their basic training possibilities. This reveals another audiological problem.

Technical Audiology (electronic engineers, etc.)

At the departments of audiology, these specialists are recruited among electronic or communication engineers of the M.S. or B.A. level. There is still a need for particular medicotechnical training possibilities for these specialists, in addition to their basic engineering training. Thus, the members of this category also have to be practically trained within the established departments of audiology.

Social Workers

They have a B.A. from a university and an additional training period within a department of audiology. Even within this category, there is no particular basic audiological training. This holds true also for *psychologists.* In some of the largest departments of audiology, there is practical training for a few psychologists with the M.A. degree. There is certainly a need for regular training possibilities for psychologists participating in an audiological team. As in the U.S.A., the large departments may need psychologists also of the Ph.D. level.

LAY ORGANIZATIONS AND FAMILY INVOLVEMENT

In Sweden there are mainly two bodies of voluntary societies, i.e., the Swedish Society of the Hard of Hearing and the Swedish Society for the Deaf. They act as pressure groups in the interest of hearing-handicapped people. These societies are functioning both on the national level and on the local plane.

The Swedish Society of the Hard of Hearing has initiated institutional activities in the form of schools for hearing-handicapped preschool children, arranged hearing aid fitting facilities, and also started a center for functional training of hearing-handicapped people, young and old. According to the conception of the society, these activities have been taken over and are now run by city or governmental authorities. One main field of interest is the guidance and assistance of parents of hearing-impaired children. The society has on its staff a university-trained social worker who functions as the parents' counselor in this area. An example of its pressure group activities is the society's critical view of all existing hearing requirements in connection with different professional training programs (which have, hitherto, often excluded hearing-impaired people for "formal" reasons which often have no functional evidence).

For obvious reasons, society has backed the governmental issues on the prescription of hearing aids and other complementary special devices by the use of state grants.

The last few years have revealed several socioeconomic trends beneficial to hearing-handicapped people, for instance, vacation grants for mothers of deaf children, grants for young hearing handicapped to attend particular language training courses, etc.

The *Swedish Society for the Deaf* has also backed the particular interests listed above. This society has been thoroughly interested in one area, namely, the utilization of the sign language as a means of communication for all deaf people who are unable to communicate *only* by oral stimulation. In Stockholm the development of sign language training facilities to staff people who handle the severely hearing-handicapped patients, including sign language interpreter service to these patients, is the result of the cooperation between the department of Audiology at Sodersjukhuset and the Society for the Deaf.

RESEARCH

Both clinical interest and research have focused on the various diagnostic, therapeutic, and rehabilitative areas that have been sketched above.

The diagnostic procedures to indicate type of otosurgical correction in transmission hearing loss may be said to be rather adequate (Lundborg and Linzander, 1970). Ingelstedt and associates (1967) have performed extensive experimental work concerning the tubar function and its clinical application.

One area, in which several investigators in Sweden have been contributing for a couple of years, is impedance audiometry. Diagnostic data are derived by assessing the threshold of the stapedial reflex (Klockhoff, 1961), by means of the tympanogram (Liden et al., 1974), and by investigating the reflex decay (Andersson, 1969). Liden et al. (1974) also have studied the variations in reflex elicitation under drug influence. Klockhoff (1973) has studied the spontaneous tensor tympani activity, and Zakrisson (1974) has correlated the ears' acoustic impedance changes by direct measurements of the stapedial muscle activity by EMG. Stapedium reflex measurements have been used by Johansson et al. (1967) also as an instrument to detect individuals with particular sensitivity to noise exposure.

The assessment of cochlear versus retrocochlear test patterns in sensorineural hearing loss by means of a suitable test battery has been demonstrated, for instance, by Liden and Korsan-Bengtsen (1973). As a screening test newborns, as well as fetuses, have been exposed to pure tones for palpebral reflex elicitation by Wedenberg (1963) and Wedenberg and Johansson (1975). Preschool children have been evaluated by utilizing play audiometry by Barr (1954) and by means of the orientation reflex (Liden and Kandunen, 1969). Psychogenic deafness has been assessed by Barr (1960) utilizing different psychoacoustic tests. For assessment of central hearing loss, special diagnostic test procedures have been developed. Directional audiometry has been utilized by Nordlund (1963), revealing impaired acuity in eight nerve and pontile lesions, and Korsan-Bengtsen (1973) has used acoustically processed speech test materials to assess impaired speech intelligibility in auditory cortex lesions. As was demonstrated by Aniansson (1974), the social hearing acuity in noise-induced hearing-loss patients has to be assessed during everyday acoustic conditions to get a representative picture of the real handicap.

Concerning the utilization of communication instruments (hearing aids and additional special devices) in therapeutic and rehabilitative work, positive experience has been gained empirically, as described, for instance, by Lundborg et al. (1972 and 1973), but still there is a lack of the conceptual framework for the underlying processes.

Johansson and Wedenberg (1961, 1975) have developed a transposer hearing aid, i.e., a device that is modulating the nonaudible high frequency sounds into the low frequency range that is audible to the hearing impaired and this has resulted in improving speech discrimination. Constructs supported by exact scientific data are needed in all communication instruments, indicating that this area still poses an urgent challenge to research. One example in Johansson's (1971) study of nonlinear distortion in hearing aids. As is well known in the aural rehabilitative procedures, i.e., auditory training, lipreading, etc., much research is necessary to find the essential factors underlying these procedures. Wedenberg (1951, 1954) has presented the basic technique for clinical use; but only a few programs have been run dealing with the basic factors, particularly because of lack of adequately trained staff members to carry on research in this field. In noise-induced hearing-loss patients, Hasselrot and associates (1975) have been studying the significance of the use of the hearing aid, either alone, in combination with lipreading, or in a "total" program, that is, an intensive aural rehabilitative course.

A topic of general interest is Andersson and Wedenberg's (1968) study on the basis for the carriers of genes for hearing loss. The utilization of data-processing records in clinical audiology has been assessed by Lundborg (1964) and by Klockhoff (1974) in screening audiometry of noise-exposed persons.

Future developments include the utilization of ERA-ECoG as topical diagnostic tools, as was performed by Arlinger (1975) and Rosenhamer (1975). A major project is run by Liden and colleagues (1975) to find criteria for noise-sensitive individuals.

PERIODICALS ON HEARING PUBLISHED IN SWEDEN

1. Acto Oto-Laryngologica, Almqvist & Wiksell Periodical Co., Stockholm, Sweden.
2. Audio-nytt (in Swedish), Landstingens Inkopscentral, Solna, Sweden.
3. Auris (in Swedish), periodical for the Hearing Society of Sweden, Horselframjandets Riksforbund, Stockholm, Sweden.
4. Scandinavian Audiology, Almqvist & Wiksell Periodical Co., Stockholm, Sweden.
5. SDR-Kontakt (in Swedish), periodical for the Swedish Society of the Deaf, Sveriges Dovas Riksforbund, Stockholm, Sweden.
6. Speech Transmission Laboratory, Quarterly Progress and Status Report, Department of Speech Communication, Royal Institute of Technology, Stockholm, Sweden.

LITERATURE CITED

Andersson, H. 1969. Acoustic Intra-Aural Reflexes in Clinical Diagnosis, KaVe Tryck AB, Stockholm.

Andersson, H., and Wedenberg, E. 1968. Audiometric identification of normal hearing carriers of genes for deafness. Acta Otolaryngol. 65: 535–554.

Aniansson, G. 1974. Methods for assessing high frequency hearing loss in every-day listening situations. Acta Otolaryngol. (Suppl. 320).

Arlinger, S. 1975. Threshold extrapolation for N-1 latencies in auditory evoked responses. Scand. Audiol. In press.

Barr, B. 1954. Pure tone audiometry for pre-school children. Acta Otolaryngol. (Suppl. 110): 89–101.

Barr, B. 1960. Non-organic hearing problems in school children. Acta Otolaryngol. 52: 337–346.

Deafness. 1973. Report of a departmental enquiry into the promotion of research (London). Reports on Health and Social Subjects, No. 4.

Hasselrot, M., Toarsson, A., Lindström, B., and Lundborg, T. 1975. Audiological treatment of noise-induced hearing impaired persons. Scand. Audiol. In press.

Ingelstedt, S., Toarsson, A., and Jousson, B. 1967. Mechanics of the human middle ear. Acta Otolaryngol. (Suppl. 228).

Johansson, B. 1971. Non-linear distortion in hearing aids. Third Danavox Symposium, pp. 126–134.

Johansson, B., and Wedenberg, E. 1961. A new coding amplifier system for the severely hard of hearing. Proc. 3rd Internat. Cong. Acoust. 2: 655–660.
Johansson, B., Kylin, B., and Langby, M. 1967. Acoustic reflex as a test of individual susceptibility to noise. Acta Otolaryngol. 64: 256–262.
Klockhoff, I. 1961. Middle ear muscle reflexes in man. Acta Otolaryngol. (Suppl. 164).
Klockhoff, I. 1973. A tonic tensor tympani phenomenon in man and its clinical significance. *In* Tenth International Congress of Otol. Rhin. & Laryngol. pp. 187–188. Venice.
Klockhoff, I. 1974. Computerized classification of the results of screening audiometry in groups of persons exposed to noise. Audiology 13: 326–334.
Korsan-Bengtsen, M. 1973. Distorted speech audiometry. Acta Otolaryngol. (Suppl. 310).
Liden, G., and Kandunen, A. 1969. Visual reinforcement audiometry. Acta Otolaryngol. 67: 281–292.
Liden, G., and Korsan-Bengtsen, M. 1973. Audiometric manifestations of retrocochlear lesions. Scand. Audiol. 2: 29–40.
Liden, G., Harford, E., and Hallér, O. 1974a. Automatic tympanometry in clinical practice. Audiology 13: 126–139.
Liden, G., Wilsson, E., Laskinen, O., Roos, B. E., and Miller, J. 1974b. The stapedial reflex and motor reaction time: a parallel investigation of the effect of drugs. Scand. Audiol. 3: 28–30.
Liden, G. 1975. Noise studies in ship building. Personal communication.
Lungborg, T. 1964. Forsok til databehandling av audiologisk. J. Nord. Audiol. 14: 130–135.
Lundborg, T. 1971. Viewpoints on the management of retrocochlear lesions in connection with a case report. Acta Otolaryngol. 72: 413–420.
Lundborg, T., and Linzander, S. 1970. The otomicroscopic observation and its clinical application. Acta Otolaryngol. (Suppl. 266).
Lundborg, T., Lingander, S., Lindström, B., and Toarsson, A. 1972. Special devices for the hearing handicapped patient. J. Audiol. Technique 11: 82–104.
Lundborg, et al. 1973. Symposium on hearing aids. Scand. Audiol. (Suppl. 3).
Nordlund, B. 1963. Directional audiometry. Acta Otolaryngol. 56: 1–18.
Rosenhamer, H. 1975. Brain stem audiology in adults and infants. Scand. Audiol. In press.
Wedenberg, E. 1951. Auditory training of deaf and hard of hearing children. Acta Otolaryngol. (Suppl. 94).
Wedenberg, E. 1954. Auditory training of severely hard of hearing preschool children. Acta Otolaryngol. (Suppl. 110): 1–82.
Wedenberg, E. 1963. Objective auditory tests on non-cooperative children. Acta Otolaryngol. (Suppl.) 175: 1–32.
Wedenberg, E., and Johansson, B. 1975. Personal communication.
Zakrisson, J. E. 1974. Experimental studies on the function of the stapedius muscle in man. Umea University Medical Diss. No. 18.

chapter 10

Communication for Hearing-handicapped People in Austria, Federal Republic of Germany, and Switzerland

Professor Armin Löwe

In this chapter, I would like to report on the current condition of the rehabilitation of hearing-impaired children and adults in the German-speaking countries of the Western world, which are the Federal Republic of Germany, Austria, and the German-speaking areas of Switzerland (which comprise more than 70% of the total population of Switzerland).

For a better understanding of the following material, it is helpful for the reader to be aware of the fact that the author has been working for more than 25 years in almost all the areas of educational rehabilitation of hearing-impaired children and adults. With this experience, the author sees the main area of concern for rehabilitation of the hearing impaired from a teacher's point of view. None of the various professional groups which today are working with the rehabilitation of the hearing impaired has such a large part and, at the same time, such a great responsibility for the hearing impaired as has the group of teachers for deaf and hard-of-hearing children, especially as one considers the time necessary to complete this difficult task. The preceding statement should not be misunderstood and interpreted so as to diminish the necessity and the importance of the work which other groups in the area of rehabilitation of the hearing impaired are doing. On the contrary, without their cooperation, modern rehabilitation would not be possible. If the cooperation of other groups is not clearly represented in the remaining parts of this chapter, this does not present any serious problems because other chapters of this handbook written by representatives of medical rehabilitation will represent the emphasis of other groups and so, taken as a whole, will provide a good balance.

HEARING IMPAIRMENT–HEARING DISTURBANCE

Whoever writes about the rehabilitation of hearing-impaired children and adults must make several statements as to what he understands about hearing impairment, a term used today as a general term in all the German-speaking countries. It is used and understood to designate all kinds and grades of medically irreversible problems in hearing. Medically reversible hearing problems are designated as hearing disturbances. One can summarize it very quickly. Hearing impairment is permanent. Hearing disturbances, on the other hand, are merely transitory problems or problems not yet fully diagnosed. Then it can be said that the general concept of hearing impairment means, therefore, a slight hearing loss as well as complete deafness and implies always two aspects–the impairment of the sense function of hearing and that of the impairment of language or spoken communication.

PRELINGUAL DEAF AND POSTLINGUAL DEAFENED

It has become common to subclassify the concept of hearing impairment into two or three areas respectively. These groups are the deaf and the hard of hearing, and that group that falls between these two. With deaf children, there are two different groups. In the *first group* of children to be considered, earlier designated as deaf and dumb, are the children who have gone through a phase in early childhood in which they were deaf and dumb more or less. This condition is avoidable today. Nevertheless, many children are still afflicted with this because their hearing problem was recognized only at a later stage. They were, therefore, not treated for it and not brought into an environment where they could be helped with hearing and speech education. This group is composed of children who are either deaf from birth or lost their hearing before they began to speak. Therefore, they are also called prelingual deaf children.

With the foregoing remarks in mind, it becomes clear that, within the classification of deafness, the point in time at which the hearing impairment occurred is a very important criterion. The same is also true of less severe cases of hearing impairment.

VARIOUS LEVELS OF HEARING LOSS

With prelingual deafness, a normal development of speech and language is not possible, but these may occur with hard-of-hearing children because of their residual hearing. The main difference between deaf and hard-of-hearing children is the way in which both groups of children perceive speech. Deaf children pick it up mainly through seeing, whereas, hard-of-hearing children pick it up mainly through hearing. With these remarks, it has already been stated that deaf children are not completely deaf and that hard-of-hearing children need some lipreading for the perception of speech. From a teacher's point of view, it is certainly difficult to narrow down the concept of residual hearing. Braun (1969) says that there are either totally deaf children or children who have some hearing left. This means then, in view of that fact that there are only very few deaf children who do not have some residual hearing (pure vibration cases), that almost every deaf child should be designated as a child who has residual hearing and should be treated as such. It seems to me, therefore, to make more sense to speak of deaf children respectively with or without residual hearing and to separate deafness from those with lesser degrees of hearing losses. One can divide them into slight, moderate, or severe categories as follows: slight hearing loss, the average hearing loss in the frequency area of 500–2,000 Hz is not more than 30 dB; moderate hearing loss, the moderate hearing loss occurs in the same frequency area as above and is from 30–60 dB; severe hearing loss, the loss occurs as above and is from 60–90 dB.

Up to this point we have only spoken of hearing-impaired children whose problems are, of course, much more difficult to solve than those of hearing-impaired adults. We can only allude to the many people who have hearing problems because of age, and we may also allude to the ever increasing number of adults who have acquired hearing problems because of noise damage.

DEFINITION OF AURAL REHABILITATION

The term rehabilitation of the handicapped, in the narrower sense, is understood today in the German language as the recapturing of the already formed physical or psychic function which has been lost by the cause of the handicap. In ever increasing measure, the concept of rehabilitation is used in a broader sense and implies also the attainment of a capability by means of special efforts and special training. It would actually be more correct to designate this as habilitation.

The task and goal of rehabilitation is the attainment of physical, psychic, and social well being in spite of the handicap. Then if one applies this rehabilitation concept to the group of hearing-impaired people, it can very easily be recognized with the reattainment of spoken communications ability on the one hand and with the teaching of spoken communications ability to people who do not yet possess this ability. Such a broad definition of a rehabilitation concept includes the provision of hearing aids, as well as all measures for the maintenance of speech or the acquisition of speech, as well as the pedagogical, psychological, social, and mental care of the hearing-impaired person, including all necessary measures for his professional incorporation or reincorporation into society. The sum total of these measures is to be understood as aural rehabilitation and not simply one measure alone. This, however, does not exclude defining more closely any one of the above named measures.

Visual Communication; Speechreading

Visual communication is a means by which the speech process is openly visible through movements and is perceived by the communications partner. It is recognized as a spoken sign. It is supplemented by various other combinations and is understood in its meaning. One can rewrite very briefly speechreading as follows: it is the understanding of spoken language with the help of visual perception.

Auditory Communication

The goal of hearing education is an intensive exploitation of the residual hearing of hearing-impaired people in order to help them toward better spoken communication. The goal is different for deaf people than for those who are hard of hearing. It must, therefore, be specifically formulated for each group. For deaf people, the goal of auditory communication is a visual-auditive setting by which visual perception is supported by the exploitation of the still available remnants of their hearing. In contrast, auditory communication for hard-of-hearing people strives for an audiovisual setting or attitude by which the hearing, in spite of the hearing difficulties, is the chief focal point of perception. The methods which are used to reach these goals are different for postlingual deafened, elderly deaf people, and those who have become deafened as a result of their occupations than they are for those who are prelingually deaf. In order to separate them terminologically from each other, one uses the term auditory training for deaf adults and hearing education or auditory education for children.

Visual communication and auditory communication are possible only when language is already at hand. Therefore, a very important task of rehabilitation is to bring language to the hearing-impaired child and to maintain the already existing ability of language in the hearing-impaired adult.

Language Development

This means the total sum of all necessary measures which contribute toward the final integration of the hearing-impaired child into the hearing world so that he will be able to understand and be able to make himself understood. It is most important that he learn to use verbal language in its spoken and written forms.

Language Maintenance

Language maintenance is the sum total of all necessary measures which will enable the adult who becomes hearing impaired to continue to use his already acquired language in the best way possible but also to understand the language or the words spoken to him by his colleagues.

HISTORICAL OVERVIEW

Two-Hundred Years of Education of Hearing-impaired Children in Germany

The education of hearing-impaired children can, with justification, be designated as the oldest special educational discipline in the world. It had taken many centuries until the connection was recognized between deafness and dumbness. Well into the 19th century dumbness was considered, in many cases, to be a medical problem which people hoped to cure with surgical methods such as the freeing of the frenulum of the tongue although, already centuries before, it had been recognized that dumbness had no anatomical causes but that it was simply the result of deafness. The single correct consequence of the recognition was that the only way a child with irreversible damage could be helped was through an educational approach. It took some time, however, until it was recognized universally as the correct method.

Heinicke (1727–1790) deserves the credit for having established in Germany the first school for hearing-impaired children. After he had already instructed, on a private basis, a great number of hearing-impaired children, he opened in 1778 in Leipzig the first state school for the deaf. He is to be thanked that the schooling of hearing-impaired children was undertaken as a public duty. Heinicke attained worldwide recognition by the introduction of his oral method. With that, he stood in contrast to the method of the French Abbé de L'Epeé who, in 1770 in Paris, founded the first private school for the deaf. In his teaching method, the hand alphabet dominated along with script and gestures.

In the first half of the 19th century, many schools for deaf children were established in Germany at teacher seminaries. The establishment of these schools was based above all on the ideas of Graser (1776–1841) and Stephani (1751–1850). Their ideas, briefly stated, were that hearing-impaired children could be promoted in a normal school situation if only every school teacher was acquainted with the method of instructing hearing-impaired children. This was said to have been attained in small schools for the deaf that were attached to the teacher seminaries. In this way, they hoped to make large independent schools for the deaf unnecessary. Because of the great class sizes at that time (approximately 60–70 children were instructed at one time in a class), the plan of Graser and Stephani did not work and had to be given up. This, however, had a very favorable effect on the education of deaf children at that time, for many of the small schools for the deaf that were attached to teacher seminaries became, in the course of time, independent schools for hearing-impaired children.

Direct Oral Association

The very fruitful, further development of the instructional reform of deaf children can be attributed to a man named Hill (1805–1874). Hill explained that language must be developed in a deaf child the same as in a normal child. He insisted, therefore, on the direct oral association, i.e., all things should be audibly spoken without the use of written language, gestures, or signs. The battle against gestures in the communication of deaf people became the battle cry of the German method which one designated as the oral method in contrast to the French method. Speech became the primary goal and it was even placed above writing. The deaf student was allowed to write only those words or sentences which he could already speak.

In 1880, the pure oral method was given general recognition at the International Congress of the Teachers of the Deaf in Milan. It was set up and used in all the German-speaking areas of Central Europe. Its most significant representative was Vatter (1842–1916). The school for deaf children in Frankfurt that was directed by him was, for a long time, visited by teachers of deaf children throughtout the whole world.

Because of the unconditional exclusion of gestures from the instruction of deaf children, there also developed countermovements. A man named Heidsiek (1855–1942) demanded the use of gestures and the finger alphabet after his study tour in American schools for the deaf. He caused many disagreements around the turn of the century with his attitude which lasted over a decade. His battle, however, was not without some success. People stayed pretty much with the oral method, but they found that there was also a place for gestures in the education of deaf children.

Global Language Acquisition and Its Predecessors

Two men, Göpfert (1851–1906) and Lindner (1880–1964), developed a method they called the writing method in which they tried to overcome the difficulties which the deaf child had in the acquisition of speech as the child attempted to learn the difficult oral method. The method of Göpfert and Lindner was not based primarily on the spoken word but rather on the written word. The hearing-impaired child first learned the language before he was taught to speak. A new way of articulation instruction was suggested by Malisch (1860–1925). In place of the very difficult instruction beginning with single sounds, he provided his comprehensive speech instruction which was further developed at a later period of time by Kern (1897 to the present). He built into his teaching method some aspects of the method of the Hungarian otologist and teacher of the deaf, Barczi (1890–1964). These methods were used widely in German schools for the deaf.

Today, the language and speech instruction for deaf and hard-of-hearing children is following the comprehensive method which has replaced the method which started with single sounds and which was connected with the name of Vatter. Two great ideas have contributed essentially to this change: namely, the so-called "auditory movement" and preschool education. Both ideas have had a lasting influence on the education of hearing-impaired children in the German-speaking countries of Central Europe from the beginning of this century.

"Auditory Movement" and Hearing Education

Toward the end of the 19th century, two otologists, Urbantschitsch (1847–1921) in Vienna and Bezold (1842–1908) in Munich, established, through the measurement of hearing, that a very considerable percentage of deaf children had a great deal of hearing ability, so much so that today we would call them hard of hearing instead of deaf. This determination started the call for special classes in schools for deaf children especially in Southern Germany, where discoveries in the area of education of hearing-impaired children were always received very well. These so called "hearing classes" were furnished and enriched with group amplifiers and, in these classes, a very intensive experimental work was started. The expectation which was promulgated by Urbantschitsch was that hearing exercises at school age would provide a very definite increase in hearing in a physiological sense. This expectation, however, was not fulfilled. The technical aids used then proved to be inadequate. Consequently, the movement started by Urbantschitsch and Bezold in German schools for the deaf gradually faded out. It is, nevertheless, an undisputed historical credit to all otologists and teachers who at that time took part in these experiments, that a new school form, namely schools for hard-of-hearing children, was already established in Germany at the beginning of the 20th century.

The development of new technical aids led very quickly, after the end of World War II, to a new hearing movement in the teaching of the hearing impaired. New tools were at our disposal, namely, audiometers instead of tuning forks as testing means as well as group hearing aids and individual hearing aids. These instruments pressed urgently for trial and use in instruction. In Germany, it was Hofmarksrichter (1900 to present), Steinbauer (1910–1971), and Braun (1926 to present) who were active as teachers at the school for deaf children in Straubing and who tested and used new hearing aids in their school and developed new paths and new ways for hearing education. Until 1960, many schools for deaf and hard-of-hearing children did not have enough means at their disposal to equip all classrooms with modern auditory training equipment. Today, in contrast, there are only a few schools in which this condition still exists. In almost every classroom we have the necessary technical prerequisites at hand for hearing education. Thus, hearing education, which originally was limited to just a few hours a week and was only listed as a special subject or special course of instruction, in many schools has now become an important principle of instruction.

Preschool Education

It was in Germany that Fröbel (1782–1852) started the first kindergarten and developed a play and work system for early childhood. In the course of the 19th century, Fröbel's idea led in many cities to the formation of kindergartens. The expectation that education of hearing-impaired children would also take over the idea of a kindergarten was unfortunately not fulfilled in Germany. There are many different reasons for this. In the 19th century the task which was more important was the introduction of mandatory schooling and the building of schools for school age children. Some of the obstacles in the way of a preschool education for hearing-impaired children were the unreliable traffic conditions of the time and the need to concentrate these children in a central place. In the 19th century, many of the causes of hearing losses were severe illnesses from which some of these children still suffered consequences. It was not advisable to separate them from their mothers and to house them in dormitories. At that time, the mandatory school age for hearing-impaired children was age 7 years. In addition, many German teachers of deaf children were opposed to preschool education for deaf children. Therefore, it called for the initiatives of otologists to bring preschool education into being, just as it had to bring about the basic idea of hearing education. Here above all, the Berlin otologist, Flatau, is to be credited for having established in Berlin, in 1895, the first kindergarten for deaf children. Otologists were also the leaders in other citities of Germany in founding this kind of kindergarten. This also holds true for the kindergarten in Vienna, which was set up in 1916 in the middle of World War I as a care center for hearing-impaired children whose mothers were working in the armament industry. This kindergarten was later developed into a modern preschool for hearing-impaired children thanks to the efforts of Viennese Freunthaller and Biffl. They were so successful that they convinced even the most skeptical teachers of the importance of preschool education. Freunthaller built the kindergarten in Vienna into a preschool that followed the lines of the mother school using new teaching materials that formed an example that was imitated in almost all of the preschools for deaf children.

Early Education

While in German-speaking countries we designate education for hearing-impaired children (4–6 years of age) as preschool education, we must also understand that early education is that educational care of children which takes place in their parents' home from the time of birth to 3 years of age. This is called "home language education." It is credited to Löwe (1922 to present), who started this early education for the first time within the German-speaking countries of Central Europe. He established this concept in many European countries. His many-sided educational initiatives led in 1959 to the opening of the first pedoaudiological guidance center for parents of hearing-impaired children at Heidelberg in Central Europe. This was the first time that a new educational idea of this magnitude was generated from within the field of special education and did not have to come from the outside (as was the case with auditory and preschool education which were started by otologists, not educators). Today almost all schools for hearing-impaired children in the German-speaking countries have guidance centers connected with them which function collaterally with the parents' work for early language development.

GENERAL DESCRIPTION OF PRESENT PROGRAMS OF AURAL HABILITATION AND REHABILITATION

Recommendation of the European Council

In 1966 the European Council in Strasburg issued, as a strong suggestion, the following measures and felt that they were very necessary for carrying out the rehabilitation and education of hearing-impaired children and adults:

1. The timely recognition and medical treatment of congenital or acquired hearing damage in early childhood during the school time and at the time of screening for entrance or for general screening in factories by otologists, by ear, nose, and throat clinics, and by audiological centers.
2. The informing and enlightening of the public as well as the advising of the parents.
3. The providing of all hearing-impaired children with individual hearing aids and the providing of schools with auditory training systems as well as with other technical aids.
4. The early education of the hearing-impaired children at home as well as their education in preschool establishments.
5. The schooling of the hearing-impaired child in a school which concentrates on the hearing impaired. Gifted students should be given the opportunity to attend further schooling which goes into greater depth.
6. The occupational preparation for hearing-impaired youth according to the degree of their education, corresponding with their knowledge and ability; occupational counseling through the general or the special counseling services which are set up for handicapped people.
7. The promotion or the furthering of the contact ability of adult hearing-impaired people with their environment; the partaking of the cultural life of the community and of their opportunities for adult education.
8. The establishment of social help centers for the counseling and supervision of the success of all measures undertaken for integration.

As the following statements show, these suggestions are considered fulfilled, for the most part, as far as the German-speaking countries of Central Europe are concerned, but we certainly cannot say that all current programs are completely satisfactory. Until the beginning of World War I, there was a special promotion only after the completion of the 7th year of life for deaf and hard-of-hearing children in the German-speaking countries. It signified, therefore, great progress when, in the time between both world wars, many of the existing schools for deaf and hard-of-hearing children had kindergartens attached to them which hearing-impaired children, upon the wish of their parents, could attend at the completion of their 4th year. Through the establishment of pedoaudiological guidance centers, which concern themselves with the "home language education" of hearing-impaired children from early infancy, it became possible, for the first time, to offer special help to these children during the first years of life. Today the education of hearing-impaired children in the Federal Republic of Germany has the following institutional structure: (a) *the outschool areas* (this is not obligatory); (b) the "*home language education*" for hearing-impaired children from their first year until their entrance into a special kindergarten or until they reach the mandatory school age; (c) *special kindergartens* for hearing-impaired children from the fourth year of life (these kindergartens are, for the most part, an integral part of schools for deaf or hard-of-hearing children; there are only very few special kindergartens which are not connected with a special school for hearing-impaired children); (d) *residential education* for all of those hearing-impaired children who, for various reasons, cannot return home daily from their special kindergarten or their special school; (e) *adult education* for the deaf and hard of hearing: (a) *school areas* (this is obligatory); (b) *elementary school* for deaf and hard-of-hearing children (4 years, from the 7th year through the 10th year); (c) *the main school* for deaf and hard-of-hearing children (5 or 6 years, from the 11th year through the 15th or 16th years); (d) *the middle school* for deaf and hard-of-hearing children (4 years—as a rule this comes after the 2nd year of attendance at the main school (13–16 or 17 years of age); (e) *the high school* for well-gifted, hearing-impaired adolescents (the duration is for 3–4 years after the successful completion of the middle school, 17–20 years of age); (11) *occupational or professional school* for hearing-impaired adolescents (3 years part-time instruction which runs parallel with the practical vocational training).

Besides these, which are open for most of the hearing-impaired children and adolescents, there are also programs for mentally retarded or physically handicapped hearing-impaired children as well as for deaf-blind children. It can certainly be deduced from this survey that there is a multitude of special programs available to hearing-impaired people for the first two decades of their lives. These programs all have as a goal the integration of handicapped people into society by making them as independent as possible.

There is a sufficient number of special schools for hearing-impaired children (most of them have also a special kindergarten and a pedoaudiological guidance center attached to them) within the German-speaking countries. In this context, one must consider the fact that the annual birth rate has sharply declined within the past few years (in the Federal Republic of Germany it has dropped from approximately 1 million births per year at the end of the 1960's to about 600,000 births per year at present). This means that the total number of hearing-impaired children has also declined.

The proportion of deaf children when compared to the total school population amounts to approximately 0.04%. The proportion of hard-of-hearing children who need a full-time special education cannot be stated so reliably. It is estimated that it is about 50–100% over the number of deaf children. That corresponds to approximately 0.06–0.08% of all school age children.

Obviously the total number of hard-of-hearing children of school age is much higher than 0.08%. Thanks to early discovery and early treatment and, not in the least, thanks to new hearing aids, it has become even more possible for an increasing number of hard-of-hearing children to partake of instruction at a regular school. These children in the regular school, however, receive no supplementary special education because, in most of the states of Germany or of the cantons in Switzerland, one finds special education only in special schools but not yet in the regular schools. (In the German-speaking countries that belong to the Western world, the education is not the responsibility of the federal government but of the single states.) The recommendations which appeared in 1974 from the Educational Commission of the German Education Council (of the Federal Republic of Germany) entitled "Zur pädagogischen Förderung behinderter und von Behinderung bedrohter Kinder and jugendlicher," suggest very strongly that special educational methods be applied in the standard school system in order to provide in this manner the successful schooling of hard-of-hearing children in regular classes in an ever increasing number. Still, it will take considerable time before these guidelines are generally recognized. Looked at in this way, there is currently, for hard-of-hearing children of school age, no genuine educational alternative to the special school. Only in a scattered way, for example, in Vienna, Austria, and Lucerne, Switzerland, do there exist partially integrated programs for classes of deaf children in the regular school system.

Less comforting are the programs in the area of rehabilitation of hearing-impaired adults, even if it is true that in the last few years a number of so called "cultural centers for hearing-impaired adults" have sprung up in some of the larger cities which, in an exemplary manner, work for the further education of the hearing-impaired adults living in their area.

In the German-speaking countries, even the private schools for hearing-impaired children receive considerable monetary help from the state (with the notable exception of the German Democratic Republic). It might be said at this point also that the number of private schools is very small; most of them are church schools. It is, therefore, not necessary for parents of hearing-impaired children to pay for their education. This applies to state schools as well as to private schools. A certain amount of teaching and learning materials is given to them free of charge. However, the regulation for the payment of the cost of boarding of those hearing-impaired children who cannot return to their homes daily is different. While in Switzerland this cost is borne by the health insurance in its entirety, the parents in the Federal Republic of Germany are charged a fee in the amount that they would have had to spend to provide for that child if he were living at home. In the German state of Baden-Wurttemberg, for example, it costs yearly about 1,000 marks; that is, approximately $400. Parents whose income does not exceed a certain amount have the cost partly or completely waived.

After this initial general discussion, a few supplementary remarks are in order concerning the establishments and institutions whose specific tasks are not generally known outside of the German-speaking countries.

Pedoaudiological Guidance Centers

Pedoaudiological guidance centers are usually connected to a school for deaf or for hard-of-hearing children but could also be connected to a child clinic or an ear, nose, and throat clinic, as is done in Zurich. Their main task is the early advancement of hearing-impaired children who are sent to them by medical specialists (pediatricians, otologists, etc.), clinics, health offices, etc. A prerequisite for a good special early education of hearing-impaired children is, in addition to an early recognition, a very early and complete diagnosis. Therefore, as a general rule, these pedoaudiological guidance centers have at their disposal the personnel and the instrumental prerequisites for audiological as well as psychological and educational examinations.

The "home language education" is important to the early advancement of hearing-impaired children. The home language education is first carried out by the parents of the hearing-impaired small child. They are given certain guidelines, either by regular visits in the pedoaudiological center or through a special visit by a special education teacher in their home. The parents also receive written directions for carrying out home language education. The parents have other methods also at their disposal, which they receive from the pedoaudiological guidance centers (such as games or exercise material which promote language and auditory trainers or phonators for use in helping the child at home).

Middle School

In the Federal Republic of Germany, and incidentally also in Austria and Switzerland, all the nonhandicapped children attend the elementary school from their 7th to 10th years. Afterward, schooling is not the same for all children. It can be either a main, middle, or high school. While the main school trains its students for the manual and industrial professions, the middle school trains its students for the practical life with more specialized economic and social responsibility and provides them with the necessary general education. In the middle school, a foreign language is obligatory—as a rule, English. A second foreign language can also be taken as a subject of choice. The second foreign language becomes obligatory for all students who, after the completion of the middle school, wish to go into the high school.

Middle school classes also exist for deaf and hard-of-hearing children. Whoever wants to enter into such a class must have the ability to learn a foreign language in addition to the German language. Since this demand is not easy for all deaf children to fulfill, the actual percentage of hearing-impaired middle school students is much smaller than one would find among those students who have no hearing problem.

In contrast to the situation in the Federal Republic of Germany, for the students in the "oberstufen classes" of Switzerland (which are comparable to the middle school classes for the hearing impaired in the Federal Republic of Germany) it is not necessary to learn a foreign language.

High School

All those students in the German-speaking countries who have their sights set on a university or college study have to take a test called the "abitur." This has as a prerequisite a 9-year successful attendance at a high school. There are different types of high schools which vary, above all, in the language sequence. However, whether it is a matter of a natural science-orientated high school or a more language-oriented high school, the students must learn three foreign languages. Furthermore, it is characteristic of the German high schools that they more or less prescribe the curriculum for their students. It is simply not possible that a student can concentrate on those subjects which come easy to him and leave out those subjects which seem to him to be a little more difficult. He must study the full program offered at the high school.

Clearly then, it will be possible only in a very few exceptional cases for hearing-impaired children to follow the instruction of a regular high school. For a few years now there have been special high school classes for hearing-impaired youth, in North Germany, in the city of Hamburg and, in Southern Germany, in the city of Freiburg, in which hearing-impaired boys and girls who have made above average progress in the middle school are allowed to go into the 4-year additional high school program. While the high school department in Hamburg is part of a regular high school, the department in Freiburg is within the school for deaf and hard-of-hearing children.

Professional School

In the dual system which prevails in the German-speaking countries, professional education takes place in business settings as well as in the professional school. Professional schools are set up as part-time schools and are taken right along with experience. These professional schools have the responsibility of providing for the general education of the students, with special consideration for the training for their particular professional job. They also provide for the practical application of their knowledge to their professional job. In exceptional cases, and this holds true especially for handicapped children, full-time study can be arranged in place of part-time study. The full-time study is put together in connecting periods of time, for example, two times a year with each period lasting 4 weeks.

All the youngsters who are in a working situation or who are unemployed are required to attend a professional school. The professional school obligation begins at the end of the full-time school obligation and lasts, as a rule, 3 years. Hearing-impaired youth fulfill their professional school obligation, insofar as they cannot attend a professional school for youth with normal hearing in a central professional school for hearing-impaired adolescents. There is, for example, in all the German-speaking cantons of Switzerland, only one central professional school for all hearing-impaired adolescents in Zurich. This central school also has branches in some of the other large cities of Switzerland. In 1972–1973, 21 classes (a total of 120 students) were held for vocational instruction of these hearing-impaired adolescents, in the so-called "intracantonal vocational schools for hearing-impaired youth." There also existed for these 120 adolescents special learning groups for approximately 50 different occupations, including: auto painter, weaver, mechanic, baker, heating designer, furrier, flower gardener, building draftsman, upholsterer, book binder, auto upholsterer, tile layer, beautician, auto mechanic, cabinet maker, lathe operator, cook, sign painter, electrician, laboratory assistant, tapestry seamstress, machinist, painter, dental technician, florist, engine fitter, draftsman, goldsmith, machine designer, dressmaker, and brick layer.

In cases of need, even if only one student requests it, new professional classes are formed. It is very satisfying that in the German-speaking sections of Switzerland the professional education of the hearing impaired has been integrated with that of normal hearing people to a large degree. Special classes and special efforts during schooling are in no way identical with segregation from those who have normal hearing. Where it is not possible to install professional school classes for hearing-impaired youth in Swiss school houses where normal hearing people are studying, they are trying to bring students with normal hearing into the vocational schools for the hearing impaired and have them work in these schools. In this way, they try combatting this very undesirable segregation.

Auditory Training, Visual Training, and Related Courses

This survey would be incomplete if no mention were made of all the various programs and aids available for the adult hard of hearing and deaf. These programs (auditory training and speechreading courses) exist in the larger cities and are offered by different groups; for example, by hard-of-hearing organizations and by schools for the hard of hearing, by ear, nose, and throat clinics, and by hearing aid centers. Professional retraining opportunities for people who became deaf as adults and who, therefore, cannot continue in professions are available for instance, at the well known rehabilitation center at Heidelberg. For this purpose, this center employs a number of teachers of the deaf who have additional study in he field of vocational training.

DIAGNOSTIC PROCEDURES

In the German-speaking countries, the concept is well recognized that success in the treatment and education of a hearing-impaired child is greater the earlier it is begun. That means that a hearing problem present in early childhood must be diagnosed and recognized as early as possible so that the residual hearing ability can be exploited and developed for speech and language development as soon as possible.

First Examination

The etiological and diagnostic determination of a child's problems takes in various areas. As a rule, this diagnosis takes place in German-speaking countries in an audiological department of an ear, nose, and throat clinic and/or in a paedoaudiological guidance center. Therefore, a very detailed history of the child has to be collected and put together, and the child's auditory behavior must be observed. Furthermore, there are, of course, tests and examinations which must be undertaken. Finally, on the basis of these results, a diagnosis is made which is viewed as a differential diagnosis.

Great value is to be placed on detailed collection of health and personal history because of the many types of etiological conclusions that can be drawn. Along with the individual health history comes the health history of the family, including occurrence of significant diseases, the length of pregnancy, birth data, as well as the sicknesses suffered by the child in his first year of life. These all have great significance.

In the diagnosis of hearing loss, organic causes of the disease and problems in the middle and outer ear have to be excluded by medical specialists. In all cases of anomaly or history of infections, an x-ray should be taken of the petrous. Blood examinations are in order when there is suspicion of an Rh factor or the incompatibility of blood groupings, toxoplasmosis, and different virus infections. Also the vestibular test might be meaningful.

Procedure for Measuring Hearing

The methods today that are used for measuring hearing in children can be arranged according to these principles: (1) their chronological or developmental age; (2) the goal (screening or diagnostic tests); (3) the auditory stimuli employed (tone or speech audiometry); (4) the relation between the intensity of the stimulus and the threshold of hearing (threshold audiometry and suprathreshold audiometry); (5) the necessity of cooperation of the child (subjective, objective, and semiobjective audiometry); and (6) the method of accomplishment or execution.

It is not within the purview of this chapter to describe all the processes which are used today for measuring hearing in children. A survey of the more important of these processes is given in Table 1, which, however, does not include the objective and semiobjective processes. On the one hand, the only procedures regarded as objective measurements are those which result in a spontaneous reaction of the child (a reaction which is independent of his intentional body movements) and those procedures which, on the other hand, do not leave the decision as to whether the child has reacted or not to the subjective judgment of the examiners. Semiobjective measurements are those with unintentional reactions on the part of the child but where the examiner still has to decide whether the child has reacted or not and has also to interpret the reactions. This type of designation was put into use for the first time by Löwe by 1974 and is set forth as follows: (1) vegetative reflex phenom-

Table 1. Processes used to measure hearing in children

Age	Screening examinations	Diagnostic examinations
Birth–7 months	Behavior observation audiometry Newborn audiometry; nursing baby audiometry	Behavior observation audiometry Newborn audiometry; crib audiometry according to Biesalski (1973)
5 months–3 years	Screening examinations according to Ewing	Diagnostic examinations according to Ewing; COR-audiometry according to Suzuki
2½–8 years	Performance audiometry Screening examinations according to Ewing; hearing-picture test; abbreviated tone audiometry	Performance audiometry Play audiometry according to Barr; speech audiometry with word materials suitable for this age level of hearing-impaired children
6 years and older	Hearing-picture test; abbreviated tone audiometry	Tone audiometry; speech audiometry with word material suitable for this age level of hearing-impaired children

enon: psychogalvanic reflex audiometry, plethysmographic reflex audiometry, and audiopneumographic audiometry; (2) acoustical feedback reflex: measuring the impedence of the eardrum, and changes in the sound of breathing; (3) electrophysiological, objective hearing measuring processes: electroencephalographical audiometry, and electrocochleographical audiometry.

Of all the processes cited, the following have achieved a certain significance in the German-speaking countries: change in the sound of breath by sound stimulus (Kumpf, Münster); the electroencephalogram audiometry (Burian, Vienna); and the electrocochleographic audiometry (Graf and Mathis, Lucerne).

The last couple of processes can only be used, because of the great expense in setting them up, in some of the more outstanding and well equipped ear, nose, and throat clinics; the subjective tests mentioned in Table 1 are used more often. Even if special screening tests are presently being carried out with newborn children in only a few clinics, the use of special tests for children aged 6–9 months is increasing very much. Children aged 5 years and older are tested with either the hearing picture test which was developed by Heller and Löwe in Heidelberg or with an abbreviated form of tone audiometry.

All the children who have been singled out either by means of a screening test of hearing or who, for another reason, are suspected of having a hearing problem, have to be carefully examined as early as possible to determine the type and severity of an eventual latent hearing impairment. The measuring processes which are used for this come under the general designation of diagnostic examinations.

Among these diagnostic examinations, one would place the already mentioned processes of the objective and semiobjective audiometry and, above all, the following subjective processes: (1) behavioral observation audiometry without conditioned reflexes; (2) behavioral audiometry with conditioned reflexes; (3) play audiometry; (4) tone audiometry; and (5) speech audiometry.

Tone and speech audiometry with their many variations cannot only be used in child audiometry, but also with adolescents and adults as well. Since tone audiometry is independent of speech, it is today seen internationally as a more or less uniform approach as contrasted with speech audiometry. In the German-speaking countries, we have found, above all, these speech audiometric approaches successful and in wide use: the Freiburg Number Test according to Hahlbrock (1957) (for the determination of hearing loss for speech); the Frieburg One Syllable Test according to Hahlbrock (1957) (for the determination of discrimination loss for isolated speech); and the Marburg Sentence Intelligibility Test of Niemeyer and Beckman (1962) (for the determination of discrimination loss for connected speech).

The previously named speech audiometric tests are of course only conditionally usable for hearing-impaired children, because the word material of the Freiburg One Syllable Test and also of the Marburg Sentence Test is exclusively designed and set up according to phonetic points of view and is not oriented around the vocabulary of children. Therefore, authors like Beckmann (1959), Biesalski and associates (1973), Jacobi (1957), and König have developed special speech audiometric tests for children. Up to this point, it has not been possible to use these tests generally.

Psychological Examination

Next to audiology, psychology has made the most significant contribution to the differential diagnosis of hearing-impaired people. This holds especially true for children. We will be thinking first of all of intelligence tests. These should be given especially in the case of children with a great hearing loss, and should only be given with the aid of nonverbal performance tests since the weaknesses which will show up in the verbal intelligence area do not designate or signify a primary intelligence defect by many hearing-impaired children. On the contrary they are the consequences of the impaired hearing.

It is to the credit of a man named Heller (1973) that special evaluative norms for hearing-impaired children in German-speaking countries were developed for some of the special tests of intelligence for hearing-impaired children.

Clinical experience has shown that hearing-impaired children have a percentage of cerebral damage greater than the norm. This damage does not always show up in neurological examination. But only at times do deviations from norms show up in special speech and psychic mental functions. Therefore, for example, a disturbance in the visual motor Gestalt function can lead to indications of central nervous system damage and to a speech defect caused by this central nervous system damage.

REHABILITATIVE PROCEDURES

Language Instruction

If, in the German-speaking countries of Central Europe, the goal in the education of deaf children is the far reaching integration of the deaf people who can speak into the hearing world, then it only logically follows that the educational goal in teaching the hard of hearing cannot be construed as being narrower, but must be construed as much broader, and with good right. The teaching methods for the hard of hearing, therefore, strive for a complete oral integration of their students into the German language community.

Of course, I am not trying to say that the deaf and the hard of hearing are to be looked at as a unified group and to be talked about in that way. Hearing-impaired children differentiate themselves from each other in exactly the same way that hearing children differentiate themselves from each other. Therefore, it cannot be overlooked in this connection that some of the hearing-impaired children in addition to impaired hearing and the resulting handicaps show still further handicaps. Approximately 30% of all hearing-impaired children are classified as multiply handicapped. The teachers of deaf and hard-of-hearing children must, therefore, be aware of that and be prepared to use alternate teaching methods to compensate and to treat this problem, namely: (1) integrated programs for those deaf and hard-of-hearing children for whom such programs are possible; (2) segregated programs for those deaf and hard-of-hearing children for whom such programs are necessary; (3) pure oral oriented programs for all the deaf children who can be advanced in this way; and (4) combined programs for a minority of deaf children who cannot be advanced sufficiently in a pure oral program.

These few remarks show that, in the German-speaking countries, there is always a strong effort made to offer a good oral education to as many deaf and hard-of-hearing children and adults as possible. However, combined programs also exist for the extremely multiply handicapped deaf children—programs which are labeled "total communication" in other places and are demanded for all deaf children and even still for many hard-of-hearing children. Almost all teachers for the deaf and hard of hearing in Germany object to this as a measure which hinders integration.

The above-named goal of rehabilitative language and speech instruction which is in the family, continued in special kindergartens, etc., is started still in the forefront of all our work in the elementary schools. It takes a broad area and is designed so that the deaf child can learn to speak so that his speech can be understood by those in his environment. This becomes possible when the child speaks in a normal pitch with appropriate intensity of voice, and with a good articulated and rhythmic dynamic structure in sentences correctly formed.

In the nearly 200-year history of education of deaf children in Germany, many paths to this goal have been tried in order to reach more or less completely the goal of good oral language. We may here refer to the publications of Schumann (1940), Kern (1958), and Kröhnert (1966) which have taken issue with the development of the different teaching methods. The language and speech methods of the present have been influenced above all by Kern (1958) (Heidelberg) and Schuy (1955) (Euskirchen). Both methods, the comprehensive language instruction according to Kern and the very constructive process according to Schuy, were, of course, developed at a time in which there was no early education for hearing-impaired children. They are, therefore, no longer applicable everywhere where there is a preschool education for the deaf child.

Although they were developed at a time when deaf children entered school without any language and speech and when no auditory training equipment was available, the basic ideas of both methods are still important for the first language and speech development, as well as for the later building up or extension of language.

If one would like to state a marked difference between the constructive method according to Schuy (1890–1965) and the comprehensive teaching method according to Kern (1897 to present), then one would have to see that the constructive method in its original form only offered to the deaf child the first spoken word when the articulatory prerequisites had been fulfilled, while the comprehensive method took precedence of language before the articulation work started. Since the advancement of comprehension of spoken language gets assigned a higher value in the "home language education," as well as in the kindergarten education, than does the advancement of any early articulation, many of the concepts of the comprehensive teaching method have crept into the work of the teachers of the deaf who are more oriented toward the constructive method of teaching, and vice versa for the emphasized global beginning in the early education of the deaf child which made possible the acceptance of some of the ideas of the constructive method in the school work of some of the teachers who prefer the comprehensive method. In this way the realization of preschool education has contributed to the fact that the confrontation of these two methods, which has existed for two decades in the education of deaf children in Germany, today is considered to be over.

Lay people believe that when deaf children have learned to speak words and sentences distinctly that they are no longer dumb, and they have total control of language. That is, however, an erroneous conclusion. Before a deaf child can speak properly, he must be fluent with the word contents and the structure of the language and both of these skills are only accomplished after a language-building process which takes many years to accomplish. Therefore, it is the opinion of many German teachers of the deaf that the language or the extent of their language knowledge has to be limited. They represent the viewpoint that the deaf child can only be offered a part of the richness of the German language. The same holds true also for the word contents or the vocabulary. All of this can only be opened up for the deaf child over a long period of time.

Because it is not easy for the deaf child to master the word contents and the grammar of the German language, teachers of the deaf have been, at all times, very much concerned with the setting up of plans for the language acquisition as well as for the building up of language. These plans try to take into consideration the phonetic viewpoint as well as the viewpoints of the didactics of language instruction. As desirable as these thoughts may be, they must in no way seduce a teacher to orient himself to them exclusively for his use of language. If he does this, he restricts not only the linguistic development but also the cognitive development of the children.

In recent times the maternal reflective method which was developed by the Dutch teacher of the deaf, van Uden, has gained quite a bit of acceptance among the younger German teachers. Van Uden, who calls his reflective method also the teaching of an oral mother tongue to deaf children, intends to give the deaf child "a world of language." Therefore, he directs his energies against the constructive methods which are still in use in German schools for the deaf. Because he believes that the consequences of this method will be that the majority of the children will never attain true reading of normal literature, he rejects it heartily.

Speechreading

The essence of speechreading is the extracting of the sense of an utterance by observation of the mouth formations and movements of the speaker. For the deaf child, speechreading is a very essential means of communication. It is always to be a part of oral instruction. It is, therefore, a very important task to teach the child speechreading as early as possible. If his language education at home has started at the age of 6 months and is carried through, then such a child can, our experience has taught us, understand the first words and sentences he connects with the situations by reading lips by the time he is 12 months old.

The ability to speechread spoken language presumes an almost normal intelligence, a great vocabulary, and a good command of the structure of a language. The speechreading of unknown words is almost impossible. Also the speechreading ability is dependent too on the type of conception. Deaf children of the visual type of conception learn to speechread easier than other types.

Speechreading takes in all the visual movements of the lips, mouth, cheeks, and neck; however, the finer articulation movements in the mouth cavity cannot be seen. Therefore, a whole group of phonemes correspond to one kineme. Kinemes are visually perceivable forms of the speech organs and of the exterior mouth region. While a kineme can be described as a speech movement form which is distinguishable from other movements, the phoneme is a synonym for a speech sound. We will name the bilabial kineme as an example which corresponds to the following phonemes "p," "b," and "m." In total, in the German language we have seven or eight consonant and four vowel kinemes in spoken language as opposed to approximately 40 phonemes. Compared to phonemes, it can be seen that the kinemes are unstable carriers of information. Their instabilities result in the fact that the successive speech movement "Gestalten" are fragmentary elements of speech perception. The diffusion of its characteristics leads not uncommonly to deceptions in sounds during the transferring from the kineme area into the phoneme area. Nevertheless, speechreading is a very suitable communications method which originates from the ability of the so-called eclectic combination, which means that the sense of the context can be perceived from fragments only.

To the deaf child, speechreading is the sole path of understanding of that which is spoken to him. Many deaf children learn to speechread their first words in their early language education at home. In later articulation instruction, which is given a high place of value in the special kindergarten, the ability for speechreading is also furthered. It is constantly used with language instruction. It is integrated into each lesson. In general, nevertheless, it is not a subject area of instruction. As a rule, deaf children can speechread their parents and teachers very well. This happens not only because they get used to the mouth formations of their parents and teachers in the course of time, but also because the parents and teachers know very well with which vocabularies and with which language structures the children are familiar. They judge their speech and tend to use these words when talking to the children. On the other hand, many deaf people have difficulties with speechreading when they are spoken to in complicated sentences, with unfamiliar words, with indistinct pronunciation, or in dialect forms. Even with profoundly deaf children, speechreading gets a big boost by also using auditory and vibratory perception which they still have at their disposal. Instead of only monosensorial speech perception, many teachers of the deaf, therefore, strive to offer polysensorial speech perception which consists of feeling, hearing, and seeing to their deaf children.

Speech

The hearing-impaired child should not only learn to understand his environment, he must also be understood by his environment. Therefore, speech must be learned by him in such a way that he can speak understandably. That is the task of the first speech instruction which deaf children already get in their special kindergarten. This instruction, also called articulation instruction, tries to give correct pronunciations to the deaf child. The representatives of the constructive method teach articulation by using single sounds first, whereas the representatives of the global or comprehensive method teach complete words or begin with complete words. Both of them use speechreading, the sense of vibration, kinesthetic feelings, and any hearing ability that the person might still have for speech work. The teaching of articulation to deaf children in the preschool period should have a very high priority. This does not mean that we must demand always an exact articulation from the child, something which he is not able to do and which, if done too early, carries with it the danger that the joy or willingness of speaking will be stifled. It must be very clearly seen that the dangers which can come about by neglect of articulation work in the preschool period are no less dangerous than those caused by an articulation drill that is begun too early. If the deaf child cannot express himself at all or if his speaking is so bad that he cannot be understood by the people around him, then he always takes refuge in gestures in order to communicate. Articulation instruction must, above all, be practiced by deaf children and carried out daily and has to extend itself over the total school time, even if it achieves a greater emphasis in the preschool time and the elementary years. Speech work assumes again great importance for all those hearing-impaired children who later on attend a middle school where they must learn a foreign language.

Auditory Education

An especially valuable articulation help for deaf children has been achieved through the use of an apparatus called the fonator, which was developed by the Siemens firm and has been in use for many years by deaf children. In the aural and oral education of hard-of-hearing children, auditory trainers of different manufactures have been in use. The exploitation of the residual hearing with these devices, as well as with hearing aids, is beneficial not only for the perception of the speech of others but also for self perception, and it becomes, for the deaf child, effective in the unlocking of the auditory feedback mechanism. The sounds are brought back to their source of movement. The deaf child receives, in this manner, his own voice over his hearing aids as an acoustical or respectively vibro-tactile-acoustic sign. In connection with the kinesthetic speech movement sense, with these the child can feed back his own speech. But the child can also compare the polysensorially perceived speech of his partner through the auditory feedback of his own speech. He can compare this in a vibro-tactile-acoustic way and try to perfect his speech movements so that his feedback articulation agrees with the perceived speech pattern of his partner. The auditory feedback of articulation provides the deaf child who has residual hearing with very obvious structural aids for the perception of demands, and good articulation instruction becomes a very important concern for hearing education.

By oral communication, the deaf child, who has been properly equipped with the right apparatus, has a number of things that work for him in a very narrow functional connection. These are visual lipreading forms, kinesthetic sensations, and vibro-tactile-hearing patterns, as well as the language of the partner and also his own language.

A very important prerequisite for hearing and speech education is an optimal provision with hearing aids which generally takes place in the audiology department of the ear, nose, and throat clinics or in the pedoaudiological guidance centers. The parents of hearing-impaired children and also the hearing-impaired adults do not have to pay for these hearing aids. Since the first of October 1974, all mandatory insurance companies in the Federal Republic of Germany are obliged to pay in full for hearing aids which have been prescribed by doctors.

Unfortunately, in a number of German schools for deaf children, it is still the case that the exploitation of residual hearing of the students who attend those schools is not given proper attention despite the availability of superior auditory training equipment.

In order to simplify speechreading, as well as speech, for children, various optical helps have been developed. These can be subdivided into two large groups, namely, the manual systems and the technical aids for making speech visible and the technical aids for speech improvement (these cannot be taken up in any greater detail here).

Different Manual Systems

The use of different manual systems in the teaching of deaf people has a substitutive character. These systems try to take the place of the damaged sense of hearing and also try to minimize the difficulty deaf people have in the acquisition of speech, in learning, and in communication. Presently there are three groups of manual systems.

Kineme Supplementary Manual Systems To this group of manual systems belongs the system of Cornett which is certainly well known in the German speaking countries but which has not yet been adapted to German as the Danish mouth-hand system of Forchhammer which enjoyed a certain following during the 1930's in Germany. While cued speech is merely for the support of the speechreader, the mouth-hand system is also designed in certain respects to serve as an articulation aid.

Grapheme-Oriented Manual Systems In the course of the past several years, Geisperger in Straubing and Jussen in Cologne have been testing the use of the one-handed finger alphabet from the United States. A research paper which was presented by Jussen in 1975 actually raised more questions than it answered concerning the use of the finger alphabet in the development of speech acquisition and speech communication, for example, the problem of the incompatibility of the simultaneous offering of rhythmically different connected sounds and finger perception. This problem was not even discussed. In reality, the use of finger alphabets very strongly influences, in a negative way, the speaking rhythm of a teacher who speaks German. This speech rhythm plays a big role, nevertheless, for the exploitation of residual hearing. The child gets a bad example to use as a model for his speech. Procedures of aural-oral education, therefore, lose their value. Therefore, we are unable to report that any of the classes, which were instructed in the use of the finger alphabet as a supplementary method, had students who were able to speak any better than those in the classes instructed without the finger alphabet. It must also be emphasized that teachers of the experimental classes in which the finger alphabet was used were oriented very strongly toward developing good speech. They felt that this total communication, as taught in the United States, would only lead to a totally restricted oral communication. This concept is a total contradiction of the aural rehabilitation of hearing-impaired children.

Phoneme-Oriented Manual Systems Whereas the grapheme-oriented finger alphabets have hand signs that correspond to letters, the phonetic manual signal systems want to give to the deaf children aids for the structure of speech and, in this way, contribute to the acceleration of the speech tempo. Now here above all, we should think of the visual tactile system and of the system developed by Wolff (1971) which was constructed with reference to the initial teaching alphabet of Pitman and of a visual motor system. Of these three systems, only the phonetically oriented manual system has achieved some significance in the German-speaking countries.

In his research work which took many years, Schulte (1975) proved that the intelligibility of speech spoken by hearing-impaired people who had learned speech with the phonetic manual system was better than that of the experimental groups who did not use the phoneme signs. It could be further proved that the speech of deaf children with the phonetic manual system (PMS) could be corrected at all levels much faster and that, by the use of the PMS, more speech could be applied. Viewed in this manner we can then say that, at the present time, the PMS is the most popular and highly thought of manual system in use in Germany because it does correspond more with the goal of oral communication of deaf people than any other manual system.

Sign Language While speech is used almost exclusively in the teaching of deaf children in the German-speaking countries during the free times after instruction in the various boarding houses in a significant number of schools for deaf children, many children, when they are alone among themselves, communicate predominately with gestures or sign language. As Maesse (1935) proved, the sign language which does not conform with grammatical and syntactical rules of oral and written language has an indirect negative effect on the language of the deaf child in the sense that it puts the total adjustment of the child to the sign language process. Whoever decides that he wants to teach a deaf child oral language in the best way will have to try very hard during the time of the early childhood and the preschool language acquisition period to protect the child from these negative influences which have the effect of strongly reducing the accomplishment of the main goal of teaching oral communication. If it is not possible, because of one reason or another, to teach deaf children speech in time so that they can communicate adequately with normal hearing people as well as among each other, then these children are forced to learn a sign language which gives them a method of communicating in a very narrow circle of people only (but, nevertheless, it is a means of communication). The main goal of rehabilitation programs, however, is to give the child the ability to communicate in the world with the greatest circle of people. We cannot allow ourselves to lose sight of this as Rammel (1974) emphasizes in his book *Versuch einer Wesensanalyse* of the sign language.

Of course, there is a certain area within the rehabilitation of hearing-impaired children and adults in which a certain use of sign language must be tolerated; for example, in the education or training of mentally handicapped deaf children, as well as in the spiritual care for deaf adults.

Up to this point, in the German-speaking countries, no experiments have been undertaken to develop a systematic sign language which currently would replace the sign language by some deaf people which does not conform at all to spoken language. This was done, for example, by Gorman and Paget for the English language.

INTERPROFESSIONAL RELATIONSHIPS

A few decades ago it was incumbent only on the teachers of deaf and hard-of-hearing children to be responsible for the rehabilitation of hearing-impaired children and adults. However, today we have many professional groups who are active in this area: otologists, neurologists, audiologists, teachers, psychologists, hearing aid acousticians, linguists, sociologists, speech therapists, phoneticians, social workers, psychotherapists, physiotherapists, professional counselors, psychiatrists, parents, and, in ever increasing numbers, the hearing impaired themselves. This means that it is no longer only the teacher on whom the task of rehabilitation of hearing-impaired children falls.

Although it is necessary and desirable for all of these groups to take part in the habilitation and rehabilitation of hearing-impaired children and adults, it brings certain problems with it which have not yet been satisfactorily settled everywhere. Undoubtedly, the main problem results from the fact that there is no independent professional group of audiologists. The tasks which elsewhere are taken care of by audiologists are taken care of either by otologists (oto-audiologists) or by teachers (pedoaudiologists) in the German-speaking countries. How the tasks, therefore, are divided up is dependent more or less upon how large or how small the engagement of the audiologist is. If he feels mainly that he is an otologist, then the audiologically interested teacher must be very active in order to help with the hearing-impaired child and to get the correct aid for the child. This is not necessary in the same way when an oto-audiologist would be there who sees himself first as an audiologist and only second as an otologist.

As a result of the nonuniform interest of the too few oto-audiologists, sometimes outsiders from the area of medicine take exception with the working arrangements between otologists on the one hand and teachers of the deaf on the other hand, both of whom dutifully are fulfilling their purposes (for instance, in the area of child audiometry and in the provision of hearing aids) but are viewed as over-stepping their competence as pedoaudiologists.

On the other hand, the disinterest of many principals of schools for hearing-impaired children toward early education activities was the reason that the initiative in this field was taken by medical people. Teachers of the deaf who are not sufficiently familiar with the local conditions are then ready to designate such medical activities in the teachers' field as a transgression.

Regardless of such occasional misunderstandings between the members of the medical field and those of the teaching field, we can very happily say that very good cooperation exists among all the professional groups who work with the rehabilitation of hearing-impaired children. This holds true especially with psychologists, the otologists, linguists, and phoneticians, some of whom had been teachers of the deaf previously or sons and daughters of teachers of the deaf.

FAMILY INVOLVEMENTS

Task of the Family in Education of Hearing-impaired Child

In order to counteract the negative effects of a high degree of hearing impairment on the development of a child affected and to avoid the stunted development of these children and to give them the opportunity for mental development that normal children would have, a special education program is necessary for the hearing-impaired child already in the first year of his life. His oral education cannot be begun early enough if one wants to reach a point where such a child will one day speak understandably and will integrate into society as one who can also understand the speech of his environment.

The first goal in the early education of these children, which takes place in the parent's home, is to avoid, at all costs, the handicapping effects of the deafness. Even the deaf child is not dumb for, in his early childhood, he cries just like any other child does, but, if his crying and his babbling are not transferred in his first imitative speech, by the time he reaches his second year or during the course of his second year he becomes deaf and dumb. In addition to this, another natural system comes into play by deaf children, namely, their so-called "turned-to-face attitude." The deaf child pays very close attention, especially before the time that he begins to walk, to the expression on his mother's face when she is speaking to him. By talking to the child in a constant, lively way from earliest childhood on, he develops (even at the beginning of his second year) his first speechreading ability. It is not at all uncommon that the child first tries to imitate these words without voice and a little bit later begins to add his voice to the words that were often spoken to him.

The child's second year of life is of decisive importance for his oral development. At the latest in the beginning of the second year, preventative measures must be taken against his becoming accustomed to deafness. Almost all deaf children have some residual hearing. This is very important to use as early as possible for speech development. Referring to van Uden, the teacher often understands deafness to be something in which sound perception plays no role. Such a behavior has to be counteracted from the earliest possible moment by speaking as much as possible to the child and by giving him the best possible hearing aids.

If everything is done to prevent a deaf child in his very early childhood from becoming dumb and from getting accustomed to his deafness, then, as a general rule, the development of sign language is prevented. The deaf child can only acquire sign language if he has a partner who answers his gestures with gestures. It, therefore, follows that the child's oral development lies, to a large degree, in the hands of his parents and their counselors and it also lies in their hands whether their deaf child will develop oral or manual communication.

Very understandably, the parents will need much professional help when they want to reach the goals of the prevention of dumbness, of getting accustomed to deafness, and of a sign language. This help comes to them in the parents' counseling sessions which are part of a general program designed to help parents of hearing-impaired children. The counseling of parents is most important directly after the diagnosis. The diagnosis of deafness causes a great shock to many parents and it produces many strong emotional reactions. These reactions can immediately be directed into constructive channels. It is, therefore, the parents who need the immediate attention and not the child. They are the ones who are suffering from the hearing impairment of the child and not the child himself.

General Counseling of Parents

Next to the general counseling of the parents, the primary function of counseling is to help the parents accept the child exactly as he is. Parents also need very in-depth counseling sessions as to their roles in helping the handicapped child. The main goal is to make the parents competent to maintain an atmosphere full of language at home for the child. Every happening has to be described orally and has to be verbalized for the child at a level commensurate with his language ability. The corresponding introduction must be developed around the household, the family, and the personality of the parents. It must have a very solidly outlined short goal, but, nonetheless, a reachable goal. The successes can be achieved in small steps. In the beginning, it is by far more important to watch the progress of the parents than that of the child. The earlier parental counseling begins, the sooner it will foster a good parent-child relationship. The basis for a good parent-child relationship is the ability of the parent to converse with the hearing-impaired child orally. Also, in the case of a child who has a substantial hearing loss, a mutual understanding and respect develop, above all, through the possibility of conversations between parents and child.

Counseling of Parents in Regard to the Handicap of Their Child

In counseling parents, they must be made aware of the knowledge and abilities which they will need for the education of their hearing-impaired child at home. For the difficult task of the first oral intervention, parents of a hearing-impaired child do not only need counseling sessions which take place at regular intervals, they also need a number of technical devices which will encourage the child to speak, such as hearing aids, sound light converters, fonators, and so forth. They need speech-encouraging games and exercise material which they can get from the pedoaudiological guidance centers (the centers responsible for counseling of the parents).

While it has been said that the pedoaudiological guidance centers will be the place where the parents get counseling, it should not be construed that the counseling can only take place there. The guidance centers are the proper place to counsel parents after the first examination of the child as well as later when further examinations must be made. For the specific counseling about their child, which concerns itself especially with the questions about the possibility of speech understanding through speech-reading and through the use of residual hearing, the house of the parents is by far more suitable. If the counselor is familiar with the specific household situation of the child's family, then he can advise the parents very accurately as to how they can guide their child to his first speech understanding and, in this way, encourage him to speak. It is usually much easier for the parents of a child to imitate the exercises with the child which were demonstrated to them by the counselor in their own home than elsewhere.

Individual Counseling and Group Counseling

Along with individual counseling, which is best done in the guidance center and in the parent's home, group counseling also has very great importance. This brings the parents of hearing-impaired children together so that they can recognize that they are not alone in having a handicapped child, but that others are in the same boat so to speak. In the group counseling, parents can exchange their ideas and experiences and encourage each other to help their child according to his ability. Group counseling, therefore, should be the only counseling parents get after their introduction to the "home language education."

To supplement the individual as well as the group counseling, there are courses for parents which last about a week and take place in a family rehabilitation center which the parents attend with as many of their children as possible. This includes the nonhandicapped children also.

Many parents of hearing-impaired children tend toward a restricted pampering educational style which is meant to protect the child. But by doing this, they hamper the development of the social behavior of the child in other areas that are not touched at all by the hearing loss. It is, therefore, an important task of parental counseling to enable the parents, by directed instructions, to make a contribution to the social development of the hearing-handicapped child which would allow the child the most normal development in the nonhearing world.

While the pedoaudiological guidance centers are adequate for the counseling of the parents in the preschool time, the counseling of the parents during the school period is mostly sporadic and depends on the principal and the teachers of the school which the child attends. It is not necessary to prove that many disadvantages are connected with such a solution which lacks every planning and regularity. To get assistance here in this area is still a goal to be achieved by teachers of deaf and of hard-of-hearing children.

Counseling Station for Hearing-impaired People

In cooperation with the professional counselors and professional psychologists of the local labor office, the schools frequently provide professional counseling. The youth and adult hearing-impaired person can, after he has graduated from school, partake of counseling opportunities and, in these counseling stations for hearing-impaired persons, there are, as a rule, very experienced social workers who, in emergency situations or in cases of need, can function as an interpreter. The first counseling stations of this type were set up a few years ago. Their number is still small, but increases from year to year.

TRAINING OF PROFESSIONALS FOR FIELD OF REHABILITATIVE AUDIOLOGY

Of the various professional groups which presently are working with the habilitation and rehabilitation of hearing-impaired children, adolescents, and adults, the teachers as well as the hearing aid acousticians have their courses of study outlined most clearly. They should be presented, therefore, in quite a bit of detail.

Training Programs for Teachers of Hearing-impaired Children

The majority of the teachers on the staffs of the special schools for hearing-impaired children have completed special training programs which qualify them to teach such children. Training programs for prospective teachers for deaf and partially hearing children are offered at Cologne, Hamburg, Heidelberg, Munich, Vienna, and Zurich. Although there are some differences between the programs of these centers (especially between the Austrian and Swiss programs) there are more or less the following two possibilities available:

1. After having qualified for admission to a university at the age of 19 or 20 by successfully passing the "Abitur," any student who wants to become an elementary school teacher has to matriculate either for a "Pädagogische Hochschule" or the department of education of a university. In both cases, the student has to take part in a basic training program over a period of six semesters (3 years) leading to the first examination of the teaching profession at the age of 22 or 23. As soon as this examination has been passed, the young teacher can start teaching in a school for hearing children. He can also decide to start teaching in a school for deaf (or other disabled) children for a probationary period of between 6 weeks and a few months. There is, of course, also the possibility to teach in a regular school for 1 or for 2 years before starting a probationary period of teaching in a school for deaf children. The principal of the special school in which the probationer is teaching usually decides how soon he will be given fully paid study leave for 2 years. During this time, he will study at one of the previously mentioned training centers. After 2 years of study, he has to pass the first examination in special education which is a sort of prediploma. The final diploma is granted after 18 months of part-time teaching under the supervision of an experienced teacher and part-time seminar work. This way of study means that the students devote 3½ years to studying special education methods and that they are about 27 or 28 years old when they finish their set period of study.
2. There is also the possibility of a so-called basic study. Basic study

(lasting 4 full years) means that the prospective teacher of deaf children can start studying the education of deaf children as soon as he has completed high school education at the age of 19 or 20. During the first 2 years, his curriculum will be focused on general education and, during the 3rd and 4th year, on special education. At the end of the 4th year, he has to pass the first examination in special education. During the following 18 months he has to teach under the supervision of a tutor teacher and also has to attend seminars which are held at regular intervals. Having completed these 18 months of study, he will have to take the second examination in special education.

This second way of study is comparatively new. It is also linked with many risks. The main disadvantage is that these teachers have not only never taught children with normal hearing, but also they are not qualified to teach them if they should fail as teachers of deaf children.

The following content of curricula is not comprehensive, but the subjects listed are those which appear in the curriculum of each center providing training for prospective teachers of deaf children:

1. Special Education and Social Education: (a) theory of special education, including its historical development and its anthropological influence; history and structure of the school system for disabled children; basic and special questions relating to special education; (b) history of the education of the deaf and partially hearing (the causes and the nature of the different hearing impairments and their sequelae); special problems and methods of teaching language to deaf or partially hearing children; didactics in the education of the deaf, the partially hearing, the deafened, and the deaf-blind; special tasks in the educational and instructional promotion of gifted as well as mentally retarded, maladjusted, and multiply handicapped hearing-impaired children; (c) procedures used in vocational schools for hearing-impaired adolescents; vocational guidance and vocational placement; problems arising in classes where training for different trades is provided.

2. Psychology: (a) introduction to basic problems in general psychology, psychology of children, social psychology, psychology of learning, and psychodiagnostics, with special reference to hearing impairment in children and adolescents; (b) psychology of perception and anomalies of perception, with special reference to perception via the auditory system (major problems in psycholinguistics); special problems in psychology of personality, psychology of behavior, social psychology, psychology of learning, educational psychology, and psychodiagnostics in behavioral dis-

turbances and as related to the academic performances of hearing-impaired children and adolescents.

3. Linguistics and Phonetics: (a) basic problems in linguistics related to the development of language, its structure and use; introduction to methods and results of applied linguistics which are relevant to the education of the deaf and partially hearing; introduction to functional and descriptive phonetics, phonology, and information theory; main problems in phonics; experimental phonetics; transcription exercises; (b) applied phonetics in the education of deaf and partially hearing children; educational audiology (play audiometry, pure tone audiometry, speech audiometry, audiovisual audiometry); early registration, early identification, early assessment, and early educational treatment of hearing-impaired infants; auditory training, phonation and speech correction as provided in schools for the deaf and partially hearing.

4. Medicine: (a) anatomy and physiology of the nervous system; psychopathology and child psychiatry; pediatrics and special education; (b) anatomy and physiology and pathology of the speech and hearing organs; clinical audiology and audiometry; neurology, psychiatry, and cerebral pathology and special education.

5. Legal Questions: (a) basic and special questions concerning laws dealing with special education.

Training Program for Hearing Aid Acousticians The training or education for hearing aid acousticians terminates with a final examination that must be taken at the end of their 3-year training. The profession of the hearing aid acoustician belongs to the blue collar working class in the Federal Republic of Germany. A prerequisite for admission to the training of hearing aid acousticians is completion of the German middle school.

The education for apprentices from the Federal Republic of Germany takes place in the training academy for hearing aid acousticians in Lübeck which, in part, also trains other people from German-speaking countries. A state professional school for hearing aid acousticians is connected with this training academy in Lübeck. This central station for professional training is necessary because there are relatively few hearing aid acoustician trainees. The practical education takes place in professional businesses which are run by experienced hearing aid acoustician masters. After completion of his apprenticeship examination and after 5 years of practical experience in hearing aid acoustical work, the young acoustician can take the master examination. Only hearing aid acousticians who have passed this examination are permitted to run their own business and train apprentices.

Since the central institute for hearing aid acousticians in Lübeck has been, until now, the only one of its kind in the world, we are showing here the curriculum and the subject matter required of the German hearing aid acoustician master grade.

Professional Regulations for Master Examination of a Hearing Aid Acoustician The practical main part of the master examination consists in the carrying out of a work test. This work test includes two portions, namely, a technical measurement and a technical fitting portion.

As a work test, the following works come into consideration:

1. In the area of technical measurement, the applicant has to carry out a complete measurement of the acoustical data of hearing in the same manner as would be required to find out which hearing aid is to be recommended. The results are put down in a report. With this, the following skills and acquirements have to be pointed out: the evaluation of the acoustical data of the ear according to different methods and the testing and the evaluation of the acoustical data of hearing aids in order to select and to determine the most appropriate hearing aid.
2. In the technical fitting portion, the applicant must fit a hearing aid (this must be done with an actual case); he must take an ear impression and also make, seal, and acoustically adapt an ear mold. He is also responsible for: the production of special ear pieces, the manufacturing of repairs of hearing aids as well as function tests of hearing aids and their assessories, the testing of the comprehension of speech during the fitting of hearing aids, and counseling the hearing-impaired person for the correct use of the hearing aid.

The applicant must also know: types, characteristic qualities, application, and manufacturing of the raw and auxiliary materials, as well as their production and storage; the structure and the effectiveness of most used sources of energy for hearing aids and their accessories; preventative hearing protection; technical drawing; technical arithmetic; the basic knowledge for the calculation of offers; special professional rules; the most important DIN norms; rules for accident protection; and basic health care.

Training Needs For the others who work with the habilitation and rehabilitation of hearing-impaired children, adolescents, and adults, there are also qualifying training courses and college courses. This holds true especially for the various medical professions as well as for the priests who work with deaf and hard-of-hearing people and offer to them their pastoral help. At the present time, there exist nowhere in the German-speaking countries educational opportunities for social workers for the hearing impaired or opportunities for educational personnel in student dormitories in schools for deaf and hard-of-hearing children. To get help in this area is a very important task for the future.

RESEARCH

In the area of the otological and audiological research, there is not in Germany, nor in Austria, nor in Switzerland a place which consistently reports or gives out information on current projects. It must, however, be mentioned in this respect that the German-speaking otologists in general and audiologists, especially in their own areas of work as well as in research, enjoy a very high degree of respect in Germany and abroad. This holds true above all for the so called "subworking group of audiologists," in which many prominent members were or are active in the development of objective as well as semiobjective processes for measuring hearing.

Essentially it is easier to report on the research projects in the area of teaching rehabilitation of hearing impaired. This teaching takes place in the four training centers for teachers of the deaf. These are in Hamburg, Heidelberg, Cologne, and Munich. The centers in Heidelberg and Cologne are especially active in research.

Research at the "Pädagogische Hochschule" Rhineland in Cologne

Family Situation of the Hearing-impaired Child Evaluation of an inquiry concerning the situation of the hard-of-hearing child in school, within the family, and in his free time is being undertaken.

Development of Teaching Programs for Teaching of Deaf People The goal of this research program is the correct designing of teaching programs which will allow the more effective methods of teaching in schools for the deaf children.

Audiovisual Instruction Methods for Speech Development This concerns the production of television films which are to be used for the instruction of articulation in schools for the deaf with the assistance of instructing examples.

Sound Film Audiometry This concerns the developing and standardization of the bases and the criteria for the production of sound films to be used in the speech audiometric examination of hearing-impaired children and adults.

Games or Working Material for Groups and Individual Working Programs for Hearing-impaired Children in Their Preschool Education This group is concerned with the material for the schooling in perception ability in the area of perception of forms (material which helps to make visual connections and to understand events as they happen). The current examinations have as a goal the development of special didactic material and of adequate methods for the preschool education of hearing-impaired children.

A Selection of Research at the "Pädagogische Hochschule" in Heidelberg

Basal Speech Audiometry for Hard-of-Hearing Children (in cooperation with Professor Dr. Kloster-Jensen, University of Hamburg). The transition in running speech between a vowel and a consonant (-ip-. -na-) is reflected in the changes of the acoustic spectrum especially as an inflection of the second formant bar. The inflection is an important clue to the perception of the consonant. Attempts are being made to develop word lists for speech audiometry on a formant inflection basis (FIB), as a refinement of the traditional phonetically balanced (PB) principle.

Audiovisual Speech Audiometry for Deaf Children The standard speech audiometry is not suited for deaf children since their hearing losses are too great for understanding speech on an auditory basis only. An audiovisual speech audiometry should not only be phonetic but also kinetic and should contain very carefully selected words or rows of words. Also, the word material that is offered must be familiar to the child.

Fundamental Linguistic Structures Paradigmental and synagmental structures found in books for hearing-impaired children are analyzed.

Heidelberg Nonverbal Intelligence Test The Heidelberg Intelligence Test (HIT) is a nonverbal group test which finds itself in the area of task analysis. The research goal is a short process in paper and pencil form but does not present the problems that the previous nonverbal tests do, that is, the outlay of time and materials necessary in these former intelligence measuring processes. The HIT has in its hypothesis to determine an indication factor of intelligence by means of the mere dimensional measuring of the ability to differentiate. This test has in it the problems of identification, logic, differentiation, reproduction, relations, and creativity.

ORGANIZATIONS AND ASSOCIATIONS RESPONSIBLE FOR HEARING-HANDICAPPED CHILDREN, ADOLESCENTS, AND ADULTS

In the Federal Republic of Germany, as well as in Austria and Switzerland, there are many associations which are concerned with the rehabilitation of hearing-impaired people. Some of the more important of these organizations will now be described.

Organizations and Associations in the Federal Republic of Germany

All of the organizations or units which are confronted daily with the question of rehabilitation of the hearing impaired are amalgamated into the German Society for the Rehabilitation of the Hearing Impaired. The only exception would be the professional group of otologists who are, of course, also active in the rehabilitation of hearing-impaired people.

German Society for the Rehabilitation of the Hearing Impaired, Inc. The German Society for the Rehabilitation of the Hearing Impaired, Inc. was founded in 1954 as a working group for the unitary promotion of education for the deaf and hard of hearing, as well as for the care of the deaf and hard of hearing. Today, in 1975, the following member clubs or units, which are all organized nationwide, belong to it:

(1) The German Association for Deaf Adults; (2) The German Association of Hard-of-Hearing Adults; (3) The German Association for Teachers of the Deaf; (4) The German Welfare Association for Hearing-impaired People; (5) The Association of Catholic Priests for the Deaf; (6) The Association of Protestant Pastors for the Deaf; (7) The Association of the Parents of Deaf Children; and (8) The Association of the Parents of Hard-of-Hearing Children. The German Society for the Rehabilitation of the Hearing Impaired represents the interests and the wishes of the hearing impaired as well as of those organizations that concern themselves with the assistance to the above named people. It coordinates the work of its member units and explains to the public about the special living conditions of the hearing impaired. It also coordinates the work of its member units and explains to the public about the special living conditions of the hearing impaired. It works with its member organizations for the development of education and continuing education as well as for the publication of magazines or literature in a simple language for hearing-impaired children and adults. It influences the passing of laws that affect the hearing impaired. The German Society for the Rehabilitation of the Hearing Impaired is also the publisher of the magazine *Hörgeschädigte Kinder* (1975 is the 12th year of publication and it has a circulation of approximately 5,000). The address is: The German Society for the Rehabilitation of the Hearing Impaired, D-2000-Hamburg 52, Bernadotte Street 126.

Member Units of German Society for Rehabilitation of the Hearing Impaired The German Association for Deaf Adults was founded in 1950. This is the so-called interest group of the German deaf organizations and cares for the economic, social, professional, and cultural interests of all deaf people in the Federal Republic of Germany. The number of its members in the 11 states is around 18,500, with 450 local clubs.

To this German Association for Deaf Adults are also connected member organizations such as the German Deaf Sport Organization founded in 1910 with approximately 5,000 members in over 100 sport clubs and also the association of the Catholic Deaf People founded in 1925 which has approximately 80 clubs and includes approximately 2,500 members. The German Association for Deaf Adults is a member of the World Federation of the Deaf. It publishes the *Deutsche Gehörlosen-Zeitung* monthly (1975 is the 103rd year of publication and the magazine has a circulation of around 8,000).

The German Association of Hard-of-Hearing Adults is smaller. While the overwhelming majority of German adult deaf people belong to the German Association for Deaf Adults, only about 5,000 adult hard-of-hearing people consider the German Association of Hard-of-Hearing Adults as representative of their interests. This small membership is a very good testimony to the fact that, in a very high measure, the adult hard of hearing have been rehabilitated and integrated into the hearing society of the Federal Republic of Germany. The approximately 5,000 members of the German Association of Hard-of-Hearing Adults are members of approximately 60 clubs which are brought together in eight state associations.

The German Association of Hard-of-Hearing Adults is also the editor of a monthly journal called *Schwerhörige und Spätertaubte* (in 1975, in its 27th year) and sees, as its main task, the care of the hard of hearing and those who have become deaf in later life. It organizes, among other things, courses for lipreading and social parties and get-togethers.

The Association of German Teachers for the Deaf was founded in 1894. It has 10 state units which have approximately 650 members. The total number of teachers of the deaf in the Federal Republic of Germany currently amounts to about 1,525. This group includes teachers for the deaf and the hard of hearing who are active in teaching. The purpose of the Association of German Teachers for the Deaf is the promotion of the educational system for deaf and hard-of-hearing children, as well as an avenue for communication among those teachers who are active in the Federal Republic of Germany in schools for deaf and hard-of-hearing children and, of course, the protection of their professional interests.

The Association of German Teachers of the Deaf arranges a national meeting every 3 years at which actual questions are discussed concerning the education of hearing-impaired children. It is also the publisher of the quarterly magazine *Hörgeschädigtenpädogogik* (1975 is the 29th year of publication; its circulation is approximately 1,200). While this quarterly magazine predominately is directed at the teachers of the deaf and hard of hearing, the magazine that is also published by the Association of German Teachers of the Deaf, called *Das Bunte Blatt,* is meant for hearing-impaired children (1975 is the 24th year of publication).

The Association of German Teachers of the Deaf is connected as a member unit to the European Federation of Associations of Teachers for the Deaf to which also belong the associations of teachers of the deaf of the following European states: Belgium, Denmark, Finland, Great Britain, France, Luxemburg, the Netherlands, Norway, Portugal, Sweden, and Spain. The European Federation of Associations of Teachers for the Deaf was founded in 1968 and has its headquarters in Brussels. Its tasks have been formulated as follows: (1) promotion of research in the area of education of hearing-impaired children and adolescents, and (2) the coordinating of corresponding efforts of the national deaf associations representing the teaching interests of hearing-impaired children to society. The European Federation of Associations of Teachers for the Deaf arranges a meeting every 2 years to which each member association cannot send more than 6 delegates. The information stemming from the national associations and from the public meeting is published in a report.

The German Association for the Welfare of the Deaf is a loose association of different regional welfare units for the hearing impaired which maintains in the different states of the Republic approximately 30 youth, old age, and care homes, and recreation homes for the multiply handicapped and contains about 1,800 beds.

The Association of Catholic Priests for the Deaf in Germany is comprised of all of the Catholic priests in the Federal Republic of Germany who are active either mainly or secondarily in administering pastoral help to the deaf. This association publishes, for its members as well as for all teachers who instruct religious subjects in schools for deaf and hard-of-hearing children, a quarterly magazine called *Mitteilungen zur Gehörlosenseelsorge.* Besides this, it is also the editor of the monthly magazine, *Epheta*, which is for Catholic deaf people (1975 is its 27th year of publication).

To the Association of the Protestant Priests for the Deaf in Germany belong almost all Protestant pastors who work with deaf people in Germany. This association publishes a monthly Protestant magazine entitled *Unsere Gemeinde*. It is for adult deaf people and this publication is in its 23rd year in 1975.

The Association of Parents of Deaf Children was founded in 1961 and there are 36 parent groups with approximately 2,500 members.

The Association of Parents of Hard-of-Hearing Children was founded in 1965 and represents approximately 3,000 parents of hard-of-hearing children.

The Professional Association of the German Ear, Nose, and Throat Doctors in the representative of ear, nose, and throat doctors who are in Germany in private practice. This unit has a membership of approximately 2,200 physicians. Its address is D 2430 Neustadt-Ostsee, Schiffsbrücke.

The German Society for Ear, Nose, and Throat Doctors and for Head and Throat Surgery was founded in 1922 by the amalgamation of the German Otological Society, which was founded in 1892, with the German Throat Physicians Society, founded in 1894. Its address is D-7500 Karlsruhe 1, Wendtstr, 9. Its purpose is the promotion of the scientific and practical ear, nose, and throat therapy and head and throat surgery. Further tasks are the protection of the unity of these special areas of ear, nose, and throat treatment and the connection with their adjacent medical specialties, and with the foreign specialist societies, as well as the continuing education in their own area of specialty. At the present time this organization has a membership of around 1,700 ear, nose, and throat physicians.

The Association of German Audiologists has existed since 1949 and consists of otologists, physiologists, and other scientists who actively research in the area of audiology. It is connected to the previously named German Society for the Ear, Nose, and Throat Doctors. This organization has approximately 75 scientists as members from the German-speaking areas of Central Europe.

The Federal Guild of Hearing Aid Acousticians is a governmentally established body and has existed since 1966 with approximately 550 members.

The Union of the Hearing Aid Acousticians is a privately run supplement to the previously named guild and has its headquarters in Düsseldorf. It has been in existence since 1960 and has, at present, approximately 540 members.

Organizations and Associations in Switzerland Similiar to the Federal Republic of Germany, there exists in the German-speaking portion of Switzerland a parent organization which covers all the other organizations which work with the rehabilitation of the hearing impaired. This parent organization has the name "Swiss Union to Help the Deaf" and has its headquarters in Berne, Switzerland. To this organization the following special organizations belong: (1) The Society of Swiss Ear, Nose, and Throat Doctors; (2) The Swiss Group of Social Workers for the Deaf; (3) The Swiss Association of Teachers of the Deaf; and (4) The Ecumenical Association for Priests and Pastors Who Administer to the Deaf.

While the main task of those four specialty units contained in the Swiss organization for help to the deaf is concerned above all with the rehabilitation of the deaf, the group of Swiss hard-of-hearing organizations is concerned with the rehabilitation of the hard of hearing and, along with this, belongs to the Swiss Society of Phoniatry and Audiology. The purpose of the Swiss hard-of-hearing organizations is the support and promotion of the help to the hard of hearing in all areas of their private and public life. Their publication called *Monatsblatt der BSSV* has approximately 8,500 subscribers.

Organizations and Associations in Austria Similiar organizations and associations to those that exist in the Federal Republic of Germany and Switzerland do not yet exist in Austria.

PERIODICALS ON HEARING IN AUSTRIA, FEDERAL REPUBLIC OF GERMANY, AND SWITZERLAND

In the Field of Audiology

1. Zeitsch. Hörgerate-Akust. (J. Audiol. Technique), Published bimonthly by Median-Verlag, D-6900-Heidelberg 1, Hauptstr. 64.
2. Der Hörgeräte-Akustiker (Official Organ of the Federal Guild of Hearing Aid Acousticians) published monthly by the same publisher.

In the Field of Education of Hearing-impaired Children and Adolescents

1. Hörgeschädigtenpädagogik (Official Organ of the Association of German Teachers for the Deaf), published quarterly by Julius Gross Verlag Heidelberg, Verlagsbüro K. Wolff, D-6909-Dielheim, Lindenweg 1.
2. Hörgeschädigte Kinder (Official Organ of the German Society for the Rehabilitation of the Hearing-Impaired), published quarterly by Verlag Hörgeschädigte Kinder, D-2000 Hamburg 52, Bernadotte Street 126.

In the Field of Otology

1. Arch. Oto-Rhin-Laryng./Arch. Ohren-, Nasen, Kehlkopfheilkunde, published in single issues, four of which normally constitute one volume (about two volumes per year) by Springer-Verlag, D-1000-Berlin 33, Heidelberger Platz 3 (in the U.S.A., Springer-Verlag, Inc., 175 Fifth Avenue, New York, N.Y. 10010).
2. HNO (Official Organ of the Society of German ENT-specialists), published monthly by the same publisher.
3. Oto-Rhin.-Laryng./Zentr. Hals-Nasen-Ohrenheilkunde sowie deren Grenzgebiete, published in single issues, six of which normally constitute one volume (about 2 volumes per year) by the same publisher.
4. Laryng., Rhin., Otol. ihre Grenzgebiete, published monthly by Georg Thieme Verlag, D-7000-Stuttgart 1, Postfach 732.
5. Monatsschr. Ohrenheilkunde Laryng.-Rhin. (Official Organ of the Society of Austrian ENT-specialists), published monthly by Urban and Schwarzenberg, D-80000-Munich 2, Pettenkoferstr.18.
6. ORL J. Oto-Rhin.-Laryng. (Official Organ of the Society of Swiss-ENT-specialists), published bimonthly by Verlag S. Karger A.G., CH-4011-Basel, Arnold Bocklin-Str.25.

LITERATURE CITED

Alich, G. 1960. Zur Erkennbarkeit von Sprachgestalten beim Ablesen vom Munde. Published by the author, Bonn.

Baar, E. 1957. Sprachfreie Entwicklungstests für taube, schwerhörige und sprachlich gestörte Kinder im Alter von 1–7 Jahren. Karger, Basel.

Barr, B. 1954. Pure tone audiometry for preschool children. Acta Oto-Laryngologica (Suppl.) 110: 89–101.

Beckmann, G., and A. Schilling. 1959. Hörtraining. Georg Thieme, Stuttgart.

Bender, L. 1938. A visual motor gestalt test and its clinical use. Amer. Orthopsych. Assoc. Res. Mon. 3, New York.

Benton, A. 1961. Der Bentontest. Georg Thieme, Stuttgart.

Biesalski, P. et al. (eds.). 1973. Phoniatrie und Pädoaudiologie. Georg Thieme, Stuttgart.

Braun, A. 1969. Hören als Lernproblem fur resthörige Kinder. Hörgeschädigre Kinder, Kettwig.

Burian, K. 1970. Die objektive Hõrschwellenbestimmung im Rahmen der Erfassung frühkindlicher Hörstörungen. *In* H. Asperger (ed.) 4. Internationaler Kongress für Heilpädagogik. Osterreichischer Bundesverlag, Wien.

Deutscher Bildungsrat. 1974. Empfehlungen der Bildungskommission zur pädagogischen Förderung behinderter und von Behinderung bedrohter Kinder und Jugendlicher. Klett, Stuttgart.

Ewing, I. 1960. Screening tests, diagnostic tests, parent guidance. *In* A. Ewing (ed.) The Modern Educational Treatment of Deafness. University Press, Manchester.

Ewing, A., and E. Ewing. 1971. Hearing-impaired Children under Five. University Press, Manchester.

Frostig, M., and D. Horne. 1964. The Frostig Program for the Development of Visual Perception. Follett, Chicago.

Griffiths, R. 1954. The Abilities of Babies. University Press, London.

Hahlbrock, K. 1970. Sprachaudiometrie. 2nd Ed. Georg Thieme, Stuttgart.

Heller, K. 1973. Intelligenzmessung. Neckar-Verlag, Villingen.

Heller, K., and A. Löwe. 1972. Heidelberger Hörprüf-Bild-Test (HHBT). Neckar-Verlag, Willingen.

Jacobi, H. 1956–1957. Kinderaudiometrie. H.N.O. 6, 1.

Jussen, H. (ed.). 1968. Sprachanbildung bei Gehörlosen. Marhold, Berlin.

Jussen, H. 1974. Schwerhörige und ihre Rehabilitation. Klett, Stuttgart.

Jussen, H., and M. Kruger. 1975. Manuelle Kommunikationshilfen bei Gehörlosen. Das Fingeralphabet. Marhold, Berlin.

Kern, E. 1958. Theorie und Praxis eines ganzheitlichen Sprachunterrichts für das gehörgeschädigte Kind. Herder, Freiburg.

Kröhnert, O. 1966. Die sprachliche Bildung des Gehörlosen. Beltz, Weinheim.

Kumpf, W. 1970. Veränderung des Atemgeräusches als Indikator für Hören. Georg Thieme, Stuttgart.

Langenbeck, B., and E. Lehnhardt. 1970. Lehrbuch der praktischen Audiometry. 4th Ed. Georg Thieme, Stuttgart.

Leiter, A. 1955. Leiter International Performance Scale. Stoelting, Chicago.
Lesemann, G. (ed.). 1966. Beiträge zur Geschichte und Entwicklung des deutschen Sonderschulwesens. Marhold, Berlin.
Löwe, A. 1965. Haus-Spracherziehung fur hörgeschädigte Kleinkinder. 2nd Ed. Marhold, Berlin.
Löwe, A. 1972. Moderne Hilfen fur Gehörlose und Schwerhörige. Keimer, Munchen-Neubiberg.
Löwe, A. 1974. Gehörlose, ihre Bildung und Rehabilitation. Klett, Stuttgart.
Löwe, A. 1974. Kinderaudiometrie. Marhold, Berlin.
Löwe, A. 1975a. Früherfassung, Früherkennung, Frühforderung hörgeschädigter Kinder. 2nd Ed. Marhold, Berlin.
Löwe, A. 1975b. Sprachfördernde Spiele fur hörgeschädigte und sprachentwicklungsgestörte Kinder. 4th Ed. Marhold, Berlin.
Maesse, H. 1935. Das Verhältnis der Laut- und Gebärdenspache in der Entwicklung des taubstummen Kindes. Staude, Langensalza.
Mathis, A., and K. Graf. 1975. Zu den Gütekriterien der Elektrischen Reaktionsaudiometrie. Audio-Technik, 17(25): 3–8. (Published by Bosch, Berlin.)
Neimeyer, W. 1972. Kleines Praktikum der Audiometrie. 2nd Ed. Georg Thieme, Stuttgart.
Niemeyer, W., and G. Beckmann. 1965. Ein sprachaudiometrischer Satztest. Arch. Ohr., Nas. u. Kehlk. Heilk. 180:742.
Rammely, G. 1974. Die Gebärdensprache. Marhold, Berlin.
Raven, J. 1938. Raven Adult Progressive Matrices. Manual. Western Psychol. Services, Los Angeles.
Raven, J. 1947. Raven Children's Colored Progressive Matrices. Manual. Western Psychol. Services, Los Angeles.
Rossi, E. (ed.). 1972. Gehörstörungen beim Kind. S. Karger AG, Basel.
Schulte, K. 1970. Phonembestimmtes Manualsystem. Hörgeschädigtenpädagogik 24: 291–293. (Published by Julius Groos, Heidelberg.)
Schulte, K. 1975. Phonembestimmtes Manualsystem (PMS). Neckar-Verlag, Villingen-Schwenningen.
Schumann, P. 1940. Geschichte des Taubstummenwesens. Diesterweg, Frankfurt.
Schuy, C. 1955. Ganzheit oder Aufbau im ersten Sprechunterricht. *In:* Neue Blätter fur Taubstummenbildung, Vol. 9, pp. 245–256.
Snijders, Th., and O. N. Snijders. 1959. Nichtverbale Intelligenzuntersuchung für Hörende und Taube. Walters, Groningen.
Stutsman, R. 1948. Guide for Administering the Merrill-Palmer Scale of Mental Tests. Harcourt, Brace & World, New York.
Suzuki and Ogiba. 1960. A technique for pure tone audiometry for children under 3 years of age: conditioned orientation reflex (COR) audiometry. Revue Laryng., 81 (1960) 33.
Van Uden, A. 1968. A world of language for deaf children. Instituut voor Doven, Sint Michielsgestel.
Wechsler, D. 1956. Hamburg-Wechsler Intelligenztest für Kinder. Hans Huber, Bern.

Wolff, J. 1971. Language before speech: A new phonetically-based combined system. Teacher Deaf 69: 96–114.

Zaliouk, A. 1966. Sprachliche Rehabilitation bei Gehörlosen durch ein visuell-taktiles System der Symbolisierung in einem akustischen multisensorischen Kreislauf. Unveröffentlichtes Manuskript. Heidelberg (übersetztes).

chapter 11

Communication for Hearing-handicapped People in Poland

Danuta Borkowska-Gaertig, M.D.

Cum tacent clamant
—Cícero

The results of rehabilitation and education of deaf children are often unsatisfactory for the hearing handicapped and for normal hearing individuals working with them. This opinion has been rendered by every generation for centuries.

One to two hundred years ago, it was believed that deaf persons would be able to participate normally in society if taught in special schools for the deaf. Consequently, special schools for the deaf have been introduced in nearly all countries of the world, but in none of them has it been possible to teach speech to more than only a small number.

About 30 years ago it was believed that the cause of the poor results of teaching speech to deaf children was that education was begun too late and also that deaf children were taught in schools isolated from their normally hearing and speaking peers. To improve this condition in an ever greater number of countries, early detection of hearing loss has been accepted as a principle, together with early rehabilitation of the deaf children in their homes in cooperation with specialists from outpatient clinics for hearing and speech impairment. Despite this, however, not all deaf children achieve good results in hearing and speech rehabilitation, and only a small proportion of them can learn in schools for the normally hearing.

In recent years failures in rehabilitation have been caused by methodological errors. Generally speaking, there are five speech rehabilitation methods for the children with profound hearing loss: (1) the exclusively auditory method with the use of hearing aids; (2) the audiovisual method with the use of hearing aids; (3) the visuo-audio-tactile method with reading and writing, with or without the use of hearing aids; (4) same as in

---

Some of the materials and procedures in this chapter were developed in connection with the Polish-American Scientific Research Collaboration Project No. 05-479-02, and special acknowledgment is made to Dr. Donald A. Harrington, Chairman, Speech and Hearing Section, Project Officer of the Polish-American Scientific Research Collaboration 05-479-02.

method (3) above but with use of manual language; and, (5) manual language method taught from infancy and followed by the teaching of oral speech as in method (2) above.

Usually every rehabilitation center uses one of the above mentioned methods in all cases. The cause of poor results in a given center is often an inefficient rehabilitation specialist or disinterested parents who do not work adequately with the child in the home.

It is true, however, that, from the standpoint of medical diagnosis, the deaf person still remains an unknown entity and his rehabilitation is not administered on an individual basis as it should be.

Hearing-handicapped people "cum tacent clamant"–silently cry accusing–they need a real communication system. Every one of them is in need of a communication system adequate to his abilities. The range of these abilities is quite extensive because of multiple disturbances which may be present at the input, in processing, and at the output. Not all of them can understand speech through hearing even if they are provided with an adequate acoustic gain by a hearing aid; not all of them can understand speech through lipreading even if they possess good visual acuity; not all of them can understand what they are reading even if they know the letters, etc. Even those who know the language may not be able to speak or write or, conversely, they may repeat the heard words without understanding them, etc.

In the present era, whenever new microlesions of the central nervous system, or, in other words, disabilities of learning are being discovered, a relativistic approach to these problems based on a wide knowledge of medicine, psychology, linguistics, pedagogics, and acoustic-electronics has become indispensable. The unquestionable ultimate aim of rehabilitation management is the teaching of patients with hearing loss how to communicate with others by means of hearing and speech.

The essential purpose of our efforts is, however, to teach communication so that everyone is able to express his thoughts and to feel satisfied that he understands and is understood. This very difficult task faces specialists who develop programs for diagnostic, pedagogic, and social rehabilitation of children and adolescents with hearing loss.

HISTORICAL OVERVIEW[1]

In 1817, the festive opening of the Institute of the Deaf, Dumb, and Blind took place in Warsaw. This was the first schol for deaf children and also the first special school in Poland.

---

[1] Based on material printed on the 150th anniversary of the Institute of the Deaf and Blind in Warsaw.

Rev. Jakub Falkowski (1775–1848) was the originator of the Institute and he organized a boarding school. He was in favor of the method known as "the sign language method" which he advocated for the training of deaf children. But as early as 1818, a remarkable educator of the deaf, physician, and also a distinguished lithographer, Jan Siestrzynski, M.D. (1788–1824), endeavored to introduce the oral method. He introduced the phonological method and also initiated quite a new branch of vocational training within the Institute, i.e., lithography. His lithographic workshop at the Institute was the first one of its kind in Poland. The manuscripts of his highly valuable works from 1820, entitled "Theory and Mechanism of Speech" and "On Lithography," were brought to the attention of professionals by Mr. T. Benni[2] 100 years after they were written.

After the war, in 1918, the Institute started a new period in its development.

The improvement of methods of work was influenced considerably by the Training College for Teachers of the Deaf, established in 1919, which, in 1920, became the Dr. Jan Siestrzynski Institute of Phonetics. The Institute of Special Pedagogics, founded in 1922, took over the activity of the Dr. Jan Siestrzynski Institute. Initially, the Institute of Special Pedagogics had its seat in the building of the Institute of the Deaf, Dumb and Blind in Warsaw, 3 Cross Square (Plac Trzech Krzyzy). A director of the Institute of Pedagogics, Dr. Maria Grzegorzewska (1888–1967), worked out the method of labor centers. The method proved to be quite suitable for elemental training and now is widely used by schools for deaf children.

Within the period of years from 1918–1938, the number of schools for the deaf increased to 16, and the number of pupils increased to 1,310. The first nursery school for deaf children and the first vocational school were founded during this period, although the vocational and operative training had received some attention before the founding of the school. Systematic teaching, according to the program of vocational schools, started in 1934 at the primary vocational school founded by the Institute of the Deaf, Dumb and Blind in Warsaw.

A development of education in Poland started slowly in 1945 after the tremendously destructive war.

At present, the number of pupils attending schools for the deaf is three times the number attending before the war. On the other hand, the number of schools is only one and a half times as many as before the war.

The increase in the number of schools for the deaf has brought about the further specialization of them. There is a school for mentally deficient deaf children, another one for backward deaf children, and there are also

---

[2] Tytus Benni. 1917. (Reports) Sprawordaria tx̄-73–94.

schools for hard-of-hearing children. Classes in the bigger schools are specialized according to needs. There are separate sections for the retarded hard-of-hearing children.

The development of vocational schools in the Polish People's Republic is particularly emphasized.

The nine schools are attended by 751 deaf young people. Within the 3-year course, they can attain qualifications and skills in various trades, namely, tailoring, pursemaking, artistic weaving, carpentry, locksmith's trade, draftsmanship, polygraphy, and bookbinding. Vocational training is carried on in school workshops and in plants. Combining vocational training in school workshops with practice in plants proves to be highly effective. This enables young people, guided by teachers, to establish contact with the plants in which they will find employment after they graduate. In this way they are also better able to get acquainted with the conditions of their future work.

Before children with impairments of speech and hearing enter the school, they are put through detailed examinations, both psychomedical and audiological.

Small children, presumed to be either hard of hearing or deaf, are examined by special audiological and phoniatric consulting centers which also provide them service.

PRESENT PROGRAMS OF AURAL REHABILITATION FOR PRESCHOOL CHILDREN

The Polish Association of the Deaf, in cooperation with the Mother and Child Institute which is responsible for special supervision of the problems of mothers and children in this country, and the state specialist in otolaryngology, organized throughout the country, in 1963, special outpatient clincs for children sustaining hearing impairments from infancy. Thirteen province outpatient clinics were organized: Cracow, Rzeszow, Kielce, Bialystok, Lodz, Wroctaw, Opole, Poznan, Szczecin, Koszalin, Bydgoszcz, Olsztyn, and in Warsaw where the Central Audiology-Rehabilitation Outpatient Clinic was organized at the Mother and Child Research Institute. This clinic, along with the Department of Otolaryngology and Rehabilitation Audiology headed by Dr. D. Borkowska-Gaertig, is a center for consultation, training, and scientific research.

As a result of cooperation with the Ministry of Health and Social Welfare, the Mother and Child Institute, the Polish Association of the Deaf, the Consultant for Otolaryngology and provincial health service, a Polish program for hearing care of the child was developed. The principles and methods of early detection, diagnosis, and rehabilitation of children with hearing impairment, developed at the Department of Otolaryngology and Audiology of the Mother and Child Institute, were the foundation upon which the program was established.

Upon evaluating the results of 10 years of activity of the Rehabilitation Clinics for Children with Hearing Loss and also the Central Rehabilitation Audiology Clinic and Department of Otolaryngology and Audiology of the Mother and Child Institute, it should be stressed that the diagnostic and rehabilitation services are provided in each outpatient clinic by teams of specialists: otolaryngologist-audiologist, psychologist, and logopedist using audiometric equipment, hearing aids, and amplifiers.

About 74% of the 4,193 children at preschool age registered at the outpatient clinics are using hearing aids for rehabilitation, 50% of them understand speech by means of hearing, 62% understand it by means of lipreading, and about 28% communicate by means of speech. Of those who received rehabilitation in the clinics and at home, over 1,000 children with severe hearing loss now attend schools for normally hearing children, while the remaining ones attend special schools for the deaf.

DIAGNOSTIC PROCEDURES

Early Identification of Hearing Impairments in Children

In the years from 1963–1974, investigations were conducted on hearing impairments in children in Poland by the Department of Pediatric Otolaryngology, Division of Rehabilitation Audiology, Mother and Child Institute in Warsaw. The prevalence of hearing disorders in children up to 14 years of age was evaluated on the basis of an inquiry throughout all Poland. Otolaryngological-audiological examinations were made of 10,000 school children from the Wola District in Warsaw, in 1963. Audiological tests were made of 12,000 children aged 8–12 months, 3–5 years, and 6–7 years in 1970–1971. It was found that one child in 1,000 has a moderately severe hearing impairment and 13 in 1,000 have moderately severe hearing disorders associated with infections of the upper respiratory tract, pharynx and ears, and other etiologies.

These investigations demonstrated changes in the prevalence of hearing impairments in various age groups in children and also sex-dependent differences.

A comparison of data from Table 1 shows that the total number of hearing loss cases increases significantly from the 6th year on, reaching a peak at the age of 8 years. These numbers of cases with hearing impair-

Table 1. Prevalence of hearing impairments in children 8 months–14 years of age

	Hearing impairments (%)			
Age of children	Total 1.	Conductive 2.	Receptive 3.	Ratio 2:3
8–12 months	0.54	0.51	0.03	1.7
3–5 years (mean in age groups of 1 year)	1.11	1.02	0.03	11.3
6–7 years (mean in age groups of 1 year)	1.9.	1.76	0.15	11.7
8 years	3.22	2.89	0.31	9
9 years	2.02	1.58	0.44	3.6
11 years	1.98	1.78	0.60	2.2
14 years	1.35	0.29	0.80	0.3

ments in each consecutive 1-year age group are functions of conductive and receptive damage. Conduction changes develop less frequently with increasing age but more frequently than receptive changes. At the age of 14 years, a breakthrough occurs and receptive hearing changes become more frequent than disturbances of conduction.

A significant role in this phenomenon is played by maturation of resistance processes in children connected with a reduction in the frequency of upper respiratory tract and ear infections leading to hearing impairment. Also of considerable importance, in light of these data, are the genetic investigations indicating a genetic predisposition for hearing impairment.

In a detailed analysis of the results of our investigations in Poland, it was observed that hearing impairment of conductive or conductive-receptive type is 35% more frequent in boys than in girls. This observation corresponds to genetic investigations. In our screening investigations of hearing acuity of school children, we found that the first phase of screening is failed not only by children with hearing impairment but also by 30% of normal hearing children. These children are marked in the school by their hyperactivity, disturbances of attention, and learning difficulties. Psychological examinations of learning difficulties in the so-called healthy school children aged 7–8 years reveal disorders of attention and memory, and problems with analysis and synthesis of the visual system are demonstrated by 56.3% and of the hearing system by 74% of children.

Psychoacoustic Diagnosis of the Auditory Capacity in Children with Hearing Aids

Pedoaudiology, as a science concerned with the hearing ability of children, should seek reliable data on the development and maturation of hearing ability of the hearing impaired in the process of auditory rehabilitation.

We have introduced a number of modifications into the conventional examination of hearing-handicapped people in order to obtain maximum information about: (1) the rehabilitation potential of the speech and auditory systems by means of amplification with a hearing aid; (2) localization of the lesion in the auditory system; and (3) processes of development and maturation of the impaired system of hearing and speech.

Methods and Management

1. A basic modification has been introduced in the audiological examination of so-called deaf children by using hearing aids as individually selected sound amplifiers. All measurements are carried out in each testing method with and without the hearing aid for comparison. The difference between the curves demonstrates the auditory rehabilitation ability (ARA) of a given child.
2. Audiometric determination of the auditory range has also been introduced. The auditory range is the distance between the hearing threshold curve and the curve of painful or uncomfortable hearing. Examinations with and without the hearing aid are compared in the same audiogram. This test determines the cochlear location of lesion in "deaf" children, just as the loudness recruitment test determines it in adults.
3. A modification of speech audiometry has been introduced with dB measurements and also percentage measurements for determining the understanding of the sounds from the acoustic environment, understanding of verbal commands, and repetition of single words. The curves with and without hearing aids are compared on the same audiograms. This method permits one to determine the localization of hearing impairment in the range of socially useful sounds, differentiating between agnosia, word deafness, and visuoauditory aphasia.

Control examinations are used for comparing hearing acuity in children studied by means of acoustic stimulation through comprehensive rehabilitation, with a more or less successful application of the hearing aid.

Comparative examinations should be carried out at intervals of several days or weeks, and later every 1, 2, or 3 months for establishing the range of frequencies heard and the intensity level in testing with and without a hearing aid plus audiometric determination of the hearing range calculated by the gain effected with the hearing aid. A comparison of these results enables the processes of development and maturation of the impaired hearing and speech system to be assessed. All reactions to meaningful stimuli are assessed in percentages and decibels as in classical speech audiometry, using only different symbols for ambient sounds, speech understanding, and word repetition, with the results of examinations with the hearing aid marked by means of thick lines as shown on Figure 1.

These methods have been used for evaluation of 108 children undergoing rehabilitation with hearing aids from early childhood from 2–8 years. The rehabilitation management was conducted by parents under the direction of specialists from the Central Audiological Rehabilitation Clinic, Research Institute of Mother and Child. The children were divided into three groups according to the severity of hearing loss.

Results The following hearing loss was found in these children: group 1–16 children 20/40–60 dB; group 2–28 children 50/60–80 dB; and group 3–65 children 80/90–120 dB.

In the evaluation of these groups, it was observed that all 108 children reacted to pure tone audiometry and showed a gain of from 15–65 dB at 1,000 Hz when using hearing aids. The value of the gain depends on individual abilities, degree of hearing loss, and power of the hearing aid. Sixteen children demonstrated pain reactions with narrowing of the hearing range at medium, high, or all frequencies. Among them, three children demonstrated a *bell-shaped curve* in testing with and without hearing aids (Figure 2). Four children (Figure 3) could not tolerate nonlinear distor-

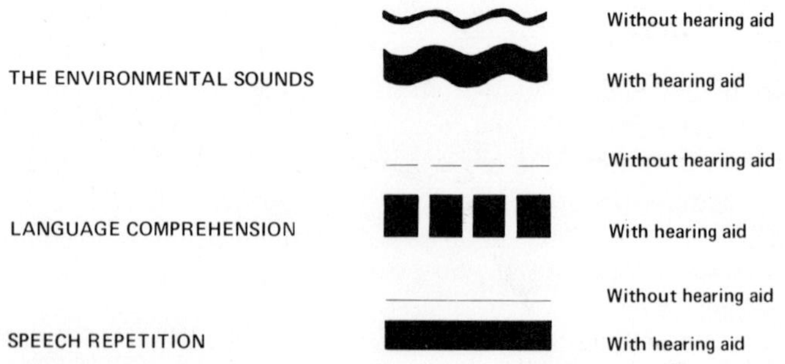

Figure 1. Assessment of reactions to stimuli by children with and without aids. Figure 1 is a key to Figures 2 to 7.

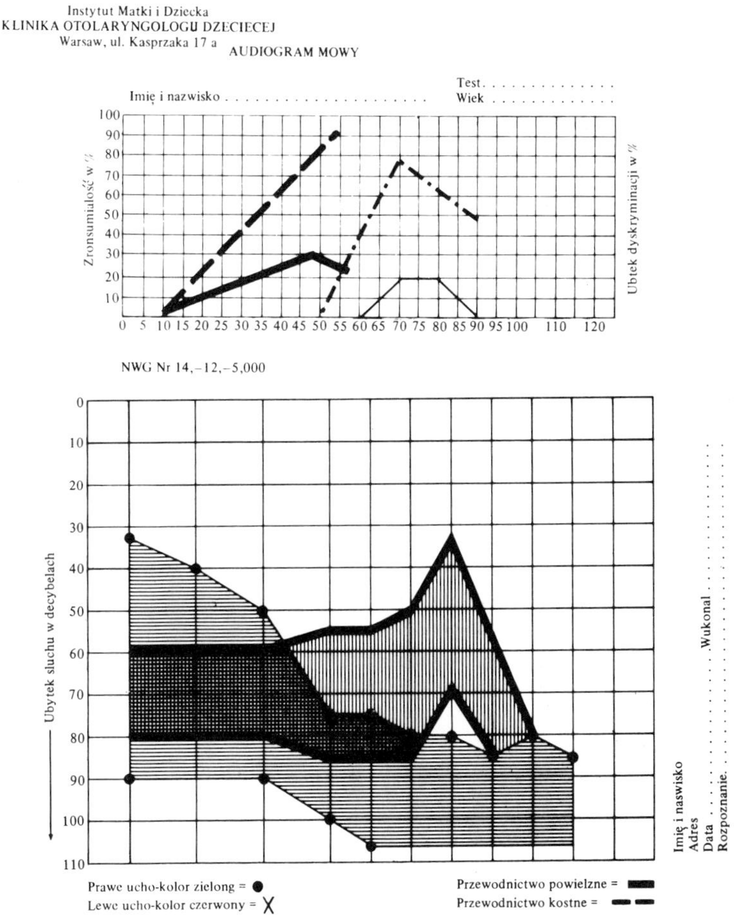

Figure 2.

tions of audiological equipment transmitting sounds, but showed no pain responses when a properly adjusted hearing aid was used without compression, and 11 children reacted with pain to distortions of the hearing aid (1) because of nonlinear amplification or (2) when the microphone on input received sounds with intensities exceeding 60 dB, or (3) when the hearing aid amplifier was working at its peak efficiency (Figure 4). These disturbances were most numerous in group 2 where (1) 85 children recognized meaningful sounds, but 23 of them recognized these sounds only by means of the hearing aid (group 3) (Figure 5). (2) 67 children understood

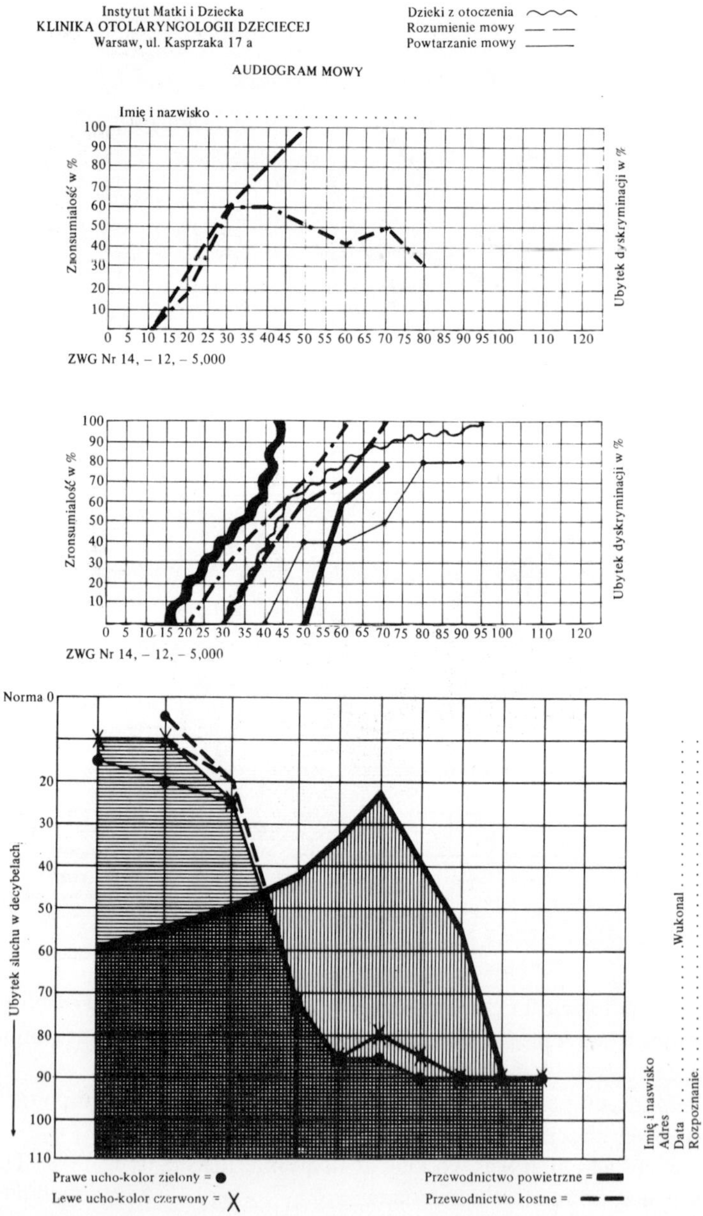

Instytut Matki i Dziecka
KLINIKA OTOLARYNGOLOGII DZECIECEJ
Warsaw, ul. Kasprzaka 17 a
Dzieki z otoczenia
Rozumienie mowy
Powtarzanie mowy
AUDIOGRAM MOWY
Imię i nazwisko . . . .
Zronsumialość w %
Ubytek dyskryminacji w %
100 90 80 70 60 50 40 30 20 10
0 5 10 15 20 25 30 35 40 45 50 55 60 65 70 75 80 85 90 95 100 110 120
ZWG Nr 14, – 12, – 5,000
Zronsumialość w %
Ubytek dyskryminacji w %
100 90 80 70 60 50 40 30 20 10
0 5 10 15 20 25 30 35 40 45 50 55 60 65 70 75 80 85 90 95 100 110 120
ZWG Nr 14, – 12, – 5,000
Norma 0
20 30 40 50 60 70 80 90 100 110
Ubytek słuchu w decybelach
Imię i naswisko . . . . Wukonal . . . .
Adres
Data
Rozpoznanie
Prawe ucho-kolor zielony = ●
Lewe ucho-kolor czerwony = X
Przewodnictwo powietrzne =
Przewodnictwo kostne =

Figure 3.

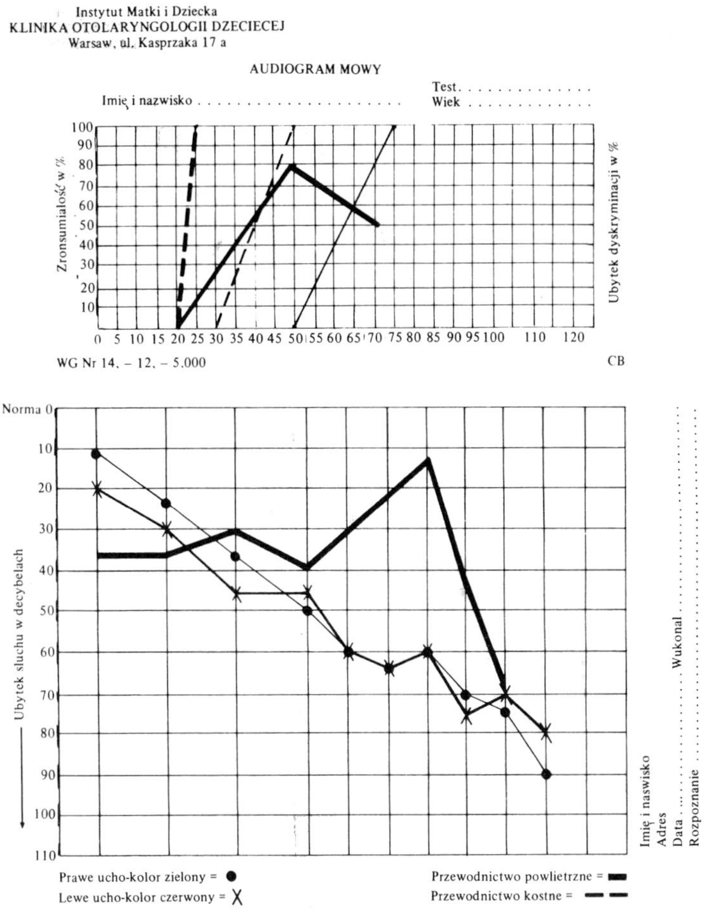

Figure 4.

speech, but did not repeat words, children from group 3 accounted for 28/64 of them; (3) 46 children repeated heard words–among them 30 from group 3; (4) nine children showed evidence of sensory aphasia disorders in the audiovisual association pathways with two of them from group 1, two from group 2, and five from group 3. In each of these groups, especially however in group 3, the application of a hearing aid facilitated speech learning and increased the proportion of learned words (Figure 6). Although some children had signs of agnosia with regard to all meaningful sounds, they retained the possibility of speech learning by vision. Some

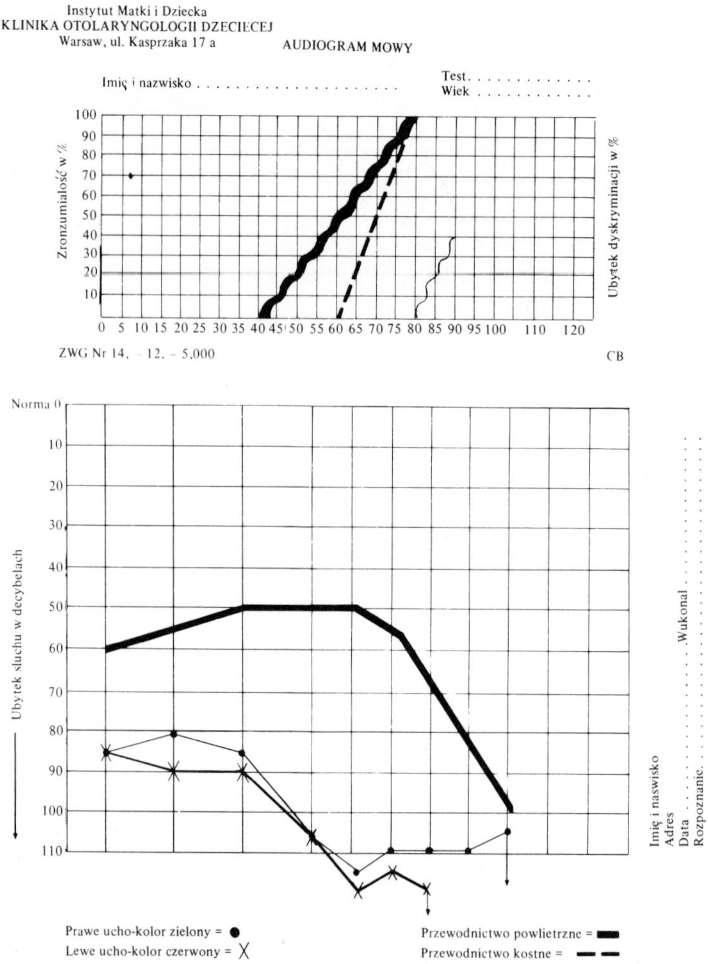

Figure 5.

children demonstrated on the audiograms difficulties in auditory learning (Figure 7).

Discussion Taking into account the most important results obtained, it should be stressed that not only pure tone audiometry, but also psychoacoustic measurements of hearing impairments are a very important and useful method in child audiology. Switching on an individual hearing aid into the audiometric measurement system, one can recognize and

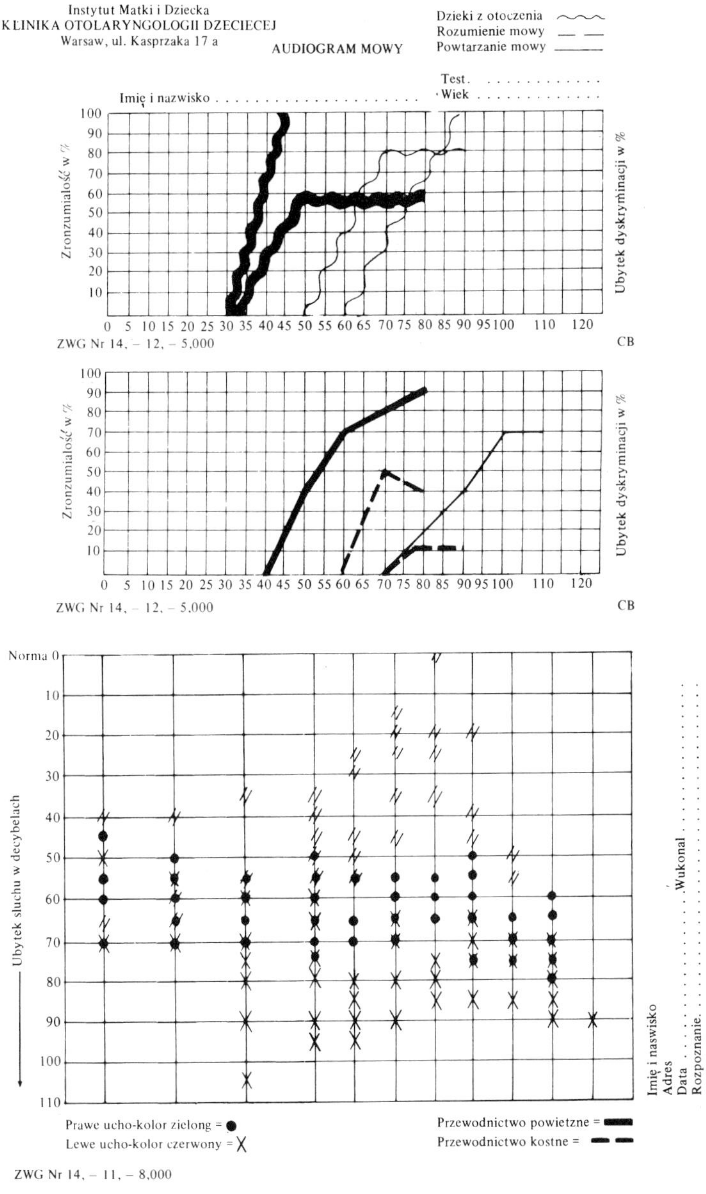
Instytut Matki i Dziecka
KLINIKA OTOLARYNGOLOGII DZECIECEJ
Warsaw, ul. Kasprzaka 17 a
AUDIOGRAM MOWY
Dzieki z otoczenia
Rozumienie mowy
Powtarzanie mowy
Test
Wiek
Imię i nazwisko
Zronzumiałość w %
Ubytek dyskryminacji w %
100
90
80
70
60
50
40
30
20
10
0 5 10 15 20 25 30 35 40 45 50 55 60 65 70 75 80 85 90 95 100 110 120
ZWG Nr 14, – 12, – 5,000
CB
Zronzumiałość w %
Ubytek dyskryminacji w %
0 5 10 15 20 25 30 35 40 45 50 55 60 65 70 75 80 85 90 95 100 110 120
ZWG Nr 14, – 12, – 5,000
CB
Norma 0
Ubytek słuchu w decybelach
10
20
30
40
50
60
70
80
90
100
110
Prawe ucho-kolor zielong =
Lewe ucho-kolor czerwony =
Przewodnictwo powietzne =
Przewodnictwo kostne =
ZWG Nr 14, – 11, – 8,000
Imię i naswisko
Adres
Data
Rozpoznanie
Wukonal

Figure 6.

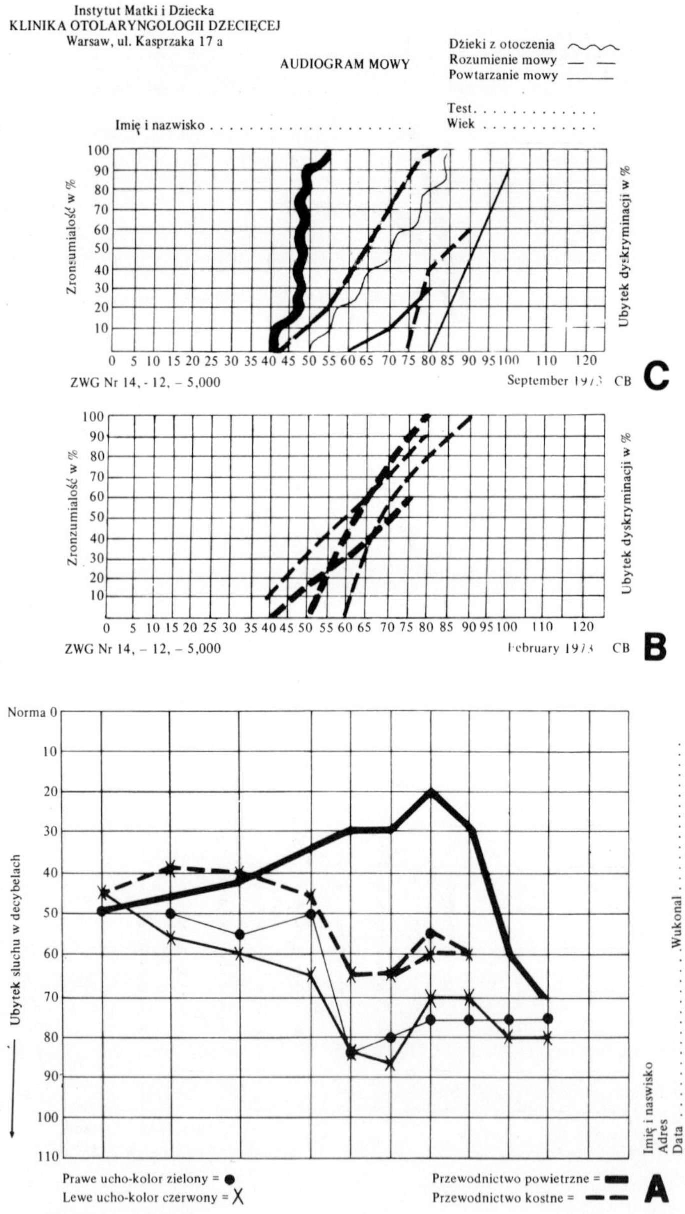
Instytut Matki i Dziecka
KLINIKA OTOLARYNGOLOGII DZIECIĘCEJ
Warsaw, ul. Kasprzaka 17 a
AUDIOGRAM MOWY
Dżieki z otoczenia
Rozumienie mowy
Powtarzanie mowy
Test
Wiek
Imię i nazwisko
Zronsumiałość w %
Ubytek dyskryminacji w %
100 90 80 70 60 50 40 30 20 10
0 5 10 15 20 25 30 35 40 45 50 55 60 65 70 75 80 85 90 95 100 110 120
ZWG Nr 14, - 12, - 5,000
September 1973 CB
C
Zronzumiałość w %
Ubytek dyskryminacji w %
ZWG Nr 14, - 12, - 5,000
February 1973 CB
B
Norma 0
10 20 30 40 50 60 70 80 90 100 110
Ubytek słuchu w decybelach
Imię i naswisko
Adres
Data
Rozpoznanie
Wukonał
Prawe ucho-kolor zielony = ●
Lewe ucho-kolor czerwony = X
Przewodnictwo powietrzne =
Przewodnictwo kostne =
A
ZWG Nr 14, - 12, - 8,000

Figure 7.

differentiate the localization of the impairment, the levels of maturation, and the rehabilitative ability not only of the hearing but also of the entire auditory system.

Davis and Silverman (1970)[3] suggested that the relation between various measures of distortion in a hearing aid and the ability of an impaired listener to receive information is not fully understood. We try to explain these facts by means of new clinical methods with hearing aids and our technical advice concerning the acoustic coupler.

REHABILITATIVE PROCEDURES

Development and Rehabilitation of Hearing in Children with Profound Hearing Loss

Our own observations, as well as those of others, indicate that the process of integration of acoustic stimuli can mature in parallel with the maturation of the cerebral cortex, its hearing centers, and association pathways if hearing is trained by means of acoustic stimulation.

When the possibility of development of responsiveness to acoustic stimuli and hearing improvement was observed in children after hearing rehabilitation, we concluded that all children aged 1, 2, or 3 years, showing low responsiveness to acoustic stimulation or even failing to respond to all acoustic stimuli in the first examinations, should be treated a priori as only retarded in the development of hearing and not as completely deaf.

It happens, sometimes, that a child fails to respond to acoustic stimuli in the first examinations because of emotional disturbance or developmental retardation. Only after longer exposure to acoustic stimulation during repeated hearing acuity tests or by means of hearing aids, does the child begin to manifest hearing responses.

In view of these observations, trials with hearing aids should be made in children manifesting responses to loud acoustic stimuli, as well as in those who do not respond even to very loud sounds, in order to provide them with an opportunity for development and utilization of their residual hearing.

A hearing aid may be prescribed by an audiologist as early as possible after establishing the diagnosis of hearing loss, if no pediatric, neurological, or psychiatric contraindications exist. Binaural hearing aids are to be used,

---

[3] Hallowell Davis and S. R. Silverman. 1970. Hearing and Deafness, p. 306. Holt, Rinehart and Winston, New York.

and periodic determinations of hearing acuity with and without the hearing aid should be made at intervals of 2–3 months. The child may use the hearing aid intermittently or all day long when awake.

When the child possesses a hearing aid chosen and checked by the audiologist, special hearing exercises are started. The program is planned so that the impaired hearing ability of a hard-of-hearing child can develop similarly to that of a normal hearing child. In this way, a child with hearing impairment begins to learn hearing not from the most complex and difficult sounds constituting speech, but from the easiest and most meaningful ambient sounds, e.g., a spoon striking a mug, slamming of a door, crying, and laughing, etc.

The aim of the program of rehabilitation of impaired hearing ability is to exercise and develop the physiological integrative processes of hearing perceptions in the period of growth and development of the child.

The program of development and rehabilitation of hearing in children aged 6–24 months, 25–36 months, and 37–48 months is described below.

Summary of Principles of Development and Rehabilitation of Hearing in Children from Ages 6–48 Months

I. Passive coding of auditory notions
   A. Subconscious recognition of meaningful auditory notions and nonmeaningful voices
      1. Human and animal voices
      2. Toys and various objects of daily use
      3. Ambient noises
   B. Exercises for development of associations connected with acoustic stimuli:
      1. Associating auditory signals with objects, persons, toys, or pictures
      2. Associating auditory signals with the rhythm, pitch, and timbre of produced sounds and acoustic stimuli
      3. Associating auditory signals with vibrations of air pressure of sound waves and other waves (sound-producing objects), e.g., a radio set, and of their own osseocartilagineous system or that of another person, associating resonances by palpation
      4. Associating auditory signals with verbal commands with or without visual control (lipreading)
      5. Sounds differing in rhythm
      6. Sounds of different intensity of vibration-resonances differentiated by palpation
      7. Sounds differing in intensity
      8. Sounds differing in vibration frequency (pitch)
      9. Sounds of different timbre and melody
      10. Sounds constituting verbal commands (with and without lipreading)

II. Active reproduction of coded auditory notions (decoding)
   A. Reproduction of rhythms on toys, instruments, record players, and tape recorders by means of own organs of motor activity and own voice
   B. Reproduction of resonance vibrations (by palpation) of sound-producing objects (acoustic pressure, musical instruments, radio set, etc.), reproduction of vibrations of their osseocartilaginous system by means of own larynx and upper airways
   C. Reproduction of ambient sounds—human voices (crying, laugh, singing, screams, words) and animal voices
   D. Reproduction of intensities by modulation of radio set, tape recorder, amplifier for hearing rehabilitation or own voice
   E. Reproduction of frequencies by means of sound-producing toys, objects from the surroundings, and musical instruments, or by own voice
   F. Reproduction of verbal commands

Design of Program for Optical Rehabilitation of Children with Profound Hearing Impairment Developed on the Basis of Our Own Investigations[4]

The inception of this kind of investigation has been stimulated by the necessity of focusing greater attention on the visual information channel, which, by contrast to versatility and the carefully investigated auditory channel, thus far failed to receive sufficient consideration, despite the fact that the scanty data in the literature on this problem indicate a higher number of deviations of the optic organ among deaf children than among those with normal hearing.

In the Ophthalmologic Clinic of Pomeranian Medical Academy in Szczecin, a number of basic ophthalmologic studies have been performed, namely, examinations of visual acuity for distance and proximity, evaluation of anterior segment and the eye fundus, examination of refraction after a 3-day long atropinization, binocular vision, and fixation, as well as examination of the direction of squint and function of the optic organ, in the evaluation of visual spatial localization, and the time of conscious reaction to light stimuli. The above examinations covered the hard-of-hearing and deaf children whose ages ranged from 7–12 years, and the results of the studies were analyzed in groups comprising children with good or bad lipreading on the basis of a 10-degree scale developed by the Children's Otolaryngological Clinic of the Mother and Child Institute in

---

[4] Credit in this section is given to Dr. G. Remlein-Mozolewska of the Ophthalmologic Clinic of the Pomeranian Medical Academy in Szczecin which is headed by Dr. Hab. T. Baranowska-George.

Warsaw. The control group designed for functional examinations consisted of children with normal hearing placed in respective age groups, the total being 213 subjects.

It appears from the studies that the factors hampering lipreading in children with severe hearing impairment are: (1) deviations from the standard within the optic organ (mainly refraction anomalies and squints; thereafter, pigmentary degenerations of retina); (2) almost inadequate visual spatial localization; and (3) prolongation of conscious reaction time.

Hence, special attention should be centered upon these three factors, and an attempt should be made to institute, as early as possible, rehabilitation treatment and exercises, so that, when the child has reached the age at which he begins intensive learning of lipreading, optimal conditions will prevail.

The following is a proposal for a rehabilitation program directed toward the respective deviations.

Suggested Exercises for the Youngest Children–4 Years of Age and Below

1. For this age group, the most suitable games would include playing with building blocks of different shapes which the child may arrange according to colors and size, constructing simple little houses, etc.
2. Colored ringlets with holes in the middle, which should be mounted onto a stand with a stick according to color and/or size.
3. Folding railway with wooden elements, with little cars of varied construction and content.
4. Ball playing (necessarily colored)–catching, pointing, rolling to marked places, etc.
5. Drawing. Tiny hands are still unskilled so, depending on the age, an attempt may be made to paint over circles outlined by the therapist; a thick brush and one or two colors of paint should be used. Here, the brush seems to be more appropriate than colored pencils, because there can be a thicker handle and no special strain is required to make a colorful blot as compared to painting by means of colored pencils, which is generally harder.
6. Dressing and undressing dolls, as well as teddy bears, with opening buttons and press-studs, walking the dolls along paths (requiring the following of a proper direction), pulling the toy trains along previously drawn track with some marshaling and transloading stations on the route, etc.
7. Exercising on a plank with numerous holes, into which the child should place the endpieces of the sets, e.g., rural farmstead, a forest with animals, little towns, etc.

Suggested Exercises for Older Children 4–7 Years of Age

1. Use blocks of smaller dimensions, namely, all sorts of building construction, arranging of blocks (the smaller the better). On the basis of our observations at the clinic, it can be ascertained that the children are able to accomplish quite amazing things when they are supplied with appropriate materials in adequate quantities.
2. Mosaics (from large to very tiny ones).
3. Construction, e.g., gardener (comprising a set of gardening elements, pots, flowers, small leaves, which the children may use to compose various designs of gardens and flower-beds).
4. Sets for manipulating–little constructor.
5. Colorful cuttings placed into different patterns and pictures.
6. Drawing and painting prepared patterns.
7. Sewing–particularly embroideries, needle and crocheted needlework.
8. Moving games–walking on a bar, rollerskating, table tennis, shooting at targets, badminton, ball playing, etc.

Suggested Exercises for Children Ages 8 Years and Older

All the above mentioned activities–but of a more complicated degree; namely, drawing, handwork (requiring tinkering), volleyball, basketball, tennis, rollerskating, etc. The higher the number of exercises the better, at least 3 hours daily.

These should be viewed as suggestions only. The most important thing is, however, to respect the principle of training the child's visualmotoric efficiency. Reading books, watching films and television are not sufficient visual exercises in that respoect.

Time of Conscious Reaction

In studies being devoted to children with severe hearing defects, reaction time to a light stimulus was determined. The observations on this activity highlighted very interesting phenomena. First of all, there is a distinct dependence of conscious reaction time on the magnitude of the hearing loss. The longest reaction time was shown by deaf children (on the average $\bar{x}$ = 275 ms), the shortest, as compared with the former, by the children being partly deaf ($\bar{x}$ = 198 ms).

The reaction time behavior, depending on the age of the children, was also studied and it was found that it became shorter progressively with the increase in age in all three groups of children. Attention was also focused on the latency period in respective groups of children, which was found to be greatest in the age group from 7–10 years, but here too, the relationship of the latency period to the extent of the hearing loss was evident.

In an attempt to elucidate the phenomenon of time delay of the reaction to the light stimulus in children with impaired hearing, it should be understood that the time depends on the degree of psychomotoric efficiency. This, in turn, is affected by a whole range of external impulses with a preponderant participation of sound impulses in that process. The greater the hearing loss, the fewer the signals. Because of the rather low number of signals in everyday life, the deaf children had no occasion to work out quick reactions to external stimuli. In the group of the hard-of-hearing children, the residual hearing permits them to perceive only part of the signals, which, in consequence, is linked to a greater frequency of reaction, and, therefore, with reaction time being shorter, as compared to the deaf children.

A rapid decrease in the reaction time during the period of the first school years is likely to be associated with the termination of the isolation period to which the deaf child is often subjected until he starts attending school. Here he is with a group of equals whose company makes him feel unrestricted (except for the first period of his stay at school). During the lessons, exercises, and common games, he trains his motor skills intensively. The influence of psychomotoric efficiency, in the sense of appropriate reaction time, related to learning lipreading, seems here to be of some importance, for it is hard to imagine that a child with markedly delayed reaction time could, in an effective way, follow the relatively rapidly changing movements of the lips during speech. That is particularly evident in the pupils in whom the reaction time is the longest. It seems advisable to direct the teacher's attention to that fact and, after taking the above findings into consideration, they should slow down the pace of words spoken when teaching a deaf child.

For purposes of producing quick psychomotoric improvement in these children, it is important to introduce exercise therapy by resorting to games that demand rapid reaction from the child. In little children, all sorts of simple mobile games should be used, e.g., rolling a ball, playing tag, hide and seek, etc. In older children, physical exercises can be included, and more time should be allotted to speedy games, competition, playing ball. The most ideal, in this case, is the "between two fires" game, volleyball, and basketball. Moreover, table tennis, table football, juvenile football, as well as a number of other games, are excellent.

One very important thing should be emphasized, namely, the problem of dealing with social withdrawal in children with severe hearing loss in the early period of childhood.

All of the above mentioned problems of optic rehabilitation of a deaf child should be taken into consideration and dealt with before the child enters school. Stated simply, time must not be wasted for improving the visual motoric coordination at the period when the child is to be concentrating his attention on very difficult tasks, namely, that of acquiring the ability to learn lipreading, and, in addition, the mastering of general school materials.

Program of Diagnostic Language Rehabilitation (Bnierzchowska)

I. Annex 1
  A. Tests and exercises
    1. Language tests (annex 1 in Polish—at the author's)
    2. Language exercises for children with particular difficulties in understanding of language signals (annex 2)
    3. Audiomotor and visuomotor rehabilitation (annex 3)
    4. Auditory training (a set of exercises prepared by Dr. Borkowska-Gaertig, M.D.)
    5. Visual training (a set of exericses prepared by Dr. G. Mozolewska, M.D.)
    6. Improving the function of speech organs by means of logopedic methods
  B. Sequence of tests and exercises
    1. For children passing the language diagnostic rehabilitation tests (annex 1)
      a) Audiomotor and visuomotor rehabilitation (annex 3)
      b) Auditory training (I.A.4.)
    2. For children failing to pass the test of differentiation of letters and simple inscriptions (I.A.1.)
      a) Visual training (I.A.5.)
      b) Audiomotor and visuomotor rehabilitation (annex 3).
      c) Exercises in discrimination between graphic signs (from the set of exercises for dyslexic children)
    3. For children who failed to pass the test of reading simple utterances from the lips (I.B.1.)
      a) Language exercises for children with particular difficulties in understanding verbal signals (annex 2)
      b) Visual training (I.A.5.)
      c) Audiomotor and visuomotor rehabilitation (annex 3)
      d) Improvement of speech organ functions by logopedic methods, if necessary
    4. For children who failed to pass the test of auditory differentiation of simple speech signals (I.B.1.)
      a) Language exercises for children with particular

difficulties in understanding language signals (annex 1)
  - *b*) Audiomotor and visuomotor rehabilitation (annex 3)
  - *c*) Auditory training (I.A.4.)
  - *d*) Visual training (I.A.5.)
  - *e*) Improvement of speech organ functions by logopedic methods, if necessary
5. For children with difficulties in verbal expression
  - *a*) Logopedic exercises increasing the efficiency of the organs of speech
  - *b*) Audiomotor and visuomotor rehabilitation (annex 3)

II. Annex 2 (kinesthetic visual language exercises for children with particular difficulties in understanding of language signals)

A. Naming of activities performed with objects of everyday use

1. Demonstration of manipulations while encouraging the child to imitate hair combing (comb), drinking (mug), eating (spoon), washing oneself (soap or sponge), cutting (plastic knife), and perambulating (toy pram)
2. Introduction of the names of activities (on labels, by lipreading, by means of earphone) and introduction of various ways of adding words (gradually), in the following sequence: she combs her hair + movement with the comb; she drinks + movement with the mug; she eats + movement with the spoon; she washes her hands + movements with the soap or sponge; she cuts + movement with the knife; and she perambulates + movement with the toy pram
3. Naming activities with pointing to the person performing them: the teacher combs her hair, drinks, eats, washes her hands, cuts, perambulates the doll; the doll combs her hair, etc. (with demonstration); the teddybear combs his hair, etc.; child's name combs his hair, drinks, etc. while pointing to the child as the person who performs these activities, in a mirror, if necessary
4. Naming the person performing the activity, the activity itself, and the object to which the activity is related:

Performer	*Activity + manipulation*	*Object*
the teacher+	combs (with a comb) +	hair
the teacher +	drinks (from a mug) +	milk
the teacher +	eats (with a spoon) +	soup
the doll +	drinks (from a mug) +	milk
the doll +	cuts (with a knife) +	bread

the doll +	perambulates (in a toy pram) +	teddybear
the teddybear +	eats (with a sppon) +	soup
the teddybear +	washes (with soap) +	his hands

B. Naming sounds produced with toys
1. Rings the bell + movement with the bell
2. Blows the trumpet + blowing the trumpet
3. Taps the drum + drum tapping
4. Knocks + knocking with a wooden block

C. Naming of the sounding toy
1. (bell) + rings the bell + manipulation with the bell
2. (trumpet) + blows the trumpet + manipulation
3. (drum) + taps the drum + manipulation
4. (block) + knocks + manipulation

C. Introduction of other activities and names of objects
1. the bird, the airplane, the fly, the butterfly flies + movement carried out with the toy first by the performer, then by the child
2. the fish swims, the boat is afloat, the ship is afloat, the duck swims (movements performed with corresponding toys—always in water)

D. Questions and answers
1. What is something doing?
   a) What is the teacher, teddybear, doll doing? + movement with an object (comb, mug, spoon, soap, knife, pram); answer: combing her hair, drinking, eating, washing, etc. (in one word)
   b) What is the teacher doing? + manipulation (trumpet blowing, bell ringing, drum tapping, block knocking); answer: blows the trumpet, rings the bell, taps the drum, knocks
   c) What does the airplane, bird, fly, butterfly do? + manipulation with a toy; answer: flies
   d) What does the fish, ship, boat, duck do? + manipulation; answer: swims or is afloat
2. Who is combing his hair, drinking, eating, washing, perambulating? + manipulation with the toy; answer: the teacher, the doll, the teddybear or the name of the child
3. Who or what is flying, swimming? + manipulation; answer: the airplane, the bird, the fly, the butterfly, the fish, the boat, the ship, the duck (with imitation of the activity)
4. What is ringing, trumpeting, drumming, knocking? + manipulation; answer: the bell, trumpet, drum, block
5. What is the teacher combing? + manipulation; answer: her hair; what is the teacher drinking? + manipulation; answer: milk; what is the teacher eating? + manipulation; answer: soup (etc.); what is

the doll drinking? + manipulation; answer: milk; what is the doll eating? + manipulation; answer: soup; what is the doll washing? + manipulation; answer: her hands (etc.); what is the teddybear drinking? + manipulation; answer: milk; what is the teddybear eating? + manipulation; answer: soup; what is the teddybear perambulating? + manipulation; answer: doll (etc.)

6. Questions related to one sentence—what is the teacher doing?; answer: combing her hair, drinking; who is combing her hair, drinking, eating, etc.?; answer: the teacher, the doll, the teddybear, the child's name; what is the teacher combing, eating, drinking?; answer: her hair, soup, milk, etc.

III. Annex 3

A. Audiomotor and visuomotor rehabilitation of children with residual hearing

1. Rising and sitting down at a sound signal (rapid drum tapping—rising, one tap—sitting down)
2. Marching at varying pace (swiftly or slowly) to the rhythm of drum tapping
3. Standing on toes at a high pitched sound or whistle; squatting at a low pitched sound (e.g., blowing the horn)
4. Lateral inclinations of the trunk to the rhythm of slow drum tapping
5. Walking a line drawn on the floor
   a) Normally, to the rhythm of drum taps
   b) With one foot put closely in front of the other
   c) With eyes closed (aided, if necessary)
6. Similarly walking a line forming a circle drawn on the floor
7. Jumping into the circle drawn on the floor at a signal, tapping a triangle, or striking cymbals
8. Jumping out of the circle at a signal different from the former one
9. Marching
   a) With both arms raised at the signal "one-two" and dropped at "three-four"
   b) With alternate raising and dropping of the left and right arms
   c) With hand clapping at each step
   d) With hand clapping to the rhythms 4/4, 2/4, 3/4
   e) With marking the rhythms 4/4, 2/4, 3/4 by stamping the foot
   f) With stopping at the signal of hand clapping, drum tapping, etc.

B. Exercises of coordination of the movements of speech organs with movements of the whole body and extremities

1. Wooden block dropping, speaking "*buch*" with each block
2. Drum tapping and repeating "*bum*" with each tap
3. Rhythmic walking repeating "pa-pa-pa-pa-, ta-ta-ta-ta, la-la-la-la, ma-ma-ma-ma," etc.
4. Playing birds, flapping extended hands and repeating "pi-pip-pi-pi"
5. Rhythmic hand clapping and repeating "pa-pa-pa," etc.
6. Marching with handclapping and repeating "pa-pa-pa, ta-ta-ta-ta, la-la-la," etc.
7. Rhythmic hopping and repeating "hop-hop"
8. Rhythmic leaning sideways from the chair and repeating "ku-ku"
9. Hand clapping and repeating "pa-pa, ta-ta . . . , la-la . . . ," etc. with marking rhythms 4/4, 2/4, 3/4
10. Beating rhythms by means of hand clapping, tapping the table with the hand, drum tapping, castanets, cymbals etc., the rhythms should be visualized by means of circles, e.g., "oo-ooo-, o-ooo" etc.; the child should read these rhythms
11. Marching to the rhythm of scanned two-syllable names of children—"E-wa, Ba-sia, Ba-sia," etc. (if the children have group exercises, they scan the name of the child marching at their head)
12. Marching to the rhythm of scanned two-syllable names of children with simultaneous hand clapping at each syllable
13. The same exercise but with stressing only the first syllable of the scanned name
14. Marching to the rhythm of scanned three-syllable names of children, e.g., "E-wu-nia, An-drze-jek, Ma-ry-sia," etc.
15. Hand clapping of scanned names of children stressing the accentuated syllable—"*O*-la, *O*-la, Ma-*ry*-sia, Ma-*ry*-sia," etc.
16. Group rhythmic singing to the doll—"a-a-a, a-a-a, a-a-a"
17. Marching to the rhythm of the song (e.g., tape recorded)
18. Marching to the rhythms of the song with singing "la-la-la"
19. Marching and running to the rhythm of successively played melodies (slower and quicker)

20. Running to the rhythm of the heard melody and stopping when the melody stops

C. Exercises for coordination of hand movements with the movements of speech organs
   1. Drawing strokes to the rhythm of heard syllables, e.g., "ta-ta"
   2. Drawing of strokes or circles with simultaneous repeating of syllables—"pa-pa-pa," etc.
   3. Arranging wooden blocks on the table with pronunciation of syllables, e.g., "ta-ta-ta," etc.
   4. Putting buttons into holes with repeating syllables, e.g., "tu-tu"

CURRENT PROGRAMS OF RESEARCH

Pediatric audiology, as a new discipline, has been developing for 20 years in Poland. This specialty embraces many problems, and there are differences in its development in Europe (where the audiologists are usually phoniatrists or otolaryngologists) and in the U.S.A. (where the audiologists are usually not physicians but specialists in psychoacoustics). In the 30 years of existence of the Polish People's Republic, the foundations for development of pediatric audiology have been laid by phoniatrists, otolaryngologists, and pediatric otolaryngologists in cooperation with specialists in acoustics, electronics, phonetics, pharmacology, psychology, neurology, ophthalmology, and psychiatry.

Research in this discipline has utilized various methods, including animal experiments, clinical investigations of children using electronic equipment and otological microsurgery, and statistical population studies of children with hearing loss and children with average socially useful hearing acuity. The topics of investigations have been as follows:

1. Physiopathology of the peripheral auditory receptor apparatus in the range of microphonic currents and of the vestibular organ (W. Jankowski, S. Kossowski, J. Sekula, S. Chodynicki, J. Malecki, T. Bystrzanowska, Z. Bchenek, A. Halama, G. Janczewski, J. Pietruski)
2. Central auditory functions
   a) Directional hearing (A. Zakrzewski)
   b) Auditory understanding of speech and nonverbal ambient sounds (M. Mitrynowicz-Modrzejewska, G. Taniewski, S. Zakrzewski, S. Iwankiewicz, J. Kuzniarz, R. Kugler, D. Borkowska-Gaertig)
   c) Cortical auditory reactivity studied by means of evoked potential audiometry (W. Bochenkowa)
   d) Development of higher auditory functions in children with hearing loss using hearing aids (D. Borkowska-Gaertig)

3. Phoniatric audiological problems in children with hearing impairment (A. Mitrynowicz-Modrzejewska, L. Handzel, S. Klajman, Z. Pawtowski, W. Tluchowski, A. Pruszewicz, H. Siedlanowska-Brzosko, B. Dwornicka, B. Hnatow)
4. Surgical treatment of deafness (J. Miodonski, J. Sekula, E. Mozolewski, T. Bardadin, Z. Bochenek, B. Moszynski, J. Kus, J. Biskupska-Wiecko, Z. Szmeja)
5. Incidence of hearing impairments in children aged 1–7 years in Poland, in school children, in urban and rural children (D. Borkowska-Gaertig, B. Potyrata, Z. Rzedowska, L. Sobieszczanska-Radoszewska, J. Urbanska, A. Pruszewicz, Z. Szmeja, T. Bystrzanowska, E. Filipowski, D. Bogusz-Rozkowa) and the incidences of hearing disturbances in fetuses and newborns (A. Jasienska, B. Dwornicka)
6. The ability of children with hearing impairment to profit from rehabilitation has been studied by teams of various specialists (otolaryngologists, ophthalmologists, psychiatrists, neurophysiologists, neurologists, psychologists, logopedists, specialists in phonetics and electronics, audiological technicians, and teachers) in nationwide investigations carried out in Warsaw, Cracow, and Szczecin, at the Mother and Child Institute, Polish Academy of Sciences, Medical Academies, State Institute of Special Pedagogics, Outpatient Clinic for Rehabilitation of Children with Hearing Defects, and in nursery schools and special schools for deaf children in Michalin, Radom, Lubliniec I and II, and Srodborow. These studies were conducted in the years 1964–1973 as part of the program of Polish-American scientific cooperation (grant WA/CB3 and 05-479-2) and were coordinated by general investigator D. Borkowska-Gaertig. (Final report, 1975)
7. Development of methods for detection, diagnosis, rehabilitation-diagnosis, and hearing aid selection in children (A. Mitrynowicz-Modrzejewska, D. Borkowska-Gaertig, B. Potyrala, L. Sobieszczanska-Radoszewska, J. Urbanska). Importance of family environment and parent guidance (T. Galkowski, M. Goralowna). In addition, two devices for hearing rehabilitation were designed and produced: Audiotrainer (patented by J. Nowosielski and D. Borkowska-Gaertig) and Logocorrector (patented by J. Nowosielski, B. Wierzchowska, and D. Borkowska-Gaertig). Another device is an acoustic coupler for hearing examination through hearing aids (patented by D. Borkowska-Gaertig and J. Nowosielski). (Final report, 1975)

A film, "Detection of Hearing Impairment in Children," has been produced to increase the availability of the methods of hearing acuity examination of little children. This film is for pediatricians and otolaryngologists as they examine many children in outpatient health services. Another film, more scientific than instructive, "Psychoneurological Examination of Children with Hearing Impairment," developed by D. Borkowska-Gaertig et al., is intended for audiologists, psychologists, and logopedists working in diagnostic rehabilitation of children with hearing loss. (Final report, 1975, Borkowska-Gaertig.)

ASSOCIATIONS RESPONSIBLE FOR HEARING-HANDICAPPED PERSONS IN POLAND[5]

The Constitution of the Polish People's Republic, accepted by the Seym in July 1952, guarantees to all the citizens a range of rights. They are: the right to work (the right to employment for remuneration according to the quality and quantity of work), the right to rest, the right to health protection and aid in the case of disease or disability to work, the right to education and the use of cultural values, the right to form associations, personal immunity, protection of individual and personal ownership, and the right to social welfare.

These rights are guaranteed to all citizens without regard to their education, financial state, racial and religious differences, and without regard to various kinds of disability. Thus, the deaf in Poland have the same rights as others in the population.

The extent to which the deaf make use of these rights depends upon their individual potential as is determined by their educational and mental levels and their adaptation to life within the community. Their social position should be considered, therefore, in light of these factors.

There are two groups of deaf: the working deaf and the nonworking deaf. This division is essential when determining the degree to which social welfare services are used. The possibilities of a working man differ from those of one who does not work, but, in spite of that, in a socialist country, even the nonworking deaf get far-reaching aid and help.

The right to work in Poland is ensured by the Constitution—this also includes the deaf. An extensive revalidation activity has been conducted for more than 20 years and it aims, first of all, at enabling the deaf to be employed, and, thus, to gain access to all social goods which are accessible to any citizen who takes part in production of material goods of the State. In this way, the number of the unemployed deaf decreases systematically.

The working deaf can be divided into several categories. The category they belong to and the extent to which they make use of facilities should

[5] The material in this section is based on a paper entitled "The Social Position of the Deaf in the Polish People's Republic," prepared by the Presidential Board of the Polish Association of the Deaf and presented at the Fifth Congress of the World Federation of the Deaf in Warsaw, 1967.

be taken into account. Considering as a criterion of division the level of education (which is decisive in this specific group), the opportunities for the deaf to make use of social resources in the community can be roughly divided into the following categories:

1. The deaf having high education—graduates from colleges for the normal hearing, also graduates from special schools who have achieved a high level of knowledge and skill which permits them to make full use of social resources. Some of them reach such a high degree of revalidation that they do not feel the results of deafness; in other words, their deafness is not an obstacle in their lives. They often hold important posts among the hearing, and because of their qualifications they obtain high salaries and participate in all blessings of civilization. However, this group, in relation to the total number of the deaf, constitutes only a small percentage, estimated at 3–4%.
2. The deaf graduates of special primary and vocational schools constitute a great majority of those within the Polish Association of Deaf. The level of their adaptation to life requires further care and further revalidation. All of them, except some individuals, work in various occupations which they had mastered in schools or in vocational education conducted by the Polish Association of Deaf and other institutions interested in the problems of deafness. Most prevalent occupations in this category of deaf are: locksmithing, drafting, bookbinding, tailoring, shoemaking, weaving, and cabinetmaking.
3. The majority of the illiterate and semi-illiterate deaf are living in villages. Their level of adaptation to life in the community requires even more care and help than that of the deaf belonging to the other categories. To this category belong the majority of those who are not yet working, but, if they are employed, it is only in occupations that do not require special qualifications.

Data on the Deaf in Poland

According to data gathered by the Polish Association of Deaf on the basis of lists made of the deaf over many years, there are now 45,242 deaf people in Poland. This figure excludes those who are classified as hard of hearing. Among them are 6,000 children up to 15 years of age; 2,342 young people 16–18 years of age; and 35,901 adults above 18 years of age.

The deaf in Poland have their own organization—The Polish Association of Deaf—which completes the tasks assigned by the State and understands that the Constitution ensures to all citizens comprehensive development and care. These tasks are carried out by the Association with financial and moral support of the State authorities. The Ministry of Health and Social Welfare executes the supervision of the accomplishment of these tasks with respect to welfare services to the disabled. The Ministry of Education is responsible for special education. A range of other ministries collaborates very closely in the fulfillment of the above mentioned tasks. Moreover, The Polish Association of Deaf cooperates with various institutions, first of all, with national councils, working cooperatives for the disabled, and trade unions.

According to the state, as of December 31, 1966, the Association had 17,314 members, with an increase over the last 4 years of 5,125 persons. Approximately 60% of the total number of the deaf in Poland are living in the country, often very dispersed. This is why the Association is still an urban organization, grouping, first of all, the deaf who are living in big groups, in towns, and who are mostly graduates from special and occupational schools for the deaf that are available exclusively in towns.

The number of deaf from rural areas who remain in towns is still growing and is increasing in the number of places they fill in the schools and boarding houses. These children, after graduating and gaining occupations, most often remain in towns because of the availability of employment to further revalidate themselves as they live within the community.

The Association has 99 regional centers in the country which are located in towns. The activity of a center covers one or several communities, which permits helping, in certain cases, the deaf living in villages.

Realization of the Right to Work

According to 1966 data (latest available to the Association), the number of employed deaf in Poland was 15,267 persons.

Considering the number of deaf already cited as being above 18 years of age, i.e., at a productive age, one can calculate that the employed deaf constitute 42.5% of this number. However, one should not forget that, among the deaf over 18 years of age, there are many who have reached the pension age or are already pensioners. There are those, especially married women, who have satisfactory financial conditions and do not have to work for a living.

Attention is being paid in Poland to the solution of the problem of making productive the deaf who live in villages, especially young people who were not placed in special schools. They have had neither the advantage of other forms of education nor have they acquired an occupation. This is one of the most difficult and important problems with which the Association is dealing. This problem has forced the Association to search for a solution. This has led to organized educational programs in villages which have provided general and occupational education preparing the deaf to work in occupations connected with agriculture.

Deaf children in Poland are authorized to learn not only in special schools. If the child's mental level permits, the educational authorities do not object to placing those children and young people in normal primary schools and secondary and high schools as well. According to our incomplete data, there are approximately 1,000 deaf children who are learning in normal primary schools, 40 children in secondary vocational schools, and 13 deaf students studying at the universities.

The Polish Association of Deaf has initiated a significant program of care of deaf children of preschool age. Its aim is to teach the gifted deaf children lipreading and receptive and expressive oral language. The idea is to raise a large group of children to a level that would enable them to learn in schools for hearing children.

This action, conducted by the Association with the help of Province Rehabilitation Clincs for children with hearing defects, is based, first of all, on the education of parents who work most closely with the children. Medical, psychological, and logopedic care are ensured for children by the above mentioned clinics, as well as help for parents. The number of clinics in Province cities is now 14, and 1,875 children are under their care. The long range aim of the Association is to have all normally developed deaf children at preschool age under the care of these clinics.

However, there is an additional problem, namely, that of organizing care for underdeveloped deaf children, for deaf and dumb children, and for those whose age exceeds that of the preschool child.

The Association, in collaboration with the State authorities, undertakes also the ensuring of educational possibilities for adults. Since 1949, illiteracy among the deaf has been virtually eliminated by means of courses organized in primary education and evening schools. Approximately 500 adult deaf are attending 40 evening primary classes.

Vocational education is conducted in special vocational schools for the deaf under the guidance of the Ministry of Education. However, not all graduates from primary schools attend these schools.

In addition to the development of education, vocational training is also conducted by the Ministry of Health and Social Welfare in Wrotaw in the center of Invalid Training, with about 85 places and in Cracow with about 85 places. The working cooperatives for the invalid conduct vocational training, applying a class system which includes several hundreds of deaf employed in working cooperatives for the invalid. The deaf improve their qualifications according to the work done in the given cooperative, mostly tailoring, shoemaking, joining, being locksmiths, etc.

Apart from these, the Association is conducting professional training in revalidation centers, organized in the Association's production institutions. This training is conducted by various systems starting with the classes of several months up to 4 years of training. The deaf are simultaneously employed in the institution. This provides new occupations for the deaf, most often in the field of artificial material processing, metallurgy, electronics, and occupations connected with agriculture. They benefit from the right to medical care, rest, and social welfare services.

All working people in Poland have social insurance, the purpose of which is to give financial help in cases of special need such as disease, work inability, old age, family increase, and so on. In Poland the number of insured people is about 20 million. The general trend is to insure all citizens. Nonworking family members are also insured.

In this system, all those insured are entitled to medical care free of charge. The deaf have indeed the same privilege if they are employed, or if they are insured because of other reasons, being family members, pensioners, and so on. Hard-of-hearing persons, especially children, take advantage of an additional privilege. The insurance agency provides them with hearing aids, free of charge. After having reached the age of a pensioner (women at 60 and men at 65 years), the deaf get pensions according to the regulation which pertains to all workers. If the deaf person becomes disabled, he obtains a disability pension, provided he has worked for 5 years during the last 10 years before losing the ability to work.

In the case of work disability not being preceded by the obligatory period of work, the deaf person gets allowances from the State fund allocated for special help. The deaf, similar to other working citizens, take advantage of vacations as do working people, sanatoria, and all other forms of rest and health improvement which are accessible to working people. Rest holidays are given to the deaf according to regulations.

Legal Rights of the Deaf

The deaf in Poland have the same right to legal action as others, except individuals who are indicted by a valid court sentence. In Poland there are very few known cases of deaf being deprived of legal action by means of indictment. These cases usually are those deaf who are severely mentally retarded.

The deaf, just as other citizens, are entitled to vote and take part in all other political, social, and legal acts.

The penal and civil codes of Poland guarantee the deaf the presence of public defenders and translators in court trials. The Polish law protects the interests of the deaf.

The driver's license for the deaf in Poland is regulated by special rules.

Right of the Deaf to Use Cultural Resources

The Polish Association of Deaf conducts large cultural and educational programs in order to provide the deaf with wide availability of cultural achievements. In 95 houses of culture and trade union halls, cultural shows of various kinds are organized in which the deaf often take part as performers. This is done to help them become acquainted with the cultural aspects of life. To facilitate understanding, there are always qualified cultural and educational workers and translators of gesture language present.

A network of sports clubs spread over the country permits the deaf to take part in competitions which they organize. Tourism also is of great interest to the deaf.

ACKNOWLEDGMENTS

The author wishes to acknowledge the following collaborators for their contribution to this chapter: L. Sobieszczanska-Radoszewska, M.D., Z. Rzedowska, M.D., I. Urbanska, M.D., A. Rola-Janicki, M.A., D. Potyrala, M.D., J. Nowosielski, Sc.D., G. Remlein-Mozolewska, M.D., Dr. B. Wierzchowska, and Dr. J. Wierzchowski.

chapter 12

Communication for Hearing-handicapped People in the Arab World

Jamil I. Toubbeh, Ph.D.,
Salah M. Soliman, M.D., Sc.D.,
and James T. Yates, Ph.D.

Rehabilitation programs in the North African and Middle Eastern Arab countries are in their infancy. Limited rehabilitation has been practiced, but the concept of total rehabilitation–concentrated effort against the entire spectrum of disabilities–is relatively new. Rehabilitation programs are developing secondarily to basic medical care and only after a firm modern educational process has been established. By contrast, rehabilitation in Western nations developed more often in concert with these endeavors. Consequently, rehabilitation programs in general, and those for the hearing handicapped in particular, have been subject to strong influences and biases implicit in the philosophy and training of medical and educational professions and practitioners.

These conditions, however, have become both an asset and a liability. Limited only by their awareness of Western programs, local practitioners have accepted the best in these systems while rejecting those precepts and methodologies unadaptable to local use. On the other hand, there is a deficiency of experience and an absence of a large body of trained professionals.

Programs in the various countries have many similar characteristics both in approaches and methodologies. However, there are numerous differences, some subtle, some obvious. That such differences exist should not surprise anyone who considers their geographical, ethnic, political, philosophical, and economic variances. These differences in concept and approach among the rehabilitation specialists make direct comparison of the programs difficult. Therefore, the authors have chosen to discuss the countries separately.

Discussion will center on Tunisia, Egypt, Lebanon, Syria, and the United Arab Emirates. Contacts and exchange of information with the latter three nations have been sparse because of a number of factors. Therefore, the description of their activities will be limited.

TUNISIA

Essentially, rehabilitation programs for the hearing handicapped are located in Tunis, in two centers, commonly administered by the Association Tunisienne D'Aide Aux Sourds-Muets (ATASM). Its philosophical guide holds that effective integration into society can only be accomplished when the hearing handicapped communicate through aural-oral means within their environment. The process develops communication skills, emphasizing speech, socialization, and stabilization of the emotional concomitants of the hearing impairment. Presently there is little effort to provide vocational training. Plans for the near future include vocational preparation, but the scope of training will be somewhat broader than that traditionally thought appropriate for the hearing handicapped.

The decision to delete vocational training in the initial stages of program development stems from another, more basic philosophy. Since the program for the hearing handicapped was to be entirely new, there were few resources available: physical facilities, trained personnel, and equipment were virtually nonexistent. Consequently, major efforts would concentrate on younger patients with the idea that, once a strong habilitation program was firmly established, the facilities and expertise developed would become the firm base for expanding service to all ages.

Historical Overview

Before ATASM's creation in 1970, coordinated rehabilitation programs for the hearing handicapped had been virtually nonexistent. Sporadic services could be obtained through the Ear, Nose, and Throat (ENT) Department of the Charles Nicolle Hospital in Tunis. Available services were limited in scope, and they were confined to those patients presenting themselves for treatment.

In October 1, 1970, ATASM founded the School for the Deaf in Bordo, comprised of a kindergarten. During that year, preparatory classes were added, enlarging enrollment to 50 students. In November 1972, a Deafness Research Center was established with support from the Rehabilitation Services Administration, United States Department of Health, Education, and Welfare, Washington, D. C. under the Public Law 480. This center accommodated two kindergarten and two preparatory classes of 40 students. In May 1972, a section for professional training of women was created to serve 20 deaf teenage girls. At the same time, a club was established for deaf adults in the Medina (old city) of Tunis, bringing together 40 deaf adults for participation in therapeutic sports and related activities. Except for this program, no structured habilitation program for the adult deaf is available in Tunisia.

Program development has been hampered by many problems, some unique to this nation. There was, for example, no indigenous model on which to build and there were virtually no trained professionals. Furthermore, Tunisians' attitudes regarding handicaps of any kind made identification and remediation difficult. These and other problems, too numerous to mention, inhibited initiation of needed programs. Once the initial efforts had been made, however, it was necessary to resolve a basic problem of education—the language of the country.

Tunisia is a polyglot society. Although Tunisian Arabic is the dominant language, it is a dialect specific to Tunisians. Classical or modified classical Arabic is the written language and the language of the media. Modified classical Arabic is the spoken language of the educated in Tunisia, as it is in the Arab World at large. French, which is widely spoken in the country as a result of years of colonial government, may be considered as dominant as Tunisian Arabic. This multiplicity creates obvious problems in the education and preparation of the acoustically impaired.

There has been extensive debate as to which language set would permit the hearing handicapped to function best. While a preliminary choice has been made to allow the program to get underway, the issue has not been fully resolved. Teaching the hearing-handicapped Tunisian one speaking set that could cut across at least classical or modified classical Arabic and Tunisian dialectic Arabic presents a formidable task. It was decided that the most promising approach would be to combine classical and Tunisian dialectic Arabic. Deaf educators opted for the Tunisian dialectic Arabic for the first 3 years of rehabilitation (preschool age) as a foundation for classical Arabic. However, since an acoustically impaired child's intellectual and social development would depend on his ability to read and write, classical Arabic would also be taught because it is the language of written communication. Once a linguistic foundation has been established, more complete dialectic Tunisian Arabic would be superimposed on the classical. Those phonemes which are nonexistent in classical Arabic would be introduced with dialectic Tunisian.

Obviously, the chosen approach excluded French. Should a decision be made at some later date to include French as an essential language, the task of rehabilitation will be further complicated. The question's resolution will depend upon the findings of research that will look into the integration of the present enrollees into society.

Program Overview

Current emphasis is on habilitation of the young hearing handicapped. Although program expansion will eventually reach the entire country, present activities are centered on metropolitan Tunis. Only a small segment of the Tunisian population of over 5 million now receives the wide range of services needed.

Regional hospitals and maternity clinics provide medical, obstetrical, and pediatric services. They are also the primary referral sources for suspected hearing impairments in these outlying regions. Unfortunately, audiological and otological facilities do not exist generally in these settings. There is not a well developed referral system to the better equipped hospitals and clinics of Tunis. The widest range of services is provided by hospitals in the Tunis metropolitan area where most of the ENT specialists are situated. Consequently, the hearing-handicapped population of Tunis receives better care than is available in the regional medical centers which serve the other governorates (Sfax, Medenine, Kef, Jendouba, Beja, Kesserine, Kairaouan, Gafsa, Gabes, Sousse, Nabeul, and Bizerte).

Identification

A limited mobile screening program is identifying children with hearing handicaps. Initial efforts were confined to Tunis, but the program is being expanded to include outlying regions. In addition, routine neonate screening is performed at Charles Nicolle Hospital, Avenue Mohammed V Hospital, and Children's Hospital of Tunis.

The mobile screening program is of great importance since many children are born outside of hospital or clinic. Because midwivery is common even in metropolitan Tunis, a system of total neonate and early infant screening is not now possible. Identification efforts are further hampered since medical help, particularly from otologists, is not sought until the problem is so severe that it cannot be ignored. This reluctance to reveal and seek help for both medical and educational problems impedes services to all handicapped.

Additionally, many people seek help from nonprofessional sources. Herbs and sulfur springwaters are considered by many as superior to medical treatment. This practice is not uncommon in North Africa and throughout the Middle East.

Evaluation and Diagnosis

Once the child has been identified as suspect of having hearing loss, he is referred to Charles Nicolle Hospital or the ATASM Deafness Research Center. Charles Nicolle Hospital has complete audiological and ENT facilities. In addition to the neonate-infant screening program, this hospital is the primary diagnostic and medical treatment center for medical problems associated with hearing impairment. A small staff of audiologists and orthophonists provides hearing evaluation and diagnosis and preliminary speech and language evaluation. No ongoing speech-hearing-language services are provided at this hospital or at Children's Hospital of Tunis.

Audiological and speech and language examinations are also performed at the ATASM research center where a small, but well equipped audiological suite is located. A cooperative arrangement between the two centers assures maximum use of available equipment and personnel. Language and speech evaluation is possibly the weakest link in the chain of services at present.

Rehabilitation Services

ATASM is composed of two interrelated units, one research oriented, the other training. Together they focus on the needs of preschool and school-age children. They serve metropolitan Tunis, but they are considered to be the first phase of an overall program which will encompass all of Tunisia. Students are seen on an outpatient basis, and the overall program is similar to educational activities in the public school systems.

Those students having mild hearing loss or whose hearing loss was incurred after lingual development was rather advanced may be placed in special classes in the public schools of Tunis. Three such classes are taught by specially chosen teachers of the regular school system who are assisted by language resource personnel.

Expanded Services

During 1974, two minibuses were purchased and equipped as mobile test centers. Each contains equipment for basic hearing, screening, and otological examinations. Although not fully operational, the mobile hearing laboratories form the nucleus of the nationwide program of identification and service. During 1974, the mobile units traveled 2 months in each of the Sfax, Medenine, Kef, and Jendouba governorates.

In 1974 a residential school for the hearing handicapped was organized outside the city of Tunis. This school will be considered as an expansion of the present ATASM facilities in the city. Vocational education and adult programs will be included as a part of the total program for the hearing handicapped.

Training Program Goals

The emphasis in training is on habilitation. This process begins at about the age of 6 years at the kindergarten level. Training includes:

(1) observation and training in lipreading (20 minutes per day); (2) reading (35 minutes per day), including identification of alphabets, words, and sentences; (3) writing readiness (30 minutes per day), including identification of geometric shapes and letters, tracing, copying, and dictation; (4) arithmetic readiness (20 minutes per day) for preparation for modern mathematics; (5) religious instruction (15 minutes per day), including prayer, development of good moral and ethical habits, body cleanliness, and identification of religious holidays; (6) art and drawing (25 minutes per day), including cutting and pasting, modeling, weaving, free painting, coloring, and copying of shapes; (7) physical training and rhythmic dance (20 minutes per day), including balancing exercises, dexterity games, and "free" movement; (8) auditory and speech training (30 minutes per day), including attention to noise, training in identification of human voice, and language of music.

A total of 4 hours of training is required. Before each daily session, students are checked for cleanliness. A 30-minute break is allowed.

Courses for upper classes (grades 1 through 3) place greater emphasis on oral language, socialization process, and civics. During these years, formal writing is initiated. Classical aural Arabic is introduced along with Tunisian dialectic Arabic. All subjects studied at the lower levels are amplified, and, upon reaching the third grade level, students are expected to achieve a basic understanding of language. Once the basic linguistic precepts have been established, dialectic Tunisian is expanded. This step is presumed not to interfere with the student's basic knowledge and understanding of the classical Arabic base.

The syllabi for the kindergarten through grade four are set forth by the Ministry of Education, with minor modifications to adapt them to the special needs of the hearing handicapped. These constitute an amplification and modification of the syllabi used in classroom instruction with children of normal hearing. Religious instruction, for example, is expanded to include not only prayer but also learning to recite verses from the Koran and education in community living (which includes respect for property and traffic accident prevention). Physical training is expanded to include structured dance lessons. Observation, expression, and lipreading are enlarged to deal with subjects related to the home environment, the street, and the school.

Types of Support

The Charles Nicolle and Avenue Mohammed V hospitals are government supported. Both are large general hospitals with a wide range of medical and support services. Although both have departments of ENT, only Charles Nicolle Hospital has a full range of audiological services at present. Plans call for expansion of diagnostic and rehabilitative audiology at this hospital, depending on the acquisition of audiologists and orthophonists.

The School for the Deaf of ATASM is supported by federal sources through a system of referrals and by private subscription. The Research Center of ATASM is partly supported by the Rehabilitation Services Administration of the U. S. Department of Health, Education, and Welfare through grants under Public Law 480 and by private funds. The school and research center are converted rental homes with fairly adequate office, classroom, test rooms, and playground space. It is inevitable that, as more hearing handicapped are identified and demand for services increases, these facilities will require expansion. As they are incapable of enlargement, such growth will necessitate relocation.

Diagnostic Procedures

At present, all extra medical diagnostic services are provided at Charles Nicolle Hospital and the ATASM Research Center. Both have reasonably well equipped audiological centers, as well as facilities for sociological, psychological, language, and speech evaluation.

At Charles Nicolle Hospital, two sound-treated suites with appropriate audiological equipment form the nucleus of the Audiology Department. A diagnostic audiometer, a conditioned orientation response (COR), and an evoked response audiometer (ERA) are included in the suites. The ATASM center has much the same equipment, but does not have an ERA facility. Specific audiological test procedures include traditional pure tone and speech, COR, and play audiometry and special testing for site of lesion. Impedance/admittance audiometry is not yet available, but is included in future plans.

Psychological tests include Koh's nonverbal test as adapted by Grace Arthur, and Snijders Comen's nonverbal intelligence scale which is particularly suited to hearing-handicapped children. The Merrill-Palmer scale and Guermadi's phonological scale are utilized.

Sociological data are routinely collected. Early efforts were concentrated on determining complete geographical and family histories. As the program progressed, attitude scaling and surveying have been introduced for families. Investigation to date shows that parents of the deaf and hearing-impaired children are highly fatalistic in their attitude toward deafness and are over-protective. Nevertheless, in many cases, the child is completely neglected because of the large number of children in the family.

General medical and otological examinations are provided for all individuals suspected of having a hearing handicap and at regular intervals for confirmed cases. The ATASM school has a small medical department for routine evaluation. Physicians from the hospital staff rotate through this center.

Rehabilitation Procedures

The emphasis in training is on habilitation. The process begins at approximately age 5½ years with kindergarten or preschool preparation. The classical classroom approach is used in language training—vocabulary development, sign-symbol association, etc. Verbalization is used extensively. Children's responses are oral or through gesture, making use of pictures. Children's responses are monitored closely by the teacher who consistently models correctly and imparts the correct response model as reinforcement. Speechreading is encouraged and emphasized.

Amplification systems are provided for all classrooms. Both fixed (hard wire) and mobile (loop and FM) systems are available. Special auditory training sessions are routinely provided by European-trained orthophonists. Auditory training may be individual or in small groups as dictated by the student's needs.

The oral-aural approach is used while children are in school, except during play when auditory aids are removed. There is no manual communication system available at this time, and adoption of such means is not contemplated because of a strong commitment to oralism.

Orthophonists, working individually with children, provide training in sound discrimination and speech production. At this point, there is a great deal of experimentation in training methods. The basic methodology is the classical approach, but variations are applied when appropriate. The professional staff is attempting to modify speech training to coincide with the natural development of sounds—working from the earliest to the latest sounds developed.

Individual hearing aids are not available. All amplification is provided by the group auditory trainers in the classrooms. The major problems are cost and maintenance. All hearing aids, as well as other equipment, must be imported. High initial cost, plus import tariffs, make hearing aids prohibitively expensive for all but a few. But, even when the problem of economics is overcome, the problem of maintenance remains. The average family has little knowledge or appreciation of such a complicated instrument. The hearing-handicapped individual or his family is unable to care for the aid to the degree necessary to achieve normal operation. It is difficult to teach families the necessity of changing batteries, much less the proper mechanics for doing so.

Interprofessional Relationships

ATASM is directed by a board which initiates and controls policy. The board is composed of physicians, government officials, and lay members. It meets regularly to review policies and activities of the school and the center. Communication between the board and the staff of the school and the center is limited to informal meetings between individual board members and staff. Since in-depth knowledge of communication disorders is lacking among many board members and a number of the staff, there exists a serious chasm between the two groups.

Medical experts comprise a powerful group in the country and are dominant among professionals and allied health personnel working with hearing impaired. Educators also comprise a powerful group that tends to impose its philosophy. As these professionals, having various roles and responsibilities, develop greater confidence in their abilities, each asserts himself more in an attempt to influence planning and administration. This assertiveness fosters a degree of unilateral performances, thereby reducing the effectiveness of interaction among professionals.

The physical distance between the medical and educational staff and those of the school and the center accentuates the problem of administration. Center staff, however, interacts daily. They comprise a committed group whose knowledge of acoustic impairment, with its social and psychological concomitants, exceeds their formal or on-the-job training. Their impact on the more established disciplines is growing. This is attributed, primarily, to their creativity and growing effectiveness and efficiency on the job.

There is good rapport between psychologists, social workers, speech and hearing clinicians, and the various support personnel within the school and the center. Case findings are routinely discussed among these workers. Innovative approaches with regard to habilitation are evaluated and implemented, and there exists a feeling among these staff members that a strong interdisciplinary approach is necessary to resolve outstanding issues.

These observations should be studied in the light of existing needs in

Tunisia vis-à-vis the severe shortage of rehabilitation personnel. Medical professionals are just beginning to realize the importance of habilitation in general and rehabilitation of the hearing handicapped specifically. The demands for medical and restorative services exceed the supply of medical professionals who can render these services. Their involvement in the habilitative and rehabilitative services, however negligible it may be at present as reflected in the interprofessional relationships, indicates a trend of interdisciplinary cooperation. As the population of hearing handicapped is identified, educators, too, will follow this inevitable trend.

The professional preparation of the teachers of the hearing handicapped is the least advanced. Although interested and active, none has had any special training for working with the hearing impaired beyond that which is accrued through on-the-job training. Even that training is provided by professionals whose preparation and expertise are not directly in education of deaf pupils. The teachers' lack of specific training has generated a subtle feeling of inferiority which was aggravated by exclusion from staff meetings which included the psychology, sociology, audiology, and orthophonist staff. Once recognized, however, the teaching staff was included in meetings and in the decision-making process. At the same time, on-the-job training was increased in quality and frequency. Communication and morale increased greatly thereby.

Family Involvements

Involving families in the rehabilitation process is difficult. They are often large, poor, and uneducated. With so many other children and older family members demanding care and attention, the affected member is often ignored. Even when families want to help, they typically find themselves unable to comprehend the technical and educational process.

Referral agencies provide most counseling. ATASM does not provide significant follow-up. A pilot project is underway with a select group of eight families who are undergoing intensive group and individual counseling. These parents, it is hoped, will act, in turn, as counselors for others. If successful, the manpower burden will be eased and counseling effectiveness increased. An added bonus is that families may enter new family groups without generating the fear and mistrust apparent with professionals.

Professional Training

ATASM clinical staff is recruited from professionals trained in Tunisia and in Europe (principally France).

There are no formal training programs for teachers of the deaf and hard of hearing in the country. Teachers for hearing handicapped classes are recruited from among public school teachers and from public school graduates, and all instruction for working with the hearing handicapped is in the form of on-the-job training. Talent, dedication, motivation, and novel teaching techniques, as well as personal dynamism, are selection criteria. The ability to express ideas gesturally, through use of body movements, ranks high among the selection criteria.

Economics plays a major role in selection and training. Developing an indigenous program is prohibitive for such a country. Sending members abroad is also expensive, but present plans include such training of a limited number of persons, either to upgrade their training or to train them in specialty areas.

No formal training programs exist in audiology or orthophonics. Current staffs were trained in France. Medical and hearing and speech staffs impart limited knowledge and skills to paraprofessionals in operational facilities.

The pervading problem in developing training programs in audiology and orthophonics is also economic. Cost is prohibitive, and trainers are nonexistent. Although there has been discussion between the administration of the University of Tunisia and the Dean of the School of Medicine, there are no immediate plans for the establishment of such training programs. The consensus among the present professional staff is that there is a very real danger of perpetuating mediocrity should dependence on ATASM training continue.

Future Needs

All Tunisian professionals are keenly aware of the need for coordinated research which would pave the way for coordinated services. A great deal has been accomplished to date, but much more remains to be accomplished.

Future developments are contingent on financial resources, manpower, and public information. Limited financial resources constitute a major obstacle to habilitation and rehabilitation programs. Expansion depends largely on accelerated support from government and private sources.

Recruitment of qualified students does not appear to be an obstacle; rather, it is the cost of training professional workers abroad. An alternative would be the establishment of an academic program in speech pathology and audiology at the University of Tunis. This is being contemplated.

Deafness and hearing impairment go unnoticed and, therefore, are not reported. Public education programs should be expanded.

Research should proceed on such target areas as demographic studies, etiological studies, studies related to identification of the population at risk, prevention strategies, standardization of tests, the status of the adult deaf, and the development of a pretest/post-test profile to evaluate the effectiveness of present habilitation programs.

EGYPT

Historical Overview

In Egypt's 7,000 years of recorded history, one experiment aimed at defining some of the variables of speech and language acquisition is worth mentioning. In the 7th century B.C., Pharaoh Psammetichus ordered two newborn infants abandoned in the wilderness under distant supervision. His aim was to learn from their first verbal utterances which language and, thus, which nation was the oldest. This experiment in feral living revealed man's language to be the product of his environment, since the two infants' only utterances were those of the surrounding creatures.

Most of the details of Egypt's ancient civilization and achievements were lost when Caesar burned the library at Alexandria and, thus, according to Bernard Shaw "the memory of man." No information is presently available about any historical programs for the hearing handicapped.

In the early 1900's, parents of deaf persons in Cairo organized themselves in a clublike organization. They met weekly. Mainly a social gathering, it provided emotional and psychological support. Its members communicated through a sign language system. Gradually, membership increased, and the Ministry of Social Affairs began to support its meetings through payment of rent and utilities. Eventually, it gained full sponsorship by the Ministry, and, in 1956, the group formed the Egyptian Association for the Deaf and Hard of Hearing. It has become the most extensive vocational rehabilitation program for the hearing handicapped in Egypt.

Aural Habilitation and Rehabilitation

Several official organizations offer programs for aural rehabilitation: the Ministry of Education, the Ministry of Social Affairs, the Ministry of Public Health, and the Ministry of Higher Education.

The Ministry of Education, through its Special Education Department, conducts classes for school age children (6–18 years) in the public schools of most governorates. There are no programs for preschoolers in Egypt. In metropolitan Cairo, there are classes for first to eighth graders in nine schools with a total enrollment of 878 (357 girls and 521 boys). Several have only one class while others have as many as 19.

Alexandria's enrollment is 409. Enrollment in other governorates' schools for which data are available is as follows: Gharbia, 12 (1 class); Kafr El-Sheikh, 63 (7 classes); Qualyoubya, 6 (1 class); Menoufiyya, 162 (17 classes); Dakahlyia, 204 (22 classes); Damietta, 23 (3 classes); Sharkya, 156 (15 classes); Giza, 27 (4 classes); Fayoum, 116 (14 classes); Beni Souif, 93 (10 classes); Menia, 84 (9 classes); Assiout, 115 (13 classes); Sohaj, 63 (7 classes); and Quena, 8 (1 class).

Most of these schools have programs for habilitation and rehabilitation. Hearing aids and auditory trainers' use is hindered by the lack of spare parts and maintenance.

The Ministry of Social Affairs has one center for children and young adults. It is vocationally oriented, although habilitation has been emphasized recently. Services include medical, audiological, sociological, psychological, educational, and vocational areas. Hearing aids and auditory trainers are used.

The center is jointly sponsored by the Ministry of Social Affairs and the Rehabilitation Services Administration of the Department of Health, Education, and Welfare of the United States under Public Law 480. It is housed in the Egyptian Association for the Deaf and the Hard of Hearing and has an enrollment of over 250 girls and boys, ranging in age from 10–18 years. The facility provides in-patient services for a segment of the student enrollment. It houses the most active program for the total habilitation and rehabilitation in the country.

The Ministry of Public Health has recently established a hearing and speech center which provides diagnostic and educational services on a day care basis for hearing-handicapped children. Teachers here are not as qualified as those from the Ministry of Education. They were recruited from among social workers and health nurses and received 6 months of training by an audiologist. Short courses in audiology, neurology, speech therapy, psychology, and educational techniques with the hearing handicapped formed the basis of their training.

This center provides urgently needed guidance and training to its clients, but the quality of services rendered leaves much to be desired.

The Ministry for Higher Education supervises Egypt's seven universities. In 1973, the University of Ein Shams (25 years old) in Cairo established a hearing and speech center in the Department of Otolaryngology, Faculty of Medicine. The center provides audiological, speech and language diagnostic evaluation, treatment of acute and chronic otolaryngological conditions, and speech and language therapy. In addition, pediatric, neurological, opthalmological, medical, and psychiatric services are available. Availability of broad medical services makes the Ein Shams center unique among other similar programs.

In the educational field, the School of Medicine initiated in 1974 a master's degree program in audiology. Although enrollment has been limited to graduating medical students, graduates from other disciplines will be included. In 1972, a 2-year program in speech pathology will open to graduates from a variety of disciplines. Student selection will be made from various geographical areas to ensure services distribution throughout Egypt.

The preceding discussion signals factors to which Egyptian specialists must address themselves: (1) there exists no central agency or national organization to coordinate the overall activities of each ministry; (2) community involvement is still embryonic; (3) the distant and remote areas of Egypt have limited resources and manpower; and (4) there exists no program to serve the preschool hearing handicapped—a serious shortcoming. Unless this deficiency is remedied, the hearing handicapped will continue to face formidable problems in later life.

Diagnostic Procedures

Referrals are made to schools, centers, or institutes by either private physicians or other professionals working in public health clinics.

At Ein Shams University, otolaryngological examinations precede audiometric testing. Routine pure tone and speech testing, Bekesy, impedance, and GSR audiometry are available. As of this writing, EEG audiometry is not provided, but its purchase is being considered. Speech tests have been developed for discrimination tests in Arabic, and development of Arabic word lists for obtaining Speech Reception Threshold (SRT) is underway. (There are a few pure spondee words in Arabic.)

Clients served in the various centers are also referred, when necessary, for general medical examinations and ophthalmological and psychometric evaluations. The Wechsler Intelligence Scale for Children and Stanford-Binet tests, adapted for the local language and culture, are generally used in psychological assessment. Other tests are currently being adapted for testing the nonverbal child. Language and speech development tests are absent primarily because of the dearth of professional manpower in speech pathology.

Rehabilitative Procedures

Aural education stresses speechreading and signing. Auditory training, utilizing electronic trainers and hearing aids, was introduced in 1970. Except for the limited number who could obtain hearing aids to date, most hearing-handicapped persons have not been trained with electronic amplification. The barriers to this system continue to be economical and technical.

Regulations for importation of hearing aids, auditory trainers, and audiological equipment have been liberalized by the Egyptian government during the last 3 years. Also, a number of professionally trained people have returned from Europe and the United States. And also, public awareness has been awakened to the special problems of the hearing handicapped. These developments point toward the establishment of viable programs.

Development efforts have been made toward a system of fingerspelling. This idea is still new in the Arabic-speaking world, and cooperation is being sought with various Arabic-speaking countries to standardize the system.

Interprofessional Relationships

In Egypt, the typical aural rehabilitation institute uses team effort. The team includes a physician, psychologist, otolaryngologist, audiologist, speech pathologist, deaf educators, rehabilitation counselors, and social workers. Usually a physician heads such a rehabilitation program, with an administrator assisting him. Weekly meetings are usually held to discuss individual problems. These meetings are chaired by a physician in charge of the program.

Family Involvements

The role of the family varies widely according to economic level, rural or urban background, and sex of the disabled. Children and young adults are considered economic assets by parents in rural areas, and sons are valued more highly than daughters because inheritance or property is greater for sons. Because education tends to have less value in rural than in urban areas, the hearing-handicapped child of a rural family may be accepted "as he is" until puberty, when help in vocational training becomes important. Among urban families of average or above average income, educational achievement is important for all children. As a general rule, these families tend to seek help for their children in terms of speech and language development.

Comparing the Egyptian society with other Western societies, the former appears to be more accepting of the handicapped population, particularly the young disabled. In Egypt, the hearing-handicapped child is at ease in large social groups and is under less pressure to achieve language skills at the preschool age. This social acceptance is, in and of itself, a major handicap to the child, who, later in life, has to demonstrate capability to survive without prior education in the rudiments of language.

Training of Professionals

There are three programs for training professionals. Each meets the needs and academic standards of the professionals involved. They were developed in an attempt to meet the demand and the right of every child to develop, in his early years, maximum competence in communication, listening, speaking, reading, and writing.

The first audiology training program, initiated in 1974, was organized by the Ein Shams University School of Medicine. It leads to a master's degree and is designed for medical graduates only. During the 2-year course, candidates must complete two examinations, one after each year of study. Its objective is to prepare medical specialists to head the various rehabilitation programs throughout Egypt.

A second training program is administered by the Ministry of Education, Department of Special Education. Students are primary school teachers with a 2-year college degree. A number, however, are high school graduates. Rehabilitative audiology is taught during 1 academic year. Candidates take final written and oral examinations. Upon completion, graduates are assigned to primary schools as speech therapists and educators of the deaf in selected special classes. Attempts now are underway to upgrade the program by enrolling only college graduates.

A third program, administered by the Ministry of Social Affairs, is designed specifically for teachers of the deaf at the Egyptian Association of the Deaf and Hard of Hearing, a vocationally oriented rehabilitation school.

Ein Shams University staff operates in all three programs. While the curriculum is essentially the same, it is modified in density and detail from one to the other course. The staff recognizes the deficiencies and pitfalls of each, particularly in the absence of a system for evaluating effectiveness and the degree of practical competence of the graduates.

Broadly speaking, the curriculum includes basic anatomy and physiology of the ear, nose, and throat, acoustics and psychoacoustics, and statistical methods. The clinical courses include principles and diagnostic audiological procedures for infants, children, and adults; causes and types of deafness; treatment and rehabilitation techniques; normal and abnormal speech and language development; principles of hereditary deafness (including a course in basic genetics); hearing aids; psychology of the hard-of-hearing and deaf persons; and methods of investigation and referral.

Research

Research activities are conducted by various organizations actively involved with the habilitation and rehabilitation of hearing-handicapped individuals, outstanding among which are the research activities that are jointly sponsored by the Egyptian government and other governments.

The Departments of Audiology and Otolaryngology of Ein Shams University School of Medicine are engaged in two research projects. The first studies a hospital-based model for delivery of speech and hearing services to communities. It is co-sponsored by the Egyptian government and the Maternal and Child Health, Division of Clinical Services, Department of Health, Education, and Welfare of the United States, under Public Law 480. Its objectives are: (1) to develop a hospital model for delivery of audiology and speech services to infants and preschool and school children with hearing impairments; (2) to evaluate the effectiveness of the model in the early identification, follow-up, and treatment of children; and (3) to evaluate the effectiveness of the model in the prevention of conditions leading to hearing impairments and more severe sequelae.

A second project, co-sponsored by the Egyptian government and the Indian Health Service, Medical Services Administration of the Department of Health, Education, and Welfare of the United States, also under Public Law 480, focuses on otitis media in rural Egypt. Its objectives are: (1) to determine the epidemiology of otitis media in selected sites; (2) to train and evaluate locally based paraprofessional personnel in the delivery of services; (3) to develop and evaluate the effectiveness of a health education program on otitis media prevalence; and (4) to determine possible effects of otitis media on the development of speech and language.

Agreements have been reached between the Rehabilitation Services Administration, Office of Human Development, Department of Health, Education, and Welfare of the United States and the Department of Social Rehabilitation of Egypt to initiate three major, long-term research projects which will focus on: (1) investigation of the relative merits and effectiveness of aural versus manual communication systems; (2) replication in Egypt of facets of on-going research in Yugoslavia on the verbo-tonal method; and (3) a multinational conference, to be followed by multinational research, on communication disorders of central origin. The first project will be of particular significance to both rehabilitation professionals working with the hearing handicapped in Egypt and in the Arabic-speaking world at large.

The objectives of this research project will include: (1) identification, through survey, of sign vocabulary used by the deaf in Egypt; (2) construction of a standard sign vocabulary based upon the results of the survey; (3) comparison of the effectiveness of aural-oral home training and sign-manual training in development of language; and (4) identification of an optimal approach of language training procedures for education of the deaf in Egypt.

PROGRAMS IN OTHER ARAB COUNTRIES

Several other Arab governments are attempting to improve upon programs or to initiate new programs. In most, however, it is not financial resources that hinder development of viable habilitation and rehabilitation delivery systems, but the dearth of professional manpower to implement programs of the various ministries of health, education, and welfare and of the private institutions. This is particularly true in countries bordering the Arabian Gulf—Saudi Arabia, Kuwait, Qatar, and the United Arab Emirates. Professionals, primarily medical practitioners, are aware of manpower shortages and are attempting to resolve them. There exists a move in the Arab World to encourage Arab professionals working in the Western countries to contribute toward the establishment of viable habilitation and rehabilitation programs in the Arab World. Arab professionals, it is felt, are sensitive to the needs of the Arab people, are well versed in the culture of the area, and present no linguistic barriers. Arab Americans are beginning to respond to Arab governments' pleas.

LEBANON

Like Tunisia, Lebanon is a polyglot society. The strength of Western, particularly European, influence is reflected in Lebanon's academic institutions—American, English, even Armenian. Unlike Tunisia, however, Lebanon has retained its identity as an Arab country. Arabic, dialectic as well as classical, is the dominant language. Colonialism, in other words, did not have the same effect on the Lebanese language as it had on the Tunisian.

Lebanon has traditionally served the hearing handicapped, but services have been limited and are often beyond the financial reach of the average Lebanese. There is no structured delivery system; rather, delivery is by private, profit-making or charitable, nonprofit organizations. The central government renders assistance to the indigent, but it is limited relative to needs.

The authors have been able to identify four institutions: the Lebanese State School for the Deaf and the Blind at B'abda; the Armenian School for the Deaf and Blind at Nahr; Father Anderec's School for the Deaf at 'Alai; and Father Robert's School for the Deaf at Jounieh.

The Lebanese State School for the Deaf and Blind was established by the wife of ex-Prime Minister Kamil Chamoun. Its facilities are reasonably well equipped, and the institution accepts school age children from 5–17 years old. Its teachers are either European or British trained. It has limited vocational training facilities, and its method of teaching is classical (vibrotactile and lipreading).

The Armenian School for the Deaf and Blind is equipped with a locally constructed sound-treated room for testing. Auditory training equipment is available. It provides vocational training for its school-age population, and the teaching methods are similar to those used in the Lebanese School at B'abda.

Father Anderec's School for the Deaf is a private enterprise and caters primarily to the children of the affluent in the Middle East. It has adequate facilities and training instruments. Training methods are similar to those used in the schools already described.

Father Robert's School for the Deaf is another private institution which receives funds from charitable institutions as well as from the government. Its principal is a dynamic person who travels extensively through Europe with his dance troupe of deaf students. Teaching methods employed are classical. Its population ranges in age from 6–17.

The American University of Beirut offers audiological services to all ages through its Department of Otolaryngology. Audiological facilities are limited, and there is no academic program for training of professional or subprofessional personnel. According to Dr. Salah Salman, Chairman of the Department of Otolaryngology, the potential for initiating an academic program in audiology is strong, and funds can become available if the issue of professional manpower to administer such a program is resolved.

Currently, Lebanon is serving not only its own population of hearing handicapped but also those of other Arab countries. The capacity to absorb clients from abroad is limited, however, and Lebanese medical professionals often refer these clients to Europe for comprehensive services.

Hearing aid dealers in Lebanon are involved in the delivery of services.

They perform routine audiometric testing and prescribe and dispense a wide range of hearing aids, including imports from the United States, Europe, and Russia.

SYRIA

The Ministry of Labor and Social Affairs administers Syria's programs. There are also two associations for deaf–mutes, with head offices in Damascus and Aleppo, which support activities in behalf of the Syrian deaf and act as their advocate. They receive substantial financial assistance from the government.

Movement toward increasing and updating service delivery suffered severe setbacks as a result of the October War of 1973. The newly constructed and well-equipped School for the Deaf at Mazza outside Damascus was bombed and the government was forced to reopen the old school at Souk Saroujah in old Damascus, shortly after the war, to accommodate the 83 residents and 41 nonresidents of the devastated school.

At least five schools serve the hearing handicapped. Besides Damascus, there are schools in Aleppo and Latakia. They all emphasize vocational education, although habilitation is stressed at the elementary levels.

UNITED ARAB EMIRATES

The United Arab Emirates constitute a union of seven emirates (Abu Dhabi, Dubai, Sharjah, Ajaman, Um al Qaiwain, Ras el Khaimeh, and Fujairah) bordering the Arabian Gulf.

The citizens of the United Arab Emirates are presently experiencing ambitious and widespread domestic development programs, including office complexes, apartment blocks, luxury hotels, and schools. There is no industry in any of the emirates, and the primary source of income is revenue from petroleum. At Defense Hospital, Abu Dhabi, Dr. Nabil Sabbagh, Egyptian-trained ear, nose, and throat specialist, stated that there is a tremendous shortage of manpower to deliver health services to the population of the emirates. He indicated that government officials realize that there is a need for progressive health programs, and that he personally favors the idea of establishment of hearing and speech centers in various emirates in the union.

Preliminary observations made by Dr. Sabbagh point out the high incidence of hearing impairment among the population which he attributes to negligence, heredity, and consanguinity. Cultural barriers prevent medical practitioners from the delivery of needed services to certain segments of the population. Public education, he feels, should be strongly emphasized in any program development plan.

The authors are aware of the existence of other programs for serving the hearing handicapped in Saudi Arabia, Kuwait, and Jordan. Descriptive materials on these programs could not be obtained, however. Kuwait, for example, has extensive programs in specialized schools for serving special target groups of handicapped and low achieving students. Saudi Arabia has similar programs.

In Jordan, a new medical complex has been established in Amman to serve the health needs of the population. This complex contains up-to-date facilities and highly trained health practitioners. Furthermore, a new medical school has been established in the country, but enrollment is limited.

Outside the city of Amman, in the town of Salt, an educational institution serves the needs of a small number of hearing-handicapped persons. Its training focuses on vocational preparation.

AURAL REHABILITATION: A DEFINITION

Generally, Arab rehabilitation workers define aural rehabilitation as a process through which behavior of an acoustically handicapped individual is modified to permit acquisition of language and facilitate its oral expression. Its objective is to allow maximum functioning within a specified social and cultural environment. The process develops articulation, reading, and writing.

The degree of commitment to oralism is exemplified by the fact that there is not a uniform system of manual communication in the Arab world, although a limited system of indigenous signs has developed among the deaf in certain groups.

While professionals agree that the goal of aural rehabilitation is integration of the hearing handicapped into society, the procedures through which this integration is accomplished differ from a group of professionals in one country to those of another. Integration in Tunisia is defined primarily in terms of linguistic/academic competence and, secondarily, in terms of ability to earn a livelihood. Hence, the emphasis in Tunisian programs is on habilitation.

In Egypt, Syria, and to a lesser extent Lebanon, the trend has been to provide socioeconomic adjustment. Therefore, the emphasis is upon vocational training. In these countries, rehabilitation workers view rehabilitation as the adjustment of the hearing handicapped to linguistic disability in order that he may function within his environment. As a result of the dichotomy between habilitation and rehabilitation, the aim of rehabilitation of the aurally handicapped adult is primarily vocational, while programs for the younger hearing handicapped stress language training and development of speech, reading, and writing skills.

SUMMARY

Philosophical, cultural, and economic differences among the various Arab countries have influenced current practices with the hearing handicapped. Tunisian rehabilitation workers reflect the French traditions, while their counterparts in Egypt, Lebanon, Syria, and other Arab countries reflect a mixture of European and United States traditions.

During the initial phases of program development, Tunisian professionals elected to place primary emphasis on the young hearing impaired. This direction in program development may be attributed to Tunisia's limited resources and the desire on the part of professionals working in a new field to demonstrate to the Tunisian public and responsible governmental agencies the feasibility of integrating this disabled population into society. Prospects for habilitating and rehabilitating the young disabled are far more promising than for the older group of handicapped persons.

There is another, more tangible reason for focusing on the young. It allows professionals to establish a firm philosophical and theoretical foundation on which an expanded delivery system can be based. Linguistically, Tunisian educators are moving in the direction of emphasizing Arabic as the primary language of Tunisia. The Tunisian, rather than the French, cultural identity is being re-emphasized. Arabic is presently stressed in schools, with French as a second language. With stress upon the former, it is hoped that the young of Tunisia will grow up with primary exposure to the national language. Thus, when Arabic is re-established as the basic language set, many of the problems facing professionals today will be eliminated. The issue of which language to teach and how many languages are essential for total integration of the hearing handicapped into society will be moot points.

In contrast to Tunisia and the rest of the Arab world, Egypt has a long tradition of service to the hearing handicapped. Egyptian institutions of higher learning train specialists to work with this population. Graduates of these institutions serve the disabled in special schools in the various governorates. Ein Shams University in Cairo has initiated the first program in audiology in the Arab world. This program will prepare medical audiologists to administer rehabilitation programs throughout the country.

While it would appear that the level of provision of services in Egypt is quite high, this is not wholly true. Although relatively extensive services do exist and have existed for some time, there is lack of coordination and absence of a unifying concept. Five governmental ministries maintain programs for the hearing handicapped. There appears to be no mutually accepted philosophical base, nor is there a vehicle for integrating the various programs and services. There is, furthermore, no obvious continuity between habilitation and rehabilitation. A similar gap exists between education and vocational training programs.

It is difficult to predict the form and scope of the delivery system for rehabilitation services which will evolve in Egypt. At present, rehabilitation of the hearing handicapped is the responsibility of medical practitioners—a concept which is at variance with practice in the Western world. The eventual plan, which is to train medical audiologists to head the various programs throughout the country, will further consolidate the control which medicine has in this area.

It remains to be seen what types of supportive personnel these medical professionals will choose to implement the programs and what types and levels of training will evolve. A very real question remains to be answered: will the medical practitioner be able to broaden his scope to appreciate the needs of the hearing handicapped beyond the medical aspects of rehabilitation?

There is a wide variation in the level of development of rehabilitation programs among Lebanon, Syria, and the United Arab Emirates. Lebanon, for example, shares similar problems with Tunisia—its programs are relatively new and the country has a polyglot population, although Arabic is dominant. The majority of available services are provided through private centers which employ Western methods with varying degrees of success. Syria, on the other hand, has developed a government-sponsored program and can boast of two associations for the deaf. Syrian schools for the deaf emphasize vocational rehabilitation for the adult deaf and classical educational programs for the young hearing impaired.

Rehabilitation for the hearing handicapped is virtually nonexistent in the United Arab Emirates at present. The need, however, is recognized in official circles and programs will, undoubtedly, be developed in the near future.

CONCLUSIONS

Long years of foreign domination, first by the Ottomans and then by Western countries, brought Arab creativity to a standstill. Between the 8th and the 12th centuries A.D., Arabic was as much the universal language of culture, science, and diplomacy as Latin was to become in the Middle Ages. There was a time when a Western scholar felt as much at home in an Arab environment as an Arab felt in a Western environment. European scholars studied in Arab universities. Cordova, Damascus, and Baghdad were the cultural centers of the then known world. European medical schools were modeled after Arab schools, and medical texts included, among numerous others, the famous works of Ibn Sina and Al-Razi. Al-Razi's text on the diseases of the eye, ear, and nose is a classic document on the subject.

The Arabs have a long tradition of empathy with and service to the sick and disabled. Here is a story many a young Arab hears from his father or grandfather which illustrates, to some degree, the tradition of the Arabs in this regard.

> A cripple enters a shop and meets a blind man. "I will never be able to reach the Calif's palace to attend the feast because of my disability," he tells the blind man.
> "I can't either," the blind man retorts, "I can't find my way."
> The shopkeeper listens, then says: "Both of you can attend the Calif's feast, if each is willing to help the other. The blind man can walk; the cripple can see. The former can use the legs of the latter, and the latter the eyes of the former."
> So the blind man carried the cripple on his back, and both were on their way to the Calif's palace. Before reaching the palace, however, they stopped at another shop to rest. There they told their story to two other men who happened to be seated outside the shop. One man was hard–of–hearing, the other deaf-mute. The two, apparently, had also received a verbal invitation to attend the Calif's feast but neither one was able to communicate with the other nor were they able to reconcile their differences. The shopkeeper did not intervene to help. So, while the blind man and the cripple were able to attend the feast, the hard-of-hearing and the deaf-mute remained behind.

This story illustrates a number of rather unique points about the Arab's outlook on disability. The Calif's treatment of the disabled, reflected by the invitation, demonstrates the interest that rulers had in the welfare of all their citizens, including the disabled. The first shopkeeper's advice to the blind man and the cripple should be of interest to modern rehabilitation workers. In effect, the shopkeeper, the counselor, intervened only to help the two disabled help themselves. The hard of hearing and the deaf mute did not receive such advice. Finally, the story teller possessed unique insights into the problems that hearing impaired face in life. Without assistance to these disabled, he concludes, they cannot function normally in society.

Arabic literature abounds with stories of this nature. The purpose of citing it is to indicate that, although structured programs for serving the disabled in the Arab world are still in their embryonic stage, we can expect rapid developments in this area in a very short period. One of the major obstacles to this development is lack of trained manpower to initiate programs to serve a spectrum of disabilities, including the hearing-handicapped. Tunisia and Egypt are well on their way to developing such programs. With adequate financial resources, we can anticipate within the next few years development of viable service systems in these two countries. Lebanon, Syria, Kuwait, Saudi Arabia, the United Arab Emirates, and Iraq should follow suit. In all of these countries, the question which is being asked is not why there should be programs to serve the disabled but, rather, how such programs can be implemented. The conceptual foundation for such programs exists within the Arabic tradition.

ACKNOWLEDGMENTS

The authors wish to express their sincere thanks to the following individuals and organizations for their extremely useful contributions: Association Tunisienne d'Aide aux Sourds-Muets, 108 Rue de Yugoslavie, Tunis, Tunisia; Mr. Toufic Abou Chaer, Second Secretary, Syrian Embassy, Washington, D. C.; Egyptian Association for the Deaf and Hard of Hearing, Zamalek, Cairo, Egypt; Hamadi Fayala, M.D., Medecin L'Colonel de l'Aviation, Hôpital Militaire, Tunis, Tunisia; Mohamed Abdel Hamid Hamzawi, Undersecretary, Ministry of Social Affairs, Cario, Egypt; Mr. Jamil Hassany, Chargé d'Affaires, Embassy of Kuwait, Washington, D. C.; Salah Eddin El Homossany, M.D., Director, Department of Social Rehabilitation, Cairo, Egypt; Mr. Adel Iskander, National Association of Hearing and Speech Action, 814 Thayer Avenue #201, Silver Spring, Maryland; Nasser Kotby, M.D., Ph.D., Assistant Professor of Speech Pathology and Otolaryngology, Faculty of Medicine, Ein Shams University, Cairo, Egypt; Diran Mikaelian, M.D., Associate Professor of Otolaryngology, Jefferson University Hospital, Philadelphia, Pennsylvania; Aly El Mufty, M.D., Dean, Medical College, Ein Shams University, Cairo, Egypt; Nabil Sabbagh, M.D., Department of Ear, Nose and Throat, Defense Hospital, Abu Dhabi, United Arab Emirates; Mohamad Saffouri, M.D., Head, Department of Ear, Nose and Throat, Ministry of Public Health, P.O.B. 5, Kuwait; Salah Salman, M.D., Chairman, Department of Otolaryngology, American University Hospital, American University of Beirut, Beirut, Lebanon; and Khaled Tahhan, President, Arab Federation for Organs of Deaf, P.O.B. 4320, Damascus, Syria.

chapter 13

Communication for Hearing-handicapped People in Israel

Judith F. Borus, Ph.D.
and Jerome Reichstein, Ed.D.

The development of both the modern State of Israel and the field of audiology occurred at about the same time–just after World War II. As tens of thousands of North African, Asian, and European Jews poured into the country, a variety of centers and services were opened to deal with their many problems. An unusually high percentage of the immigrants were handicapped in one way or another, including a large number with hearing problems. It was fortunate, in a way, that no audiological center had existed in Israel before this time because, in order to establish new speech and hearing centers, all new equipment had to be obtained–at a time when excellent equipment was finally available. As a result, there are no really antiquated facilities in Israel. Nothing is older than the State–the oldest center, the Speech and Hearing Department at Hadassah Hospital, is less than 25 years old.

Israel is a remarkable country in many ways, one of which is that it is a country composed of immigrants. Even today, less than half of the population is native born. The total population of 3,400,000 is composed of 2,900,000 Jews and 500,000 Arabs and other minority groups. The men and women who parented the field of speech pathology and audiology in Israel were all immigrants–mostly from Europe, but also from Iraq, South Africa, the United States–truly from all over the world. The majority, however (or perhaps the most influential of them), came from Europe and brought with them the ideas and ways of their backgrounds. For this reason, speech and hearing services in Israel are patterned after the European model.

M. Seeman (1966, pp. 439–440) describes this model (based on the organization of speech and hearing services in Czechoslovakia): "The title of specialist in phoniatrics can be attained (only) by a doctor. . . . The phoniatrist works either in the phoniatric out-patient department or is head of the phoniatric department with in-patient facilities which is attached to otorhinolaryngological departments. In phoniatric departments, there are also speech therapists. Logopedics are lectured as part of a 4-year course in defectology at pedagogical faculties. Graduates have the title graduated pedagogue. . . . According to the instructions of the Ministry of Health, the phoniatrist is responsible for treatment of disease of speech, voice and defects of hearing on a regional level and logopedists are subordinated to him and report to him on their activities."

The men who run the clinics, university departments, and research facilities in Israel were, and are, physicians almost without exception, and speech and hearing clinicians perform their duties directly under their supervision and control.

Another aspect of Israeli society which needs consideration at the outset of this discussion is the national health insurance system. Most speech and hearing services are paid for and increasingly directly provided by Kupat Holim, the largest of the national health insurance plans. Kupat Holim is the sick fund of the large nongovernment national labor organization called the Histadrut. The Histadrut is an institution that conducts a variety of activities in addition to its primary purpose, that of trade unions. (Listed among the Histadrut's trade unions are those for physicians, speech and hearing clinicians, teachers, clerical workers, and lifeguards, among many, many others.) Members of the Histadrut who choose to do so pay a relatively low monthly fee for membership in Kupat Holim. As of 1970, approximately 70% of the population of Israel, more than two million people, belonged to the Histadrut's Kupat Holim and 2,600 of the country's 5,500 physicians were employed full-time by it. The remaining 30% belonged to other much smaller sick funds or did not belong to a sick fund at all.

More than half of the Histadrut's funds are allocated to the Kupat Holim division. Kupat Holim provides comprehensive medical care, including treatment by a physician or other; medical specialist (nurse, physical therapist, etc.) either at a clinic, hospital, or at home; hospitalization benefits; medical appliances, including hearing aids; any drugs the physician might prescribe; regular doctor's visits (at his office, at the patient's home, or in the hospital); and rehabilitation therapy, including regularly scheduled speech or language therapy and aural habilitation or rehabilitation.

Patients who are members of Kupat Holim may receive speech and hearing services from a Kupat Holim out-patient clinic or from a center in one of the Kupat Holim hospitals, or they may choose to go to a non-Kupat Holim hospital or clinic. In the latter case, Kupat Holim will reimburse them either wholly or in part for the services provided. In either case the patient pays only a minimum charge.

HISTORICAL OVERVIEW

Before the formation of the State of Israel in 1948, there were only limited speech and hearing services available in the country. Several pioneer otolaryngologists in Israel, including Dr. F. Gumpertz, Dr. A. Zaliuk, and Dr. M. Salzberger, were among the first to introduce treatment of speech and hearing problems into the country.

Among the earliest institutions which provided services were schools for the deaf, the first of which was opened in 1932 in Jerusalem. This was followed by a second school in Tel Aviv in 1941, and a third institution, opened in 1951 in Haifa. Today there are two other schools for the deaf in Beersheva and Nazareth. In addition to these five Jewish schools, there are two Arab schools for the deaf.

The first modern, well equipped and professionally staffed center for speech and hearing services in Israel dates from 1950, when an audiology center at Hadassah Hospital in Jerusalem was opened. (Ten years ago Hadassah moved into its new quarters.)

Hadassah Hospital's Audiology Clinic was followed 1 year later in 1951 by the opening of the Rosen-Bergman Diagnostic and Rehabilitation Center for Speech and Hearing Disorders in the ENT Department of the Chaim Sheba Government Hospital in Tel Hashomer (near Tel Aviv). The clinic was named after two Americans, Dr. Samuel Rosen and Professor Moe Bergman, both of whom planned and helped to set up the clinic. Professor Bergman, who recently retired from teaching at Hunter College and resettled in Israel, conducted Israel's first course in Audiology in 1953 under the sponsorship of the Ministry of Health. This intensive 8-week course was for ear, nose, and throat physicians and for audiometricians. It was the first course of its kind in Israel. Again, in 1954, Dr. Bergman was in the country as an audiological consultant with the U. S. Point Four program. Starting in those years and continuing until the present, he has played a very crucial role in planning and designing most of Israel's largest hospital-based speech and hearing centers.

The demand for hospital-based services such as at Hadassah and Chaim Sheba was the result of the introduction of middle ear surgery and the need for pre- and postoperative audiological assessments. Technicians were trained to perform this function. Speech therapy on any significant scale followed much later.

In the late 1950's, the first of Israel's five MICHA preschool centers was founded in Tel Aviv. These centers serve the needs of severely hard-of-hearing children between the ages of earliest infancy to 6 or 7 years.

In 1965, a medical school was opened at Tel Aviv University with some of the courses and most of the professional training being given at Chaim Sheba Government Hospital. In 1967, as part of the Medical School, a School of Communication Disorders was opened, also based at Tel Hashomer. From its inception, the school has been under the able direction of Dr. Moshe Rubenstein, M.D., an ear, nose, and throat physician.

Within the past few years, speech and hearing services have been introduced into the school systems, but very slowly. At the present time, there is a fairly well developed, but small, program in the Tel Aviv municipality Department of Education under the direction of the co-author, Dr. J. Reichstein. There is another municipal school program in Ramat Gan (a suburb of Tel Aviv), and a third newer program has recently begun with a survey of speech and hearing problems in the Lod-Ramle area. New school system therapy services are being added slowly.

Today in Israel there are over 60 programs in a variety of settings which provide services for the speech and hearing handicapped. They are staffed by more than 200 qualified speech and hearing clinicians. With a very few exceptions, the centers are well equipped and up to date in every respect (Figure 1). In addition to providing direct patient services, many of the centers carry on a full range of related activities, including the initiation of experimental programs, research, and teaching.

DIAGNOSTIC PROCEDURES

The early detection of deafness in Israel is enhanced by the fact that most infants are followed from birth until the age of 1 or 2 years (some up to 5 years of age) in Ministry of Health or Kupat Holim Well Baby Clinics all over the country. A hearing screening is performed on all infants at the age of 7 months, using devices such as the Apritone or Babytone instruments. In most of the baby screening programs, the Ewing Stimuli are used. The Babytone, used in the Tel Aviv area clinics, is manufactured and distributed in Israel by Bepex, Ltd. It produces a narrow band warble tone centering at about 3,150 Hz at intensities of 70, 80, 90 and 100 dB when held 12 cm from the infant's ear. Instructions given to the nurses are: "The test must be done in very quiet surroundings. The baby sits comfortably on his mother with his legs straddling his mother's lap. He faces away from his mother, looking at an assistant sitting opposite him. The tester approaches from behind, without shoes, bringing the Babytone to about

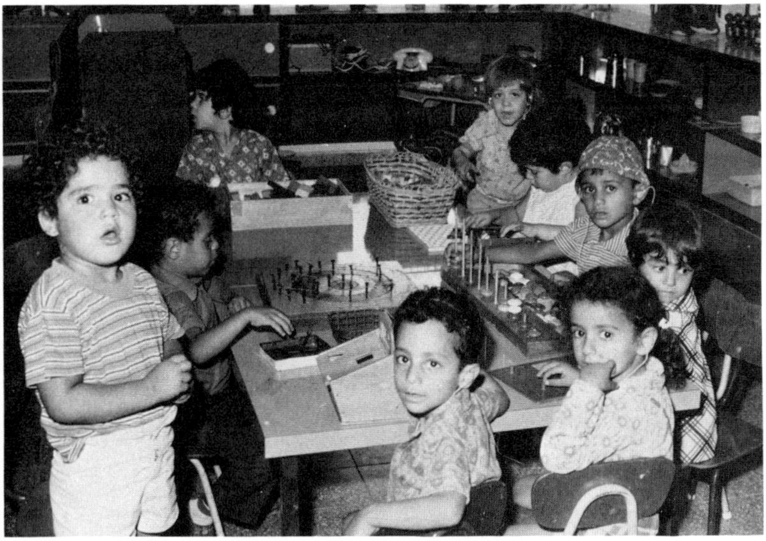

Figure 1. An example of a present-day speech and hearing center in Israel.

ear level, 30 cm away, about 45 degrees in back. Facing the Babytone directly at the ear, present a 2-second burst of tone, pressing the 70 dB switch (which means 60 dB SPL at the baby's ear according to the 30-cm calibration). At 7 months of age, the normal response is a clear turn of the baby's head in the direction from which the tone is given. If there is no response present another 2-second spurt about a minute later. Then move to the other ear. If the baby responds when the 70 dB SPL tones were presented to both sides, he is considered to have passed the test."

Babies who do not pass the hearing screening at the Well Baby Clinics are retested a few weeks later. Those who do not pass the second screening are then referred to audiological centers or to ear, nose, and throat physicians. Eventually, the vast majority of young children requiring further care is then referred by the physicians or by the diagnostic audiologist to the local MICHA center, while some go to various speech and hearing centers for their therapy and follow-up.

In many, perhaps most, school districts, all school-age children have their hearing checked by pure tone screening methods once or twice during their school careers. Those children who do not pass the screening procedures are referred to the appropriate agencies for further diagnosis and treatment.

In these agencies, the type of audiological testing done depends in large part on the equipment and expertise available and the training and background of the audiologist. In some clinics where there is a minimum of sophisticated equipment, the work that can be done with young children, hearing aids, etc., is obviously severely limited, even though there may be well trained professionals available. A few examples of well equipped audiology departments are Beilinson and Ichilov Hospitals and the Communication Disorders Department of the Child Development Clinic, all in the Tel Aviv area. In the person of Esther Kamen-Eshkol, Ichilov Hospital (a joint Ministry of Health and Tel Aviv municipality institution) has an exceptionally well-qualified audiologist who functions only in audiology (and not in speech pathology also). As a result of a viable and professional working relationship between the ENT department and the audiology department, and good equipment well maintained by first rate personnel, some excellent diagnostic work is being performed at Ichilov. In Jerusalem, the Speech and Hearing Center at Hadassah Hospital is also very well equipped and staffed. Hadassah was the first hospital clinic to offer speech and hearing rehabilitative services in addition to diagnostic evaluations. Hadassah's staff, however, all function both as speech pathologists and audiologists, performing both diagnostic and rehabilitative work in both areas.

Without doubt, the best equipped diagnostic facility in the country is the Diagnostic and Rehabilitation Center at Tel Hashomer. In addition to several two-room testing suites (all of which are equipped with console audiometers with speech channels), the center is also provided with Bekesy equipment, impedance testing units, cortical evoked audiometry, and nystagmography. The center is largely staffed by undergraduate and graduate students in the degree programs of the School of Communication Disorders of Tel Aviv University. These students work only under the indirect supervision of the faculty of the School of Communication.

REHABILITATIVE PROCEDURES AND FACILITIES

For many hearing-impaired persons, the first step in the rehabilitative process is obtaining a hearing aid. Hearing aid evaluations are performed at most hospital-based speech and hearing centers as well as at some centers not located within hospitals. Audiologists, on the prescription of a physician, fit hearing aids in these centers, and patients usually return to them to have the aids periodically re-evaluated. The patient leaves the center with a prescription to purchase a specific hearing aid. The prescription is generally taken to the office of the Sick Fund to which the patient belongs, and, eventually, the patient receives the aid. Alternatively, infants, children, and adults who need hearing aids may be referred directly to hearing aid dealers by their physicians or they may go directly themselves to the dealers.

Hearing aid dealers are found in all of the major cities. About 60% of the hearing aids sold by Medtechnica, the largest dealer in Israel, are European makes. The remaining 40% are American brands. The following brands of hearing aids are presently available in Israel: Auditone, Beltone, Bommer, Danavox, Maico, Microson, Omnitone, Oticon, Philips, Radio Ear, Siemens, Sonotone, Telex, Vicon, Viennatone, Widex, and Zenith. The cost of a typical hearing aid is from $80–$175, less than half of what it would cost in the United States, but this sum represents, on the average, about 750 Israeli Pounds, a half month's salary for many Israeli families. Because of the participation of the governmental Ministries of Health and Welfare when necessary, Kupat Holim, and other special funds, most families in Israel receive substantial assistance in the purchase of hearing aids.

In the case of infants and young children, the step which often follows obtaining a hearing aid, and sometimes even precedes it, is referral to a MICHA center. The name MICHA is derived from the Hebrew words meaning "educators of deaf children." It is an extraordinarily well organized and well run society whose purpose is the identification and education of young hearing-impaired children. MICHA deals with children from early infancy to about age 7 years (Figure 1). The first MICHA chapter, in Tel Aviv, was founded in 1953 by a small group of parents and volunteers under the leadership of Dr. Ezra Korine, M.D., an ear, nose, and throat physician who is one of the pioneers of preschool training of deaf children in Israel. MICHA borrowed heavily from the John Tracy Clinic in assisting children with their educational needs. (Finally, 20 years later, the translation of the John Tracy Clinic Correspondence Course into Hebrew has been completed and will shortly be available for general use in Israel.)

Today there are five MICHA centers in Israel, the largest and newest being in Ramat Aviv (a suburb of Tel Aviv) under the direction of Mrs. Ethel Cohen (Figure 2). The Ramat Aviv center provides educational and therapeutic services for 148 children. Forty of them are enrolled in five integrated kindergartens, three in the Tel Aviv public school system (as well as receiving certain MICHA services directly), and one each in Ramat Gan and Herzlia. Two are very young infants who are provided with home training programs. Ten come from Arabic-speaking homes and receive their instruction from MICHA in Arabic.

MICHA provides more than speech and hearing habilitative and rehabilitative services to its children. There is a preschool nursery program on the premises. Psychological services include individual testing and evaluation,

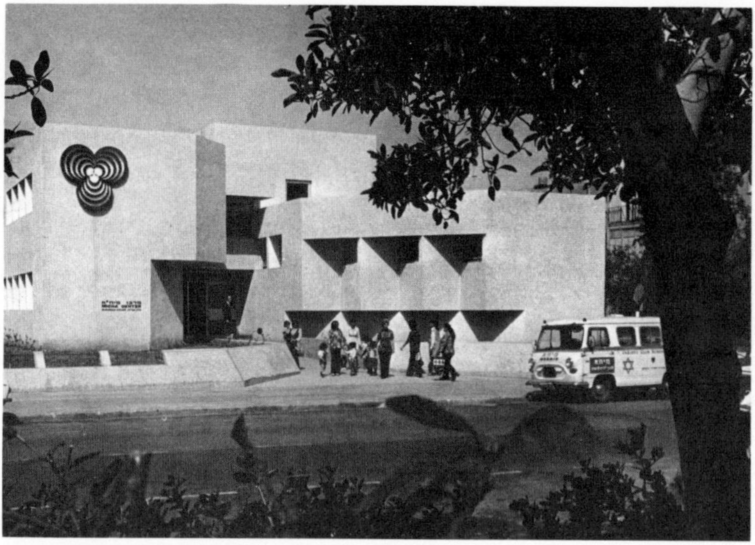

Figure 2. MICHA. Ramat Aviv's modern facility.

weekly parent discussion sessions of small groups of no more than 10 parents, and individual parent guidance and counseling sessions. In addition, MICHA provides an orientation program for public nursery school teachers who have deaf children in their classes who are involved in the MICHA programs. Arrangements have been made for these teachers to spend two afternoons a week at the MICHA center learning how to deal with the problems of the deaf child and his family. As a result of this program, nursery school teachers throughout the Tel Aviv area are slowly becoming more knowledgeable and competent in accepting and working with deaf children in their regular nursery classrooms. Also, a variety of students participate regularly in MICHA's programs, including students from Tel Aviv University's School of Communication Disorders, Bar Ilan University's Department of Special Education, and the Teacher's Seminary of Kibbutzim's senior special education students.

MICHA accepts immediately all referrals made to them. (This is partially because of MICHA's private funding sources which make it possible to avoid becoming entangled in the red tape of most government-sponsored programs and partially because of MICHA's philosophy which is based on the premise of accepting infants and children at the earliest possible age.) There is no minimum age and there are no requirements (such as no additional handicaps) for admission into the MICHA program.

Children are fitted early with binaural hearing aids and provided with intensive auditory training and continued diagnostic evaluations. Extensive parent participation and integration are intrinsic with the program.

MICHA is unique in that it provides total services to its population. Its philosophy is well stated by the Ramat Aviv director, Mrs. Cohen:

> Certainly the factors most responsible for successful oral communication seem to be the ability of the child to utilize his residual hearing with amplification, the ability to develop lipreading skill, his intelligence and motivation. Basically important is the early age at which the child is exposed to amplification and the auditory learning program. Also basically important is the consistent supportive help of parents. To ensure this support from the very start and all during the four to six years that the child is in our program, the parents are expected to attend the introductory course for parents in the evenings during the first two years. This is an 18 to 20 hour course consisting of lectures by staff teachers, psychologists, psychiatrists and guest lecturers such as otologists, audiologists and pediatricians. At many of these meetings "graduate" parents participate in panels. This is of tremendous importance for in addition to getting the scientific cold facts from the specialists, they have the opportunity to hear from other parents how they themselves worked with their childen "that it can succeed". . . . I do believe that if we have faith in the auditory approach, are able to start to work with the child at a very early age, keep the child in a hearing environment all during the pre-school years, give the parents the much needed guidance and training, our total results will be consistently better. . . . I do not believe that the simultaneous method or total communication approach, as it is now known, of teaching the deaf is valid at the pre-school level. . . . If we prejudged the ability of our children to learn to communicate orally on the basis of thei auditory thresholds, we would be denying many, perhaps most, deaf children the chance to learn to communicate orally. The fact is that many of our children with severe hearing losses are communicating orally, with pleasant and understandable speech (Cohen, 1973).

In June 1974, MICHA graduated 18 children from the Ramat Aviv program. Five went into regular public school classrooms, five entered a School for the Deaf and eight entered special unit classes of one type or another. MICHA seems to be remarkably staffed with well-trained, able, and compassionate personnel. Mrs. Cohen speaks of devotion, love, and belief in rehabilitation as the three principles which guide this modern, well established program.

Israel has a well developed system for education of the deaf. It is estimated that there are approximately 750 Jewish deaf children in Israel in the age range of compulsory schooling, 5–15 years. The current incidence of deafness is estimated at 1.2 per thousand, more among the Sephardic population largely because of intermarriage. About half of these youngsters are in schools for the deaf, while the other half are in various types of integrated programs in regular schools. Each of the four major cities (Jerusalem, Tel Aviv, Haifa, and Beersheva) has both a school for the deaf and an integration program. There is a fifth school for the deaf in Nazareth. The schools vary considerably in size. The Beersheva school serves 60 children as compared with the Tel Aviv school which has 120 students. Only the Jerusalem school has residential facilities. Most of the schools have a limited number of children in foster homes. In addition to the five Jewish schools for the deaf, there are two Arab schools, one in Nazareth and one in Bethlehem, and 18 classes scattered in villages all over the country.

The schools have a great range of students. The principal of the school for the deaf in Tel Aviv, Mrs. Chana Goldgart, reported that there are 14 classes from first through eighth grade into which children are placed according to their mental ability and degree of language comprehension. Many of the children have other handicaps in addition to being deaf (Mrs. Goldgart listed cerebral palsy, mental retardation, and brain damage as examples) and the age range in the school is 5½–16 years.

The children study subjects such as Hebrew, Bible, history, geography, nature studies, arithmetic, reading, handicrafts, agriculture, art, and music. Many of the children also receive individual and group speech and language therapy and auditory training. Most of the students attend the schools for 9–10 years and then go on to vocational courses or attend vocational high school. A few continue on to study at various colleges or universities in the country. All of the schools for the deaf give their pupils as much oral language as they can; however, gesture sign language is used in specific classes when necessary. Nearly all the classrooms in the schools for the deaf are equipped with group hearing aids, now being produced locally according to international standards by the Electronic Corporation of Israel.

There is a tendency in Israel, as in other countries, to place deaf children with multiple disabilities in schools for the deaf where a concentration of special services and attention is possible, and to refer deaf children without additional disabilities to integration programs. The first program of integration of the deaf in regular schools in Israel was started in Haifa in the early 1950's by Dr. A. Zaliuk (1954), the developer of the visual-tactile system of phonetical symbolization. Haifa now has five integrated elementary classes and one school where 15 children are scattered in different classes throughout the school. In this latter school, there are a resource room and two teachers to provide individual or small group tutoring. In Tel Aviv, there are nine integrated classes. Jerusalem and Beersheva have only individual integration with much supervision and a great deal of individual and group assistance for the children. For example, in Jerusalem, many of the integrated children come together for supplementary group lessons in the afternoons.

Hearing-impaired children (both deaf and hard of hearing) who attend school anywhere in the country are entitled to 3 hours of special tutoring from the Ministry of Education on a weekly basis if they require it. In some cases, this extra tutoring is provided by special teachers, but, most frequently, it is provided by the regular school teachers.

Many children and adults receive their habilitative and rehabilitative services from a variety of speech and hearing clinics located throughout the country. In late 1974, a questionnaire was prepared by the authors and sent to all the existing centers in Israel (outside of MICHA facilities and the schools and special classes for the deaf) which deal with the problems of the speech and hearing handicapped. Thirty-six clinics filled out and returned the questionnaire. This represents a return rate of over 90%. Of the 36 centers, five stated that they did not accept the hard of hearing or the deaf as clients. These centers are not included in the summaries which follow. The remaining 31 centers all provide rehabilitative services for the hearing impaired.

Twenty of the reporting centers are located within hospitals or clinics (such as the Kupat Holim clinics), five are separately housed speech and hearing clinics (such as the League for the Hard of Hearing Center in Jerusalem), three are programs in public school systems, and three are speech and hearing services offered to children enrolled in special schools (where the service is offered within the school, such as the Ilanot School for Cerebral Palsied Children in Jerusalem). The various centers were founded between 1950 and 1974; about half of them began offering speech and hearing services after 1970. The responding centers geographically represent the entire country, including large hospitals and clinics in Tel Aviv, Haifa, Jerusalem, and Beersheva, as well as smaller centers in these cities and in smaller towns, such as Afula, Holon, and a kibbutz in the Jezreel Valley.

Very few of the clinics differentiated between speech pathologists and audiologists. Even in large well established hospitals such as Hadassah Hospital in Jerusalem, the clinicians perform all of the functions offered by the center: speech evaluations, hearing evaluations, hearing aid evaluations, speech and language therapy, and aural rehabilitation. (In part, this is no doubt because all students in the Department of Communication

Disorders at Tel Aviv University, both undergraduate and graduate, take exactly the same coursework–whether they prefer speech pathology or audiology.)

A total of 22 full-time and 131 part-time clinicians were employed by the reporting institutions. Only 13 centers reported having any full-time clinicians. The majority employed part-time clinicians only. This rather unusual situation is probably partly because some clinicians simply prefer part-time work. In many instances, funding is only sufficient to support part-time positions. Also, graduate students in the School of Communication Disorders at Tel Aviv University are required to work part-time in the field during their 2 years of graduate study. This has probably also helped to foster both the need and acceptance of part-time work and workers.

When asked about the training and background of their clinicians, the centers reported, with only one exception, that all of the clinicians had obtained at least a bachelor's degree (or its equivalent) in the field of speech and hearing. The exception was an individual trained in Russia who, although she has a great deal of practical experience in speech pathology and audiology, did not attend a degree-granting institution. Over 90% of the bachelor's degree level clinicians received their training in Israel at the Tel Aviv University School of Communication Disorders. Less than 20% of the clinicians held master's degrees, and the majority of the master's degree level clinicians received their training in the United States. The School of Communication Disorders awarded its first master's degrees in 1974. As the University of Tel Aviv begins to graduate more of its master's degree level students, there is no doubt that the balance will shift away from United States-trained master's degree level clinicians to Israeli-trained ones.

Because so many of the centers for speech and hearing services are located within hospitals or clinics, other services are usually available to the client and to the clinician on a consultative basis. Services such as medicine, social work, and psychology are most often mentioned, although some centers also list occupational therapy, physiotherapy, and educational services as also being available within the institution. Twenty-nine of the responding centers listed one or more of these services as offered to their clients for diagnostic and therapeutic purposes.

Five of the reporting centers regularly have university students participating in their programs either as observers or as student clinicians. A total of 72 students were thus involved. (This does not include the Diagnostic and Rehabilitation Center program at Tel Hashomer, where the majority of the University of Tel Aviv students in the School of Communication Disorders regularly participate in the clinical program.) Several of the centers also reported having medical, social work, and teacher seminary students as regular participants in their programs.

Caseloads at the various reporting centers vary from 12–450 clients per week, the average being 100. A full 40% of the caseload was reported to be either diagnostic or rehabilitative work with the deaf or hard of hearing. Only one center stated that it works with the deaf and hard of hearing only. One center reported that it works with adults only, and 17 only provide services to children. Many, however, provide services to both children and to adults with any type of speech and/or hearing problem.

When specifically asked about the type of services provided, 14 centers responded that they provide the full range of services: speech and language evaluations, hearing evaluations, hearing aid evaluations, speech and language therapy with the normal hearing population, and speech and language therapy (including lipreading, auditory training, etc.) with the hearing handicapped. Seventeen centers were equipped to perform hearing aid evaluations, and 22 were equipped to carry out hearing evaluations. Cases seen for therapy were usually seen twice weekly (the range was 1–6 times a week). The vast majority (82%) were seen in individual therapy.

The amount of time taken both for therapy and for diagnostic work-ups was also investigated. Speech evaluations take from 30–60 minutes, with a mean of 55 minutes and a median of 60 minutes and hearing evaluations from 15–90 minutes, with a mean of 42 minutes and a median of 45 minutes. Hearing aid evaluations lasted from 30–120 minutes, with a mean of 80 minutes, and a median of 60 minutes and therapy from 20–60 minutes, with a mean of 32 minutes and a median of 30 minutes. The centers, then, reported that 80% of their cases are seen in individual therapy for 30 minutes twice weekly.

With regard to equipment, 14 centers reported having 23 portable audiometers, and 20 centers reported having 44 console audiometers with speech channels. It was surprising to find that there were eight centers equipped to do impedance measurements and three centers outfitted for cortical evoked response audiometry. There are 10 Bekesy units in nine locations, and five centers are equipped with a peep show or similar pediatric equipment. No operant conditioning units were reported. Various centers also mentioned neonatal testing units and auditory trainers among their equipment. These data do not appear to be unusual with regard to practices in the United States, but it should be noted that two centers that reported regular hearing aid evaluations as part of their routine activities do not have sound-treated rooms of any type. Nor does either one own an audiometer with a speech channel. One cannot help but wonder how these hearing aid evaluations are carried out. The fact, however, that these centers, under these conditions, feel compelled to provide this service, points out the extreme needs of the population and the lack of other available centers where these services may be obtained. This is certainly the case in certain parts of Israel, particularly in districts far from big city metropolitan areas.

The largest speech and hearing facility in the country, serving approximately 450 clients weekly, is the Diagnostic and Rehabilitation Center at Tel Hashomer, until recently under the direction of Dr. Ezra Korine. There are three full-time and 20 part-time clinicians employed by the clinic, all of them trained in Israel. There are also two physicians, a psychologist, a paraprofessional who performs certain administrative and audiometric duties, and an electrician on the staff. In addition, 60 students obtain supervised clinical practicum hours at this facility at any given time. The average weekly caseload consists of 150 speech and language cases (which would include all therapy cases, both with the normal hearing and the hearing impaired) and 300 audiology cases (hearing evaluations and hearing aid evaluations). The caseload is comprised of both children and adults, and virtually every type of speech, language, and hearing disorder is represented.

The average length of diagnostic and therapy sessions was given as: hearing evaluations, 1 hour; hearing aid evaluations, 2 hours; therapy, 1 hour; and speech and language evaluation, 30 minutes. The unusual length of therapy time (1 hour twice weekly) is because this is largely a university training institution. As such, students observe and participate in many of the therapy sessions, and a portion of each session is reserved for discussion of the case by the clinician and participating students. Most therapy cases are seen twice a week; 30% of them in individual therapy and 70% in group therapy. This is the only center in the country that reported seeing a majority of its therapy cases in a group setting. This was certainly not the case 5 years ago and is very likely because of the influence of American visiting faculty and staff over the past few years.

There is a steady growth in the amount and scope of speech and hearing services being offered within the network of Kupat Holim hospitals and out-patient clinics. Outstanding examples of the latter include the Zamenhoff Clinic in Tel Aviv and the Linn Clinic in Haifa. One of the newest additions is the Kupat Holim clinic in the Bet Levinstein Rehabilitation Hospital in Ranana whose extensive research, diagnostic, and therapeutic programs are under the direction of Mr. Yitzchak Schechter.

Rehabilitative processes and facilities in the country, then, are remarkably well organized and varied. The fees charged for these services are modest. Kupat Holim patients who go to a Kupat Holim Clinic for therapy pay only 3.60 Israeli pounds (about 60 cents) for treatment of nonorganic disorders and nothing at all where organic disorders are involved. Patients at the Rosen-Bergman center pay 18 Israeli pounds (about three dollars) for one session of therapy, but a good portion of this fee is usually covered by Kupat Holim and other agencies.

PROFESSIONAL AND LAY ORGANIZATIONS AND ASSOCIATIONS

There are many voluntary and public organizations in Israel that provide services to the hearing handicapped in a variety of ways. Among these are SHEMA, a Parents' Association of deaf and hard-of-hearing children; HOD, a club for hearing-impaired youth and young adults and for oral deaf and hard-of-hearing youth; the Association of the Deaf and Mute in Israel, an organization of the adult deaf; JDC-Malben, an organization which helps with the establishment of new services for handicapped children; ORT, an international organization of women dedicated to the vocational training of youth; and the Israeli Speech and Hearing Association, an organization of professionals in the field of speech pathology and audiology.

SHEMA was founded in 1967 by parents of deaf and hard-of-hearing children for the general purpose of assisting in and advancing both the education and general welfare of Israel's hearing-impaired children. The organization has six basic goals: (1) "lobbying" and pressing educational authorities for improvements in the educational system for school-aged deaf and hard-of-hearing children; (2) assisting the school programs for the deaf and hard of hearing (including both schools for the deaf and regular school classrooms into which hearing-impaired children have been integrated) with equipment and special services; (3) education of the public on the needs and problems of the hearing impaired; (4) setting up pilot programs and services; (5) helping children and parents with specific problems; and (6) fund raising.

The national chairman of SHEMA is Dr. Yehoshua Mazur. He and his organization have created an instructional media and educational resource center and hired a specialist who prepares transparencies and instructs teachers in the use of the audiovisual equipment available to them. The center has donated dozens of overhead projectors to schools and classes for the deaf and prepared thousands of transparencies to be used with them. SHEMA has a special fund for providing group hearing aids at reduced cost to schools and classes throughout Israel. They have provided a variety of special services (the cost of most of which is eventually assumed by the appropriate agencies and authorities), such as a social worker for the Tel Aviv school therapy program, speech and language therapy for every class of deaf children in the country, psychological services for the deaf children enrolled in schools in the Tel Aviv area, and teacher aides in various classes. SHEMA also has a hearing aid purchase fund. *KOL* is a magazine for parents of hearing-impaired children published by SHEMA. In summary, SHEMA often is able to step in quickly and provide special funds for equipment or services on a temporary basis until local agencies are prepared to take over. They specifically attempt to fund new services and then press the local authorities to take them over. SHEMA's plans for the future are to continue to help the school system and seek the improvement and expansion of educational and rehabilitation services and facilities for hearing-impaired children and youth.

In 1970, with the financial and organizational assistance of SHEMA, a new organization, HOD, was established whose goal was to provide social and cultural activities for hearing-impaired oral deaf and hard-of-hearing youth in the 18–25 years age bracket. The oral hearing-impaired youth is often neither assimilated by the normal hearing population, that lacks the patience needed for satisfactory communication, nor by the manual deaf who, of course, use sign language as their primary means of communication. HOD's purpose was, and is, to provide a pleasant atmosphere and draw these youngsters out of their social and cultural isolation. At the present time, there are three HOD groups. Two are in Tel Aviv–one for youngsters aged 14–17 years and one for the age group of 18–25. The third group is based in Jerusalem for young adults aged 18–25. In all, HOD has about 100 members. The groups meet weekly in local community centers and enjoy programs which include talks on areas of mutual interest, group discussions, movies, dances and ballroom dancing lessons, sports events, parties, excursions, etc.

While HOD was originally funded by SHEMA, today it is partially supported by JDC-Malben and by the Ministry of Welfare (which provides the group with speech and language services, a social worker, and a psychologist). HOD's plans for the future include expansion into other Israeli cities (such as Haifa and Beersheva) and continued work on two specific projects: convincing the Broadcasting Authority to include printed subtitles in Hebrew at the bottom of the television screen for news and certain other shows and the integration of the hearing impaired into the armed services (up until now they have not been accepted for army service in any capacity).

The Association of the Deaf and Mute in Israel, the oldest voluntary organization in the field, is the major organization for deaf adults. It is estimated that about 85% of the deaf population above the age of 20 belongs to the Association. There are nine branches, with the largest club and national headquarters in Tel Aviv. The Association has two main functions: to provide a social, recreational, and cultural program for its members and to provide a variety of professional services, such as social work services, a translation bureau, and counseling.

The Association has especially dedicated itself to improving and expanding vocational training and the occupational horizons of the deaf in Israel. Over the years, it has been instrumental in obtaining various special considerations for its members, such as the reduction of taxes and certain other fees. It played the crucial role in the creation of a vocational high school for the deaf. As for the future, like their counterparts in other countries, members are working on improving the Israeli sign language—including introducing a sign alphabet—and pressing for its use in education. They are also working on obtaining special programs for the deaf and improving the treatment and rehabilitation of the deaf-blind.

Joint Distribution Committee (JDC)–Malben is an international organization which, in Israel, works with the aged and with handicapped children. In the area of handicapped children, it does not provide direct services but rather cooperates with local authorities in establishing new services and programs. On this basis, JDC-Malben participation in service, guidance, and funding of these new programs is gradually reduced until the local institution takes over completely. The list of programs in the field of speech and hearing that JDC-Malben has helped to start includes the Tel Aviv University School of Communication Disorders, MICHA centers, SHEMA, and the Tel Aviv school therapy program.

Organization for Rehabilitation through Training (ORT) is deeply involved in many countries in the vocational training of youth. In Israel, in addition to their programs for the normal hearing, ORT runs a vocational training school for high school-aged deaf persons.

The history of the professional organization of workers in the field of speech and hearing in Israel reflects, in a very interesting manner, the growth and development of the field in general. The Israeli Speech and Hearing Association was established in 1958 by a group of speech pathologists, audiologists, and teachers of the deaf. The major purposes of the organization were to improve the knowledge and competencies and professional status of its members and to press for improvement and expansion of speech and hearing services and programs.

During the Association's early years, anyone who worked with the speech and hearing disabled could be a member. In 1964, the membership was split into two sectors, the clinicians and the teachers of the deaf. The clinicians' sector had about 50 members, about half of them well trained new immigrants from countries such as the United States, England, and

South Africa and about half who today would be considered to be paraprofessionals. The teachers' sector had about 100 members, a few of whom had been trained abroad. The majority received their training in Israel in in-service programs.

In 1968, the clinicians' sector took an important step forward when it established membership requirements which required 3 years of formal study in the field of speech and hearing for membership. In 1970, the membership requirements were strengthened to require an academic degree and, in 1971, both the degree and specific minimum coursework (based on the Tel Aviv University curriculum) were required for full membership in the Association.

In 1974, the clinicians' sector of the organization was unionized into the academic and professional sector of the Histadrut (see Introduction). This occurred in spite of the fact that the Ministry of Health had recently completed a study demonstrating that, in most countries of the world, speech and hearing clinicians are not considered to be academicians or professionals and advising against their categorization as such in Israel. The two important elements in Israel that were able to overcome this recommendation and achieve this desirable academic and professional categorization of communication clinicians (as in the United States, Canada, and South Africa) were the School of Communication Disorders of the University of Tel Aviv and the Israeli Speech and Hearing Association.

As this chapter is being prepared, the two sectors of the Israeli Speech and Hearing Association are split into two separate organizations, one for the clinicians and an entirely separate organization for the teachers of the deaf. The decision to do this was based on the fact that, whereas all speech and hearing clinicians today are academically trained, most teachers of the deaf still receive their training in nonacademic teachers' seminaries (see section below on Training of Professionals).

The new Association of Communication Clinicians has 230 members. New members of this association will have to meet both the degree and course requirements for full membership in addition to 1 year's successful supervised employment. (An American bachelor's degree qualifies for associate membership only. An American master's degree would qualify for full membership.) The Association is sensitive to the fact that Israel is still a country of immigration. Clinicians from other countries with at least 2 years of university level coursework, who are qualified to work in their country of origin, are given associate membership in the Association and 3 years in which to begin study toward a degree and completion of coursework that they are missing. In the interim, they are permitted to work under supervision.

INTERPROFESSIONAL RELATIONSHIPS

The relationships between physicians and communication clinicians are still in the developing stage (which should eventually approach equal and appropriate partnership in the management and rehabilitation of their patients). The Association of Communication Clinicians and some leading otolaryngologists are involved in efforts to change government regulations that require the directors of audiology centers to be physicians. The phrasing being sought is that the director be a worker appropriately trained and experienced in speech and hearing, whether it be a physician or an individual trained in the field of speech pathology and audiology.

Active cooperation between speech and hearing clinicians and other nonmedical professionals can readily be found. Centers located within hospitals and clinics make frequent interaction with other personnel such as psychologists, social workers, and physical therapists simpler. This type of interaction with other professionals is certainly enhanced by the fact that the overwhelming majority of speech and hearing centers in Israel is located within larger clinics or hospitals where many services other than speech and hearing are also provided. An unusual example of full, easy cooperation among professionals for the purpose of differential diagnosis and treatment of handicapped children is the Children's Diagnostic Clinic in Beersheva, under the direction of Dr. I. Ashkenazi, M.D. The clinic employs (in addition to Dr. Ashkenazi, who is a psychiatrist) a speech pathologist, special educator, teacher, nurse, social worker, psychologist, and pediatrician. These professionals have arrived at a successful working relationship with each other that appears to be unique in the country.

Clinicians who work in centers located within school systems or special schools have easy access to educators, special educators, school nurses, and psychologists. However, the recent split in the Israeli Speech and Hearing Association into an organization for clinicians only (moving the deaf educators out into an organization of their own) makes one wonder about the degree of cooperation that will exist between these two groups in the future.

TRAINING OF PROFESSIONALS

Until 1970, there were no Israeli-trained speech pathologists or audiologists. Services had been provided by immigrants who had received their training in South Africa, Great Britain, the United States or elsewhere, or by physicians who had decided to specialize in this area, or by technicians trained by otolaryngologists to fill the ever increasing need for these services. Courses in speech pathology and audiology were first offered in

1967 at Tel Aviv University through the faculty of Medicine in the School of Communication Disorders. The School was established by Professor M. Rubenstein and graduated its first class in 1970. Tel Aviv University is still the only university in Israel which offers a degree program in the field of communication disorders. The Government Ministry of Health and JDC-Malben played important roles in funding the establishment and early years of the school.

At the present time, there is a 3-year undergraduate program leading to a bachelor's degree and a 2-year master's degree program (plus thesis). Plans are underway to develop a doctoral degree program as well. The first 30 Israeli speech pathologists and/or audiologists were graduated with bachelor's degrees in 1970 and the first master's degrees were awarded 4 years later. The program accepts about 30 undergraduate and 15 graduate students each year, every year from a larger and larger number of applicants. The first non-Israeli students were admitted into the program in 1972.

The curriculum in Communication Disorders is divided into a 3-year series of required undergraduate courses and a 2-year series of required graduate courses. The first year undergraduate program consists of 10 full-year courses and three half-year courses (all courses meet for 2 hours a week with the exception of phonetics which meets for 3 hours a week). The first year of the undergraduate curriculum is composed of the following full-year courses: Anatomy, Pathology of the Speech and Hearing Mechanism, Basic Statistics, Normal Speech and Voice Development, Linguistics and Semantics, General Phonetics, Basic Audiometry, Developmental Psychology, Introduction to Research (English Language), and Articulation Disorders. The half-year courses are: General Physiology, Physics, and Physics Laboratory. The second year of the undergraduate curriculum is composed of eight full-year courses and six half-year courses, all of which meet for 2 hours a week. The full-year courses are: Ear, Nose, and Throat, Psychology of Adjustment and Psychopathology, Voice Disorders, Aphasia, Advanced Audiometry, Auditory Disorders of Children, Introduction to Research (English language), and Stuttering. The half-year courses are: Neurology, Pediatrics, Auditory Training and Lip Reading, Psychodiagnosis and Psychological Testing, Physiology of the Ear, Nose, and Throat, and Language Problems in Children. Third year undergraduates take four full-year courses and two half-year courses, all of which meet for 2 hours a week. The full-year courses are: Introduction to Instrumentation, Consulting and Therapeutic Approach, Seminar in Audiology, and Seminar in Speech and Language. The half-year courses are: Teaching Speech and Hearing to the Acoustically Handicapped and Hearing Aids. Third year seminar students are all required to write papers in both seminar classes. These are often of the research variety, particularly those in the Audiology Seminar. In addition, third year students attend six lectures in Stomatology and five lectures in Cerebral Palsy.

First year master's degree candidates take five full-year courses and three half-year ones, all of which meet for 2 hours a week. The full-year courses are: Neuroanatomy and Physiology of the Auditory System, Integrative Analysis of Clinical Cases, Phonetics and Phonology, Introduction to Linguistics, and Psychoacoustics. The half-year courses are: Genetics, Statistics, and Instrumentation. Second year graduate students take three full-year courses and one half-year course. The full-year courses are: Linguistics, Integrative Seminar in Psychology, and Psycholinguistics. The half-year course is: Nystagmography.

All students take the same courses regardless of whether they are planning to specialize in speech pathology or audiology. (As mentioned earlier, in many of the speech and hearing clinics in the country, the clinicians will be expected to perform both as audiologists and as speech pathologists.) As can be seen from the list of courses given above, the emphasis is highly medical—as would be expected since the faculty is largely composed of physicians. The School of Communication Disorders has only one full-time faculty member, Professor Moe Bergman. Classes are taught by a large part-time faculty which includes Ph.D.'s or Ed.D.'s in areas such as statistics, physics, linguistics, semantics, psychology, etc.; an American-trained woman, Margot Lapidot, with a master's degree in speech pathology, and several physicians, including Dr. M. Rubenstein, director of the School of Communication Disorders, Dr. E. Korine, director of speech pathology and audiology at the Tel Hashomer Diagnostic and Rehabilitation Center, and Dr. R. Ezrati who specifically directs speech pathology service at the Center. (In addition, there are now several Israelis with master's degrees from the school—or very close to them—who help to supervise the clinical programs.) Also, there have recently been a number of visiting professors in speech pathology and audiology from the United States, including Professors Jon Eisenson, Maurice Miller, Margaret Byrne, Judith Borus, and Moe Bergman among others.

The School of Communication Disorders is presently primarily housed in the Clore Diagnostic and Rehabilitation Center for Speech and Hearing Disorders at Chaim Sheba Hospital in Tel Hashomer. Many of the classes are taught there, and most of the clinical practicum is obtained in the speech pathology and audiology clinics there. However, since second year undergraduates must spend 200 hours in observation in a speech clinic, and third year undergraduates are required to put in 450 hours of clinical work during their senior year, and since both first and second year master's degree candidates are required to work 3 full days a week in the clinic, additional opportunities for clinical practice have been arranged at a variety of other centers in the Tel Aviv Metropolitan Area.

With regard to teachers of the deaf in Israel, most of them have been trained in special 1 year courses conducted by the Ministry of Education. During the past decade, this training has taken place first in conjunction with MICHA, Tel Aviv and, later, with the Tel Aviv School for the Deaf. Plans are now underway to set up a full-fledged university level Teacher of the Hearing Impaired training program in one of the country's universities. It is felt that the training of teachers in general in Israel will probably become academicized within the next few years.

RESEARCH

Israel has had a reputation of being a country of intellectuals. Even today, there are more physicians in Israel (per thousand population) than in any other country in the world, including the United States. Many of these physicians are heavily engaged in research. In the field of speech pathology and audiology, much of the research is carried on at the major hospitals in the country. At Chaim Sheba Hospital in Tel Hashomer, graduate students of Tel Aviv University's School of Communication Disorders are involved in animal research as well as research using human subjects. Most of the research is carried out as part of the student's degree requirements under the direction of Dr. Rubenstein or another faculty member.

Research from Hadassah Hospital in Jerusalem is usually a joint effort between the Department of Otorhinolaryngology and the Speech and Hearing Clinic. Hadassah is the only speech and hearing center in Israel where speech and hearing clinicians, employed on a regular full-time basis, are encouraged and expected to carry out research. Much credit must go to Mrs. Lilly (Bauberger) Tell, the clinic director, for her wisdom and skill in being able to accomplish this.

Both Hadassah Hospital and Rambam Hospital (belonging to the Government Ministry of Health) personnel have been extensively involved in research and study of the problem of neonatal screening and early detection of deafness. A Rambam team is studying developing more objective means of selecting out infants with possible hearing loss. Following is a partial list of some of the more outstanding recent publications from these and other centers in Israel that relate to the hearing handicapped and have been authored by Israelis.

REFERENCES

Altman, M., R. Shenhav, and M. Zeltzer. 1971. Mass Screening for Deafness in the Newborn Nursery. J. Israel Med. Assoc. 81: 535–536. (Rambam Hospital.)

Altman, M., and R. Shenhav. 1969. Mass Screening of Infants For Early Detection of Deafness. J. Israel Med. Assoc. 76: 238–240. (Rambam Hospital.)

Altman, M., and R. Shenhav. 1971. Methods for Early Detection of Hearing Loss in Infants. J. Laryngol. Otol. 85: 35–42. (Rambam Hospital.)

Altman, M., R. Shenhav, and L. Shaudinischky. 1975. Semi-Objective Method for Auditory Mass Screening of Neonates. Acta Otolaryngol. In press. (Rambam Hospital.)

Bergman, M., and J. Reichstein. 1971. Speech Pathology and Audiology in Israel. ASHA 13: 9–12. (Diagnostic and Rehabilitation Center for Speech and Hearing Disorders, Chaim Sheba Government Hospital.)

Cohen, E. 1973. Auditory Techniques in Israel. Presented at the International Conference on Auditory Techniques. February 1973, Pasadena, California. (MICHA.)

Cohen, T., A. Brand-Auraban, C. Karshai, A. Jacob, I. Gay, J. Tsitsianov, T. Shapiro, S. Jatziv, and A. Ashkenazi. 1973. Familial infantile renal tubular acidosis and congenital nerve deafness: An autosomal recessive syndrome. Clin. Genet. 4: 275–278. (Hadassah Hospital.)

Dar, H., and S. T. Winter. 1969. A genetic study of familial deafness. Israel J. Med. Sci. 5: 1219–1226. (Rothschild Hospital.)

Eliachar, I., M. Altman, W. Meyer, and R. Shenhav. 1971. Secretory otitis media and functional appraisal of the eustachian tube by measurement of acoustic impedance. J. Israel Med. Assoc. 80: 356–359. (Rambam Hospital.)

Feinmesser, M., and L. Tell. 1974. Evaluation of Methods for Detecting Hearing Impairment in Infancy and Early Childhood. Research Report. Hadassah University Hospital. Jerusalem. (Hadassah Hospital.)

Feinmesser, M., L. Tell, and R. Bilski-Hirsch. 1959. A hearing survey in the public schools of Jerusalem. Israel Med. J. 18: 59–63. (Hadassah Hospital.)

Feinmesser, M., L. Tell, A. Lev, and S. David. 1972. Routine use of cochlear audiometry in infants with uncertain diagnosis. Ann. Otol. Rhinol. Laryngol. 81: 72–75. (Hadassah Hospital.)

Feinmesser, M., L. Tell, and F. Marcus. 1963. Causes of deafness in children. J. Med. Assoc. Israel 64: 294–297. (Hadassah Hospital.)

Feinmesser, M., L. Tell, and F. Marcus. 1966. Consanguinity among parents of deaf children in the Jewish population in Israel. J. Laryngol. Otol. 80: 1253–1256. (Hadassah Hospital.)

Fried, K., M. Feinmesser, and J. Tsitsianov. 1969. Hearing impairment in female carriers of the sex-linked syndrome of deafness with albinism. J. Med. Genet. 6: 132–134. (Hadassah Hospital.)

Gumpertz, F., and L. Tell. 1966. Speech pathology in Israel. *In* R. W. Rieber and R. S. Brubaker (eds.), Speech Pathology, pp. 512–526. North Holland Publishing Company, Amsterdam. (Hadassah Hospital.)

Korine, E. 1967. Medical results of 17,000 hearing tests on school children. J. Med. Assoc. Israel 10: 261–263. (Diagnostic and Rehabilitation Center for Speech and Hearing Disorders, Chaim Sheba Government Hospital.)

Korine, E., M. Modan, and J. Fisher. 1969. An evaluation of the use of hearing aids by hard of hearing children. J. Israel Med. Assoc. 77: 471–476. (Diagnostic and Rehabilitation Center for Speech and Hearing Disorders, Chaim Sheba Government Hospital.)

Korine, E., M. Rubenstein, and D. Yance. 1975. Influence of Hypometabolic State Due to Hypothyroidism on the Latency Period in E.R.A. Reponses. Presented at the Third International Symposium on E.R.A., September 10, 1973, Bordeaux, France. In press. (Diagnostic and Rehabilitation Center for Speech and Hearing Disorders, Chaim Sheba Government Hospital.)

Miller, M., E. Kamen, and A. Miller, 1974. Hearing Aids and Audiological Services in Israel. Presented at the National Convention of the American Speech and Hearing Association. November 1974, Las Vegas, Nevada. (Ichilov Hospital.)

Reichstein, J. 1967. Integration of Deaf Children at the Pre-school Level. Proceedings of the International Conference on Oral Education of the Deaf, pp. 2038–2051. Alexander Graham Bell Association for the Deaf, Washington, D. C. (Tel Aviv Municipality Department of Education.)

Reichstein, J., and C. Goldgart. 1970. Education of the Deaf in the Municipality of Tel Aviv. Proceedings of the International Congress on Education of the Deaf, Stockholm. pp. 399–406. Alexander Graham Bell Association for the Deaf, Washington, D. C. (Tel Aviv Municipality Department of Education.)

Sade-Sadowsky, N., and E. Huppert. 1971. Research and Demonstration Pilot Project on Rehabilitation of Deaf Persons in Israel. The Association of the Deaf and Mute in Israel, Tel Aviv.

Shemer, H., M. Feinmesser, L. Bauberger-Tell, A. Lev, and S. David. 1972. Routine use of cochlear audiometry in infants with uncertain diagnosis. Ann. Otol. Rhinol. Laryngol. 81: 72–75. (Hadassah Hospital.)

Winter, S., and J. Dar. 1957. Deafness among children in Northern Israel. Israel J. Med. Sci. 3: 894–898. (Rothschild Hospital.)

Zaliouk, A. 1954. A visual-tactile system of phonetical symbolization. J. Speech Hear. Disord. 19: 190–207.

ACKNOWLEDGMENTS

The authors wish to thank the many Israeli professionals in the speech and hearing field who cooperated in the questionnaire survey and contributed to this chapter.

PERIODICALS ON HEARING PUBLISHED IN ISRAEL

1. Journal of the Medical Association of Israel, Harefuah.
2. Hebrew University of Jerusalem Medical Research Reports.
3. Israel Journal of Medical Sciences.
4. Journal of the Association of Communication Clinicians.

LITERATURE CITED

Bepex, Ltd. 1974. Instruction Manual–Babytone. Tel Aviv, Israel.

Bergman, M., and J. Reichstein. 1971. Speech pathology and audiology in Israel. Asha 13: 9–12.

Cohen, E. 1973. Auditory Techniques in Israel. Presented at the International Conference on Auditory Techniques. February 1973, Pasadena, Calif.

Gumpertz, F., and L. Tell. 1966. Speech Pathology in Israel. *In* R. W. Rieber and R. S. Brubaker (eds.), Speech Pathology, pp. 512–526. North Holland Publishing Company, Amsterdam.

Seeman, M. 1966. Speech Pathology in Czechoslovakia. *In* R. W. Rieber and R. S. Brubaker (eds.), Speech Pathology, pp. 439–457. North Holland Publishing Company, Amsterdam.

chapter 14

Communication for Hearing-handicapped People in India

Y. P. Kapur, M.D.

Before 1960, unified national programs designed to habilitate and rehabilitate the hearing handicapped in India were practically nonexistent. In the early 1960's, with the return of audiologists and speech pathologists trained in the United States and the United Kingdom, great strides were made in coping with the problems of the hearing handicapped and national interest in programs to aid these people was generated.

India, the seventh largest land mass nation in the world, occupies 1,260,000 square miles. In population, it is second with 547,000,000. The population is distributed among 19 states and 10 union territories. Eighty percent of her people live in rural areas. India is classified as a developing nation, having gained her independence from British rule in 1947.

Contributing to the complexities of this country are the facts that there are 300 recognized spoken languages, 15 major scripts, and large groups of people of various racial backgrounds all attempting to live in one nation as an integrated society.

In order to establish a coordinated program which would deal effectively with the needs of such a large, widely dispersed populace, a call was sent out to all states and union territories to bring together people dealing in all phases of habilitative and rehabilitative services to the hearing handicapped. Nationwide workshops were held to bring together these interested individuals, for information exchange, discussion of needs, and to search for possible solutions to the needs identified. These workshops led to a unified national approach to India's program of aid to the hearing handicapped. This national interest focused on establishing research and training programs, development of industries which could manufacture diagnostic equipment and aids, and the development of centers where diagnostic assessment and habilitative, as well as rehabilitative, programs for the hearing handicapped could be administered.

Training programs were established at the B.Y.L. Nair Hospital (Bombay), the All India Institute of Speech and Hearing (Mysore), and the Christian Medical College Hospital (Vellore).

Diagnostic audiometric equipment was designed and manufactured at the Bharat Electronics Firm, Bangalore, and amplification devices were developed and manufactured by the Indian Telephone Industries of Bangalore.

Because there was limited information available concerning the causes of these handicaps, and limited facilities were available for aid to these people, the public was generally unaware of this group's problems. While services for other groups of handicapped individuals (i.e., the orthopedically impaired and the blind) were well supported by both governmental programs and voluntary agencies, it can be liberally estimated that only 1% of the total amount being expended annually in assistance to the handicapped groups was being used to aid the hearing handicapped. The Social and Rehabilitative Services Agency of the U.S. Department of Health, Education, and Welfare, Washington, D.C., the Commonwealth Foundation, London, England, and the Danish Government all contributed grants to support projects and to provide funds for equipment. For the first time, the hearing and speech centers could provide counseling and training, and an interchange of programs and personnel with centers in the United States, the United Kingdom, and Denmark occurred. The resulting progress was remarkable; however, many problems soon became evident. All centers had problems of keeping patients for prolonged periods of evaluation, diagnosis, and treatment. Travel to the centers by large numbers of patients who lived in rural areas was difficult, causing problems with follow-up examinations. It then became clear that, in order to have programs of this type succeed in developing nations, the problems unique to each nation because of its geographical size, population distribution, and the level of education of the populace, as well as social, cultural, and economic considerations, must be carefully weighed and suitable approaches capable of dealing with such problems generated. It was necessary for those involved in conducting India's aid programs to: (1) introduce and establish procedures for evaluating patients in the shortest possible time; (2) develop home training programs in which patients, parents, and relatives would be involved (these home training programs are crucial for effective rehabilitation in rural areas); (3) develop materials which could be used for problem explanations, therapeutic procedures, and evaluating the gains made by treatment and therapy; and (4) evaluate methods proved effective in increasing communication between the center's personnel and the patients.

The problems involved in finding methods which provide effective rehabilitative services to handicapped individuals are not unique to India nor are they solely to the developing nations. A recent Rand Corporation report (Brewer and Kakalik, 1974) points out that, although almost 5 billion dollars a month are spent by federal, state, and local governments for programs to aid the handicapped, these programs lack both coordination and direction. The programs were found to be fragmented, uncoordinated, and lacking in responsiveness to the needs of the individual.

Development of effective programs and methods geared to the individual, workable equipment, and getting meaningful results form the essence of the great challenge for all nations attempting to provide habilitative and rehabilitative services for their peoples.

HISTORICAL OVERVIEW

The first formal school for the deaf was established by missionaries in Bombay in 1885. No records are available which would indicate that schools, as such, existed before that time, although in ancient India the deaf were taken care of by the kings. During the reigns of the Emperors Ashoka and Harsha, the deaf along with other physically handicapped individuals were given alms and protection. When India was ruled by the Muslim emperors, these same systems of assistance were continued. A large portion of the income of the State was set aside to provide for such maintenance of the disabled. Naturally, the idea of care was quite different then, but more important is the fact that these people were not ridiculed or neglected by the rulers. As an example, there is a legend in Sanskrit literature of a great sage and scholar, Ashta Vakra, who suffered from many physical handicaps. Vakra was invited to participate in a large symposium, convened by the king. All of the other invitees were scholars and intellectuals of great repute. The presence of Ashta Vakra, with all of his physical handicaps, invited ridicule even before he had opened his lips. When Ashta Vakra was asked by the king to participate in the debate, he refused, saying, "To whom shall I speak? This audience is not one of scholars and intellectuals, for they have already judged me by my skin. This is a herd of traders of hides and skins, who know nothing of the beauty of the soul and know not how to measure intellect." This rebuke struck home and there were profuse apologies tendered to Ashta Vakra. The ancient writings stated that speech was the essence of man.

The Maratha rulers and the Peshwas sometimes employed deaf people as their spies. Copies of confidential correspondences were made by deaf mutes. This shows that the deaf mutes of the time were useful citizens of society, even though they were not educated in schools. It is possible that, in ancient India, there were some Rishis and Munis (holy men) who may have tried to make the mutes speak. This is reflected in a poem in Sanskrit which states that the deaf could talk with the help and favor of Almighty God. Unfortunately, at this same time, there are also reports in the literature which indicate that stutterers were employed in the courts of kings and feudal lords as court jesters to provide pleasure and amusement at the cost and discomfort of these employees.

Bengal was the second state to take the lead in establishing formal schools for the deaf. A school was opened in Calcutta in 1893. This school, with the cooperation and support of the government, played a major role in the annals of education of the deaf in India. Deaf education subsequently made progress in other parts of India, with the establishment of schools for the deaf in Palayamkottai in 1897, Ahmedabad in 1908, Bansal in 1912, Nagpur in 1915, Dacca in 1916, Chittagong in 1923, Poona in 1924, Hyderabad in 1925, Madurai and Nanguneri in 1930, Delhi, Coimbatore, Murshidabad, and Madras in 1931, Berhampur in 1934, Patna and Indore in 1936, Sholapur, Chotta, Nagpur, and Cochin in 1937, Tiruvella and Karaikudi in 1938, Lucknow, Burdwan, Bogra, and Komla in 1939, Travancore in 1940, Jaipur in 1945, and Varanasi in 1947.

Mention must be made of the role played by the Maharaja Sayajirao Gaekwad of Baroda. It is said that, while on tour of Europe, the Maharaja met an Indian gentleman who was in Europe in search of a teacher of the deaf who would educate his deaf daughter. The Maharaja was moved when he understood the situation facing the deaf in India and, on his return to India, the Maharaja made moves to immediately start educational programs for the deaf in the State of Baroda. It is also reported that he canceled the orders for jewelry which he had desired to purchase for Her Highness, the Maharani of Baroda and, using these funds, made provisions in the budget for the education of the deaf in his state.

OVERVIEW OF RECENT DEVELOPMENTS AND PROGRAMS

There are no reliable estimates of the number of deaf persons in India; however, a conservative estimate would be that there are between 15 and 20 million deaf children and adults. Presently, India has approximately 85 schools which are providing instructional programs for the deaf. This is roughly equivalent to the number of residential American schools alone. While India's schools are capable of educating 6,000–7,000 students, the residential American schools have an enrolled student population totaling 20,000. This clearly indicates the magnitude of the problem encountered by India's hearing-handicapped individuals.

While the educational programs for the deaf are limited as to the number of individuals to whom they can provide services, their history in India, as has been previously mentioned, is very long. The development of rehabilitative services for the speech and hearing handicapped, on the other hand, has a very recent history. This is not to say that only recently has interest been generated toward providing rehabilitative services to India's speech and hearing handicapped. Concern for the rehabilitation of the handicapped in India is clearly outlined in the constitution which states that, within the limits of the economic capacity of the country, provision must be made for the disabled. It must be understood, rather, that because of extreme pressure to develop programs aimed at researching and treating the more acute diseases prevalent in India between 1947 and the early 1960's and because the economic capacity in these years was at its limit, it was not possible to make plans and expend funds for rehabilitative services in speech pathology and audiology.

Until very recently, little research had been carried out which would indicate the major causes of hearing loss in the Indian population. Furthermore, little had been done to document statistically the incidence of the different speech and hearing problems in India, and no listings of facilities capable of offering rehabilitative services to these people existed.

Deafness Research Project, Christian Medical College Hospital, Vellore

In order to meet this need, a Deafness Research Project was started at the Christian Medical College and Hospital, Vellore, South India in 1962 in collaboration with the Johns Hopkins Hospital and with support from the National Institute of Neurological Diseases and Blindness, U.S.A. (Kapur, 1966*a*). The objectives of this project were: (1) to obtain information concerning the causes of deafness in a young population, previously unstudied in India; (2) to develop valid hearing test procedures designed for the succeeding age groups; (3) to use these hearing tests on a preselected population group; (4) to develop a pool of hearing-tested individuals from which normals, for the population being studied, could be established; (5) to determine the extent, types, and degrees of hearing loss present in the population being studied; (6) to identify the diseases causing hearing loss in this group with emphasis on the role the common infectious and tropical diseases and nutritional deficiencies play in the etiology of hearing loss; and (7) to obtain the temporal bones and brains of individuals dying within this group for pathological analysis and correlation with hearing studies.

To determine the prevalence of hearing loss among the school age youth of the region, a hearing survey of the children in three schools in the Vellore area was carried out (Kapur, 1965). The children in this test group were between 5 and 14 years of age and adequately represented the socioeconomic background of the school age population in the region. The results of this study revealed that the prevalence of hearing loss among the 857 children tested was in the range of 16–18%. This is very high when compared to studies which reveal a 3% incidence in Norway, a 5–8% incidence in England, and an approximately 5% incidence in the United States.

If this 16–18% rate prevailed among all school age children in India, it would mean that there were, at the time of the study, over 14,580,000 children between 5 and 14 years with a hearing loss which required treatment, based on the Ministry of Education, Government of India's statistics indicating approximately 89,602,000 school children in the country at the time.

It was found that conductive hearing loss accounted for between 90–97% of the hearing losses detected by the study on the school children. It was known, however, that those children with a sensorineural hearing loss were not admitted to the schools, but rather they had to be kept at home and, as a consequence, did not receive any formal education or treatment.

Although the Deafness Research Project was primarily concerned with investigations and research, patients from all parts of the state began to come to the center for treatment and advice concerning their problems. This is because, at that time, there were no hearing and speech centers or other facilities in South India where people could receive proper assessment of their hearing or speech disorders or guidance regarding their medical, educational, and rehabilitative needs. It appeared that the general medical practitioners were unaware of the need for early diagnosis of these disorders and the great value of initiating rehabilitative programs immediately upon discovering an individual's handicap. Evaluation of hearing loss was not usually obtained at an early age. Ideally the child's handicap should have been recognized, and evaluation sought, when the child was 3–4 years of age. Ultimately, when diagnosis was made, the appropriate medical and surgical services which would alleviate or correct the condition were provided, but the educational and/or vocational needs of the individual were not considered. Consequently, many hard-of-hearing school age children received their education in schools for the deaf and the vocational training needs of adults went largely unattended. The parents of handicapped children and the communities where these children and handicapped adults lived were equally in great need of assistance in planning and establishing programs and services leading to constructive practices in the education and rehabilitation of persons with hearing and speech disorders.

In 1966, an investigation of the facilities available in India for the speech and hearing handicapped revealed that there was a great shortage of personnel, equipment, and number of facilities capable of providing these services (Kapur, 1966*b*). Information was obtained from 54 out of the 84 teaching hospitals affiliated with medical colleges. Twenty-two of these hospitals had undergraduate training in otolaryngology and 32 offered postgraduate training programs in otolaryngology. It was revealed that nine of these teaching hospitals did not have any audiometers. These nine included two institutions with approved postgraduate training programs in otolaryngology. In addition, there were four institutions owning audiometers which were not in operating condition. Thus, there were 13 teaching institutions, fully 24% of those responding, which could not provide diagnostic audiometric assessments. Other statistics revealed that there were 22 other teaching hospitals which had at least one audiometer inoperable, and only 10 teaching hospitals responding had a sound-treated room in which to conduct assessments. Of these 10, only four had measured ambient noise levels in the room. None of those responding had facilities for periodic calibration of the audiometric equipment at their hospitals and, furthermore, none of the centers had recalibrated their audiometers since they had been purchased, which, in some cases, had been 20 years before this study.

The Deafness Research Project conducted another survey among the schools for the deaf which were operating in 1966 (Herrick and Kapur, 1969). Of the approximately 85 schools, 40 responded to the survey and their responses resulted in the following information:

1. In one-third of the schools, the age of admission varied between 3 and 5 years, whereas in the remaining two-thirds, the earliest age of admission varied between 6 and 10 years.
2. Only one-third of the schools sampled required audiological tests before admission; slightly over one-third required otological evaluation before admission.
3. Preschool classes were conducted in only five schools reporting in the survey.
4. Fewer than 10% of the population in the schools for the deaf were fitted with hearing aids.
5. Two-thirds of the responding schools had group auditory training equipment.
6. Sixteen schools had a ratio of one trained teacher to between 20 and 99 students. Trained teachers were available on a 1:9 ratio in 25% of the schools responding to the survey.
7. The manual means of communication was used in the majority of schools.

8. The choice of a language for instruction posed a great problem. While it appeared appropriate to use the regional language for this purpose, often students attending a school came from outside the region the school was expected to serve. Administrators often selected two languages for instruction.
9. Social and vocational training programs were poorly organized in the majority of schools surveyed. Students leaving the schools faced unemployment. One-third of the schools had an employment rate of under 10% of students graduated. There are no trained vocational counselors in any school for the deaf in India.
10. The schools for the deaf have long waiting lists. One school in Madras, India, had a waiting list of 600 children.

These studies emphasized the urgent need for both making available more diagnostic and rehabilitative centers and updating those centers which were then providing services to the speech and hearing handicapped in all parts of the country.

A Hearing and Speech Center was added to the Deafness Research Project in February 1966 with the support of the Social and Rehabilitation Service (then the Vocational Rehabilitation Administration) of the United States Department of Health, Education, and Welfare. The major objectives of the Center were: (1) to develop comprehensive medical, audiological, and counseling services suited to local conditions for patients and parents; (2) to develop hearing and speech testing procedures in the Indian language; (3) to explore the possibilities of manufacturing hearing aids, using the resources of local industries and indigenous materials; (4) to develop procedures for the evaluation and fitting of hearing aids and to provide guidance to parents and patients in the use and care of hearing aids; (5) to establish a program for community education and guidance on hearing and speech problems; and (6) to determine ways to expand opportunities for persons with hearing and speech disorders and to demonstrate to local employers their capacity to perform satisfactorily on the job.

All India Institute of Speech and Hearing, Mysore

While the centers in Vellore were being developed, the National Government of India became increasingly concerned with the plight of the speech and hearing handicapped. In 1963, the Ministry of Health requested the consultative services of an American speech pathologist. This individual would be utilized to assist in formulating plans for establishing facilities for speech pathology and audiological assessment and treatment. The late

Martin F. Palmer was selected to provide this consultation and, on his recommendations, the All India Institute of Speech Pathology and Audiology was established in Mysore in August 1965. This institute was affiliated with the University of Mysore, but, uniquely, was under the administrative control of the Ministry of Health of the National Government of India. The major purpose of the Institute is to provide a training and research facility for speech clinicians and audiologists. The Institute also provides a comprehensive clinical program which offers a full range of diagnostic services, treatment, and counseling facilities for all speech and hearing disorders.

B. Y. L. Nair Hospital, Bombay

The first speech therapy clinic in India was established in the B. Y. L. Nair Hospital in Bombay in January 1963. This institution is a charity hospital, and the clinical facilities were made possible through the generous donations of a philanthropist. In 1966, a 2-year program was established at the B. Y. L. Nair Hospital to provide training for speech clinicians and audiologists.

All India Institute of Medical Sciences, New Delhi

In 1965, a Rehabilitation Unit in Audiology and Speech Pathology was established at the All India Institute of Medical Sciences, New Delhi, with the support of the Social and Rehabilitation Services Division, U.S. Department of Health, Education, and Welfare, Washington, D.C. The three main objectives of this program were: (1) to establish a prototype audiology and speech pathology unit within a research and training institute; (2) to develop hearing and speech services appropriate for use in India; and (3) to study methods for the preparation of audiologists and speech pathologists in India.

Indo-Danish Program

In September 1969, a 5-year Indo-Danish agreement was signed at the Ministry of Health, New Delhi. This agreement called for Denmark to contribute audiological equipment, hearing aids, ear mold laboratories, and supportive personnel to five centers established in India. These centers include: the All India Institute of Medical Sciences, New Delhi; the All India Institute of Speech and Hearing, Mysore; the Hearing and Speech Center, Christian Medical College Hospital, Vellore; the B. Y. L. Nair Hospital, Bombay, and the Benares Hindu University Medical Hospital, Benares, India. The agreement also provided for the training of the Indian personnel from these centers at institutions in Denmark.

Benares Hindu University Hospital, Benares

In 1970, a program in speech and hearing was established at the Benares Hindu University Hospital in Benares, India. This program, like the others previously mentioned, is involved in both training and treatment programs for the speech and hearing handicapped.

All of the centers previously mentioned have a staff which is comprised of otolaryngologists, speech pathologists and therapists, psychologists, audiologists, and social workers. Consultants in all of the specialties are available to these centers and this allows a very broad based diagnostic and rehabilitative program for the hearing handicapped. These programs are available to both children and adults. With the exception of the Institute at Mysore, all of these centers are located within major medical teaching centers. All of the centers also have association with otolaryngology programs, and the program directors at all centers are otolaryngologists. In addition to the clinical and rehabilitative services which these centers offer, all centers are active in research into communicative disorders in India.

PERSONNEL TRAINING PROGRAMS

The status of programs to aid the hearing handicapped was not known in 1966. The number of workers in the field and what was being done were also unknown. Consequently, in April 1966, the First All India Workshop of Speech and Hearing Problems was held to evaluate the work being done (Kapur, 1966*b*). The workshop brought together leading otolaryngologists, psychoacousticians, audiologists, speech pathologists, teachers of the deaf, and manufacturers of hearing aids. Hopefully, by having all groups participate, an exchange of information and discussion of needed solutions to problems could be accomplished.

It was generally agreed at this workshop that some of the major obstacles to effective programs were a lack of trained personnel, a lack of locally manufactured audiometers, and the high cost of hearing aids.

Suggestions made by members of the workshop to deal with the problem of a lack of trained personnel were:

1. That students with an intermediate education in physics and biology should undergo a minimum of 2 years of intensive training in speech and hearing therapy. This training would result in the awarding of a B.Sc. degree for the student.
2. That training for the specialized personnel be in affiliation with a teaching medical institution. Hopefully this affiliation would provide the

student with an adequate variety and volume of cases during the training period.
3. That, because of limited number of teachers available for this training, only one or two centers should be attempted at one time.

To cope with the high cost of hearing aids and the lack of locally available diagnostic equipment, the first workshop organized committees to investigate the feasibility of increasing locally available equipment and to investigate means to reduce the cost of hearing aids.

The second workshop was held in Vellore, in May 1967 (Kapur, 1967). Progress reports were submitted on the recommendations of the 1966 workshop. It was reported that training programs had been started at the B. Y. L. Nair Hospital in Bombay, the All India Institute of Speech and Hearing in Mysore, and at the All India Institute of Medical Sciences in New Delhi. However, it was noted that all programs were different. Mysore offered a M.Sc. program, Bombay a B.Sc. program, and Delhi offered a technician's course. The workshop felt that a uniform sound program at all centers was necessary and agreed to request the cooperation of the three centers in achieving this training uniformity.

The third workshop was held in January 1969 (Kapur, 1969). A review of personnel training was made, and the workshop delegates discussed the progress of the programs in existence. The success of the programs in filling the needs of the country was also discussed. The committee's conclusions were that one soundly organized program should be offered which would maximize employment opportunities for the program graduates. It was agreed again that a 2-year program leading to a diploma in speech and hearing science should be the approach taken. Admission to the program would be open to candidates holding a B.A. or B.Sc. degree from any recognized university. It was felt that this approach would allow for greater flexibility in trainee selection and would also allow students an opportunity for changes in their careers. Also, this formal program for trainees would enable the centers to request financial assistance from the University Grants Commission for nonrecurring expenditures and part of the recurring expenditures created by the administration of the programs. The workshop noted the growing interest of professional otolaryngologists in the training of speech and hearing personnel and recommended that trainees and graduates work under the supervision of professional ear, nose, and throat specialists. A request was made to the Indian Speech and Hearing Association to survey the need for trained personnel by various institutions in the country. It was also requested that a projected need of trained personnel for the next 5 years be made. The workshop also discussed the possibility of a specialty training in medical audiology for otolaryngologists who wished to have such training. Vellore and Varanasi were two suggested sites for this specialty training.

The delegates to the workshops held were of the opinion that the existing programs were inadequate to meet the country's needs. Graduates of B. Y. L. Nair Hospital Training Center in Bombay tended to stay in Bombay, the state of Manarashtra, or in neighboring Gujarat. Graduates of Mysore were local people and considered unsuitable for personnel needs in other areas. Because of linguistic problems, it was felt that local training of personnel was the best approach.

Currently, three institutes have functional programs which offer either a B.Sc. degree, a M.Sc. degree, or both degrees in audiology and speech pathology:

All India Institute of Speech and Hearing, Mysore

The All India Institute of Speech and Hearing was established by the Government of India in the city of Mysore in August of 1965. The training program began in October of 1966. It is directly affiliated with the University of Mysore (Draft Final Report of Project, 1973).

The initial class was 15 students. The training program was 3 years in duration, leading to a master's degree in audiology and speech pathology. A second course, leading to a bachelor's degree in speech and hearing, was added 2 years later. The duration of the bachelor's degree program is 3 years. Fifteen students were originally admitted to the M.Sc. degree program, but, following the introduction of the B.Sc. degree program, the M.Sc. degree program was gradually eliminated. Fifteen students are presently admitted to the bachelor's degree program annually. These students are eligible for the M.Sc. degree after 2 years of postgraduate education and training and after having completed a one-year internship.

B. Y. L. Nair Hospital, Bombay

The school for audiology and speech pathology was established in 1966 at the Nair Hospital. The Nair Hospital is the major teaching hospital of the Topiwala National Medical College, Bombay. The training program is 2 years long and leads to a degree in audiology and speech pathology. Ten students are admitted annually to the program. The program is affiliated with the University of Bombay.

All India Institute of Medical Sciences, New Delhi

A program for the training of audiometry technicians was started in June of 1966 at the Rehabilitation Unit in Audiology and Speech Pathology,

All India Institute of Medical Sciences. The course was originated because of the need for properly trained technicians at medical institutions and other centers throughout the country. The course comprises four semesters in 2 academic years to include theoretical instruction and practical training. The enrollment in the program varies from year to year (Establishment of a Pilot Rehabilitation Unit in Audiology and Speech Pathology in India, 1973).

GENERAL DESCRIPTION OF PRESENT PROGRAMS OF AURAL HABILITATION AND REHABILITATION

The programs at the Christian Medical College and Hospital in Vellore, All India Institute of Speech and Hearing in Mysore, B. Y. L. Nair Hospital in Bombay, and All India Institute of Medical Sciences in New Delhi offer habilitation and rehabilitation for the hearing-handicapped children and adults. All the programs, with the exception of the Institute at Mysore, are located within major medical teaching centers. All the centers also have association with otolaryngology programs, and the program directors are all otolaryngologists.

The history, objectives, and types of support for these centers are given in the sections on historical overview and description of training programs.

A new speech and hearing program was opened at the Benares Hindu University Hospital, Benares, India in 1970. The University is supported by the Central Government. The staff of these centers is comprised of otolaryngologists, speech pathologists and therapists, psychologists, and social workers. Consultants in all specialties are available to these centers, thus allowing a very broad based diagnostic and rehabilitation service for the hearing handicapped.

In addition to clinical and rehabilitative services, all centers are active in research into communicative disorders in India.

AURAL REHABILITATION

The term aural rehabilitation encompasses an integrated approach to the restoration of functional hearing in the hearing-handicapped individual of all ages so that he is socially and emotionally able to overcome his handicap.

This is accomplished by evaluation of the handicap and, if not medically or surgically correctable, by use of devices for amplifying the sound in suitable individuals, instruction in the most effective way to use this sound, speechreading courses, and counseling (both educational and vocational). No one person can accomplish all this. It requires a team approach by a group of professionals fully cognizant of the problems faced by a handicapped person and motivated in working closely with such individuals. The team is comprised of the patient's physician, the otolaryngologist, the clinical audiologist, the speech pathologist, the vocational counselor, and the social worker. Last, but not least, a very crucial role is played by the individual's parents and close relatives who must accept the handicap, have full comprehension of the handicapped person's problems, and participate in the rehabilitative process.

Diagnostic Procedures

Physical Facilities All centers have locally built sound-treated rooms. The ambient noise levels are below the maximum allowable level laid down ty the American Standards Association. The audiometers in all the clinics are made by Arphi, Inc., Bombay and Bharat Electronics, Ltd., Bangalore.

Assessment of Hearing Loss In the great majority of adults and young hard-of-hearing patients, the type and severity of the hearing loss is evaluated by using pure tone audiometry. Speech audiometry has been developed in a number of Indian languages–Hindi, Tamil, and Malayalam–and is currently being developed in the other Indian languages. Use of speech audiometry has its limitations, however, because of dialectical variations, as well as educational limitations and unfamiliarity with recorded sounds. Thus, voice testing has been found to be more practical. But, for very young children and infants, play testing is done using calibrated sound stimuli along the lines recommended by Ewings and Whetnall (1963).

Because of the lack of awareness among physicians and the community of the need and importance of early diagnosis, the average age of referrals is still 6 years. Very few infants are referred to the centers. However, when children are referred to the centers they are very apprehensive and nonresponsive. This is mainly because of exposure to an unfamiliar environment and unfamiliar equipment. Repeated visits by the patient and a great deal of patience and understanding by the audiologist and the team are required before a reliable hearing test can be administered. In the great majority of cases, these procedures constitute a sufficient basis for therapeutic measures whether they be medical, surgical, or rehabilitative.

In view of the relative inaccessibility of the hearing and speech centers, attempts are being made by these centers to organize field teams who conduct hearing and speech camps in the neighborhood villages and screen the entire village population. This has helped in identifying: (1) a large population group with a variety of hearing and speech disorders; (2) large numbers of cases receiving treatment and rehabilitation; and (3) increasing awareness in the community and an opportunity to provide counseling to parents. Thus community education is achieved.

Rehabilitative Procedures

Current procedures in language training, auditory training, and speechreading are in their early stages of development. Following the establishment of the hearing and speech centers and availability of diagnostic facilities, the first problem encountered was hearing aid availability. Studies at the Christian Medical College, Vellore (Kapur, 1970*b*) revealed that only 24% of persons advised to have hearing aids were able to purchase them. Forty-eight percent of the cases who responded to the questionnaire stated they had not purchased the aids because of the high cost of those available. Rehabilitation for the majority was meaningless in the absence of hearing aid availability. These findings highlighted the need for the development and manufacture of low cost hearing aids in India. Those who could purchase hearing aids were unable to get custom-made ear molds. But under the Indo-Danish agreement, ear mold laboratories were given to the centers at Bombay, Benares, Mysore, New Delhi, and Vellore. This was another major step for rehabilitation success.

Once hearing aids were available and fitted, the next problem was in keeping patients at the center the necessary length of time. This posed a problem because of socioeconomic reasons. To overcome this, attempts are being made to train parents in the use and care of hearing aids, giving speech and language therapy, and educational training. The problem is similar both for adults and children. The Vellore study pointed to factors that had contributed to success and lack of progress of home training procedures. Factors contributing to progress were: (1) use of quality hearing aids; (2) use of hearing aids throughout the day; (3) use of custom-made ear molds; (4) cooperation of parents and patient; and (5) age at which hearing loss occurred. Factors contributing to lack of progress were: (1) use of poorly made hearing aids; (2) use of the hearing aid only part of the day; (3) fitting of hearing aid without custom-made ear molds; (4) lack of enthusiasm on the part of parents; (5) age at which hearing loss occurred (those fitted at a later age showed significant lack of progress); and (6) parents concerned about the safety of the hearing aid would take the aid off when the children went out to play.

The evaluation of parents' cooperation and the success of parent training was very difficult to judge. All parents professed interest in the problem the child had, but an objective measurement of these factors has, so far, not been possible. Generally it was observed that, in cases where parents appeared to be more cooperative, the children made greater progress.

Family Involvement

Acceptance of the handicapped child both in a physical and mental sense has been one of the goals in rehabilitation of the speech and hearing handicapped in India. The average Indian family is usually ignorant of the true nature of the handicap and assumes a fatalistic attitude toward it, thus fostering a sense of helplessness in the family and in the handicapped person. Among the more affluent and educated families, the parental response is that of overindulgence. Overprotection is more common than rejection. In order to overcome these attitudes, programs in community education were undertaken by all the major speech and hearing centers. Information and education booklets were prepared stressing the need for medical evaluation, explaining the goals and process of rehabilitation, and need for parental involvement and family understanding.

Parents often expect magical cures once they bring a child to a center and very often suffer a shock when they are advised that medical and surgical therapy are not of value in the treatment of the handicap. The process of acceptance and understanding is often time consuming, and one of the major problems in rehabilitation in this area has been that of keeping patients at the centers for prolonged periods for evaluation, diagnosis, and treatment since they came from great distances and found it difficult economically to stay away from their work. The process of counseling involved a team effort by the physician, audiologist, speech therapist, and social worker.

Once the handicap is accepted and the nature of the problem and rationale of treatment to be given was explained, the method of therapy to be given was demonstrated and then the benefit that could result was discussed. This has been found to be an effective approach.

In order to carry the message further, to rural areas where 80% of Indians live, mobile exhibits have been prepared by all the centers and taken to villages, exhibitions, and state fairs. The success of this is reflected in the increasing number of cases with speech and hearing handicap being seen at the centers. Rural screening surveys have also served this purpose. However, research is still needed on the development of effective home training programs and evaluation of the results of such programs.

INTERPROFESSIONAL RELATIONSHIPS

Before 1966, the only professionals active in the field of speech and hearing handicapped were the educators of the deaf. They had an organization called the Association of Teachers of the Deaf, and they had very little to do with otolaryngologists.

At the Third All India Workshop, held in Vellore, for the first time deaf educators participated in a discussion of the problems of the deaf with otolaryngologists, audiologists, speech pathologists, physicists, and psychologists. At the same time, deaf educators were admitted as associate members of the Indian Speech and Hearing Association, making available a forum for an interprofessional discussion of mutual concerns and interests.

The first audiologists and speech pathologists in India were trained in the United States. They set to establish the same patterns of training and professional associations as in the United States. At the First All India Workshop (Kapur, 1966*a*), held in Vellore in 1966, it was the consensus that audiology and speech pathology centers should be located within medical centers and in close relationship with otolaryngology departments in medical colleges. However, the government in India, on a recommendation by the late Dr. Martin Palmer, a consultant sent to India by the U.S. Department of Health, Education, and Welfare, Washington, D. C., established the All India Institute of Speech and Hearing in Mysore. The Institute was located outside a medical center in a university setting. All other centers in Bombay, Vellore, and Delhi were located within departments of otolaryngology of major medical centers.

Discussion of the optimal location of the Institute was the subject of lengthy and, at times, heated debate at the All India Workshop held in Vellore in 1966 (Kapur, 1966*a*), 1967 (Kapur, 1967), and 1969 (Kapur, 1969) and the Special Workshop in Delhi in 1970 (Kapur, 1970*a*). There was broad agreement that audiologists and speech pathologists work closely with otolaryngologists in developing both training programs and clinical centers as this would strengthen the approach being made to the state government and the central government for recognition and support for programs for the speech and hearing handicapped. The formation of the Indian Speech and Hearing Association in 1967 provided a mechanism whereby otolaryngologists, audiologists, speech pathologists, physicists, deaf educators, and social workers could meet at the annual conference and present papers and discuss mutual problems. Thus, in India at the present time, this Association has led to better interprofessional relationships among all those working for and with the hearing and speech handicapped. This Association has led to a better understanding by otolaryngologists of the problems of habilitation and rehabilitation of those with speech and hearing handicaps, and in the majority of the states they have been instrumental in initiating and developing audiology and speech centers. Thus, there are more opportunities for audiologists and speech pathologists currently being trained. The present trend is toward a real team approach and mutual understanding and respect for the competence of each area involved in working with the speech and hearing handicapped.

Indian Speech and Hearing Association

The growth and interest in and the demand for speech and hearing services resulted in the establishment of the Indian Speech and Hearing Association in December 1967. To be eligible for membership in the Association, applicants must have either a degree or diploma in speech pathology and/or audiology from a recognized training institution in the world. Membership is also open to otolaryngologists and psychologists interested or active in the field. Associate membership is open to physicists, educators of the deaf, and acousticians. The aims and objectives of the Association are: to encourage the scientific study of the processes of individual human speech and hearing, to promote investigations of speech and hearing disorders, to foster improvement of therapeutic procedures for such disorders, to stimulate exchange of information among persons thus engaged, and to disseminate such disorders, to stimulate exchange of information among persons thus engaged, and to disseminate such information.

The association has established a Committee on Educational Standards to ensure high professional and ethical standards in the training of personnel in audiology and speech pathology. In order to maintain a close relationship with the otolaryngologists, the Association resolved to meet annually in conjunction with the Association of Otolaryngologists of India.

Growth of the Association has been remarkable. Since its inception in 1966, it now has a membership of 350. This became possible because of the better understanding of the role of the audiologist and speech pathologist in diagnosis and management of speech and hearing disorders, the development of training programs in the area, organization of workshop and symposia, and locally manufactured equipment (including audiometers and hearing aids).

The office of the Secretary of the Association is presently located at the B. M. Institute, Ashram Road, Ahmedabad, Gujrat.

All India Federation of the Deaf

Since its inception in 1955, the All India Federation of the Deaf has been devoting itself to further the welfare of the deaf in India. The aims and objectives of the federation are:

1. To rehabilitate and unite the deaf all over the country.
2. To further, protect, and promote their interests.
3. To maintain a liaison between the deaf, the public, and the authorities and to keep them informed about the state and opinions of the deaf.
4. To establish, run, and aid the institutions, libraries, welfare agencies, and associations of the deaf, helping them to organize exhibitions of their work.
5. To take such steps as may be necessary for prevention and cure of deafness, wherever possible.
6. To publish literature and official organs of the federation as may be necessary for the guidance and information of the deaf.
7. To establish and maintain homes and hostels, etc., for the aged, poor, and infirm deaf.
8. To cooperate with social organizations and institutions for solving the problems of the deaf.
9. To cooperate with social organizations and institutions in other countries and make one cause with them.
10. To have its own bodies, institutions, and economic organizations for performing its various tasks.
11. To collect data concerning the education, the legal and social position, the organizations of assistance, the professional rehabilitation of the deaf in all states of India, and to inform its members of the results achieved.
12. To help and assist schools, workshops, training centers, associations, and societies for the deaf.
13. To encourage the establishment of state, zonal or district branches of the All India Federation of the Deaf, wherever necessary, for advancing the cause of the deaf.
14. To promote the inclusion of the problems concerning the deaf among those to be dealt with at an international level in cooperation with United Nations organizations, its bodies and its specialized agencies and to carry on correspondence with other national bodies or organizations for that purpose.
15. To promote awareness among the general public of the problems of the deaf and to organize meetings for the purpose of studying the various

problems with the help of the members of the public interested in the cause.

Membership in the Federation is open to associations (societies), associations of parents of the deaf, cooperative societies, and similar other organizations.

The Federation's headquarters are located in New Delhi, and branch offices are located in the majority of the states of the Union. The Federation holds an annual conference every year.

The main current activity of the Federation is focused on establishing a multipurpose training center for the deaf in New Delhi. This center has been conceived as an integrated project which will provide educational and training facilities, residential accommodation, clinical and vocational services, an open air theatre, and other recreational centers.

The Federation receives support from the central government.

Indian Society for Rehabilitation of the Handicapped

This society is concerned with five handicapped groups: the visually handicapped, the deaf and hard of hearing, the mentally retarded, those affected by leprosy, and the crippled and orthopedically handicapped. The society, which began as a voluntary group concerned with running an occupational therapy center, has expanded its activities to encompass all the handicapped (although the major emphasis is still on the orthopedically handicapped). The society has affiliates in most states of India and sponsors programs which bring attention to the handicapped, publishes a journal called *Rehabilitation in Asia,* and works closely with the International Rehabilitation Society in New York. The Society is active in distributing literature on the developments in rehabilitation all over the world and major policy trends of rehabilitation.

The main office of the society is located c/o All India Institute of Physical Medicine and Rehabilitation, Haji Ali Park, Mahalaxmi, Bombay.

CURRENT RESEARCH

Research related to evaluation of hearing and speech disorders and in aural rehabilitation is being conducted at a number of centers in India. At the All India Institute of Speech and Hearing in Mysore (Final Draft Report of Project, 1973), the main areas of research focus are:

1. Research is being conducted on the development of speech materials in Kannada, the regional language. The study is in progress at this time.

2. Study of noise and hearing patterns in industries in Mysore City. The objective of this study is to perform noise analysis, determine noise risk criteria, and make recommendations for noise conservation.
3. Developing infant screening programs. An infant screening program was developed to identify neonates with hearing loss using varying sound stimuli. But, of a total of 2,110 infants tested, 1,578 passed the criteria laid down. The 532 infants who failed the test are being followed to determine if they have a hearing loss, and, if so, the type and degree of loss. It will also be determined if they have other deficits.
4. The Institute is also developing educational materials to provide guidance to parents of handicapped children, to organize publicity campaigns, to stimulate awareness in the community on the need for early diagnosis for the hearing handicapped, and to publicize the facilities available for rehabilitation. Studies are being conducted on the best and most efficient way to effectively educate the community.
5. The Institute has a team approach in the evaluation, treatment, and counseling of hearing and speech handicapped. Students are being trained to work as part of this team and, thus, set a future pattern for comprehensive services for these handicapped.

At the All India Institute of Medical Sciences in New Delhi (Establishment of a Pilot Rehabilitation Unit in Audiology and Speech Pathology in India, 1974), the main areas of research focus are:

1. Preparation of spondee and phonetically balanced word lists in Hindi for use in speech audiometry. Frequency count for all consonants given by Ghatage was regarded as the basis. A word list of 423 monosyllabic words and 368 most commonly used words was analyzed for syllabic construction, frequency of initial and final consonants, vowel frequency, and familiarity. On completion of the analysis, two word lists of 50 words each were prepared based on frequency counts to familiarity. Two tests of 38 spondee words each were also prepared from among words of common usage. These word lists were tested on 30 normal young adults. The optimum for Hindi words was tentatively fixed at 20 dB above the speech reception threshold. These word lists are currently in use and are being refined. Research is also being done on use of these materials for preparing word lists for articulation tests in Hindi.
2. Study on evaluation of noise and its health hazards. This is being conducted by the Noise Trauma Cell of the Rehabilitation Unit in collaboration with the occupational medicine section of the Department of Preventive and Social Medicine. Field surveys are being conducted to

measure noise levels in hospitals, industrial areas, and high density traffic centers with the objectives of determining the levels of noise, need for protecting individuals exposed to noise, and measures for noise conservation.
3. Demonstration activities mainly aimed at arousing the awareness of the community, in general, and governmental and voluntary agencies, in particular, as to the needs of the speech and hearing handicapped. The Rehabilitation Unit has also translated into the Hindi language the John Tracy correspondence course for parents of young deaf children. Publicity materials and pamphlets are being prepared to familiarize parents and the public with the problems and needs of the hearing and speech handicapped. Scientific seminars for practicing physicians and otolaryngologists are also held periodically.

At the Christian Medical College and Hospital in Vellore (Kapur, 1970*b*), the main areas of research focus are:

1. Test materials for use in speech audiometry in the Tamil and Malayalam languages (developed by the Hearing and Speech center in Vellore and published in 1971) are currently being used and being refined because of dialectical variations in these two languages.
2. A study was conducted on the "Comparative Visibility of Four Spoken Languages" (Oyer et al., 1974). The languages studied were Hindi, Tamil, English, and Malayalam. The purpose was to determine the relative visibility of these languages, to determine if there were significant variations in their visibility and, if so, the implications for rehabilitation. English was rated most highly visible, followed by Tamil and Malayalam. It was concluded that the less visible the language, the more difficult it is to lipread. The study pointed to the need for more carefully controlled studies in speechreading.
3. The other areas of research conducted by the Deafness Research Project and the Hearing and Speech Center are described under Current Overview.

The Bharat Electronics, Ltd., Bangalore, and Arphi, Inc., Bombay, have been active in manufacturing pure tone and speech audiometers. There was a great need for locally made audiometers which could be serviced and calibrated by India-based manufacturers. Bharat Electronics is a central government organization. Arphi, Inc. is a private concern. The audiometers being produced are based on specifications laid down by the three All India Workshops held in Vellore. Over 200 audiometers are produced annually, and this has made possible the development of hearing and speech centers at many centers in India.

To meet the large demand for hearing aids in India, the Indian Telephone Industries, Bangalore, a central government-sponsored concern, began research into the development of low cost hearing aids in 1967. The hearing aids were developed according to the specifications laid down by the Indian Standards Institution, New Delhi. To date, the Indian Telephone Industries have manufactured low cost hearing aids, and these are being tested by the Indian Standards Institution before they are used in clinical trials and put into large scale production. Rehabilitation of the hearing handicapped will make tremendous strides once these hearing aids are available.

RESEARCH NEEDS

In spite of the ongoing research, the needs for research into methods for providing effective rehabilitation for the aurally handicapped are great. Some of these areas are: (1) need for early detection and identification of the hard-of-hearing and deaf children (the average age for referral is still between 6–7 years); (2) suitable educational programs for preschool children with hearing and speech handicaps; and (3) research to study the role of home training programs which can play a part in the rehabilitation of the majority of cases who are unable to stay at any center for socioeconomic reasons (the factors which need special study are methods to be used for training parents and patients, evaluation of the efficacy of training programs, and the role parents can play; home training programs are crucial in providing effective rehabilitation services in the country).

PERIODICALS ON HEARING PUBLISHED IN INDIA

1. Mook Diwani, which is published bimonthly by the All India Federation of the Deaf, Connaught Place, New Delhi, India.
2. Indian Journal of Otolaryngology, which is published monthly by the Editorial Office of the Department of Otolaryngology, All India Institute of Medical Sciences, New Delhi, India.

LITERATURE CITED

Brewer, G. D., and J. S. Kakalik. 1974. Handicapped children, summary and recommendations. R-1420/1-HEW: 15–17.

Draft Final Report of Project. 1973. SRS 19-P-58134-F-01, All India Institute of Speech and Hearing, Mysore.

Establishment of a Pilot Rehabilitation Unit in Audiology and Speech Pathology in India. 1973. All India Institute of Medical Sciences, New Delhi.

Ewing, A. W. G. 1963. Educational Guidance and the Deaf Child, 21–43. Manchester Univ. Press, Manchester, England.

Herrick, H. M., and Y. P. Kapur. 1969. Education of the deaf in India. Volta Rev. 71: 492–499.

Kapur, Y. P. 1965. A Study of Hearing Loss in School Children in India. J. Speech Hear. Disord. 30: 225–233.

Kapur, Y. P. 1966*a*. Hearing and infectious diseases. Laryngoscope 76: 418–457.

Kapur, Y. P. 1966*b*. Proceedings of the First All India Workshop on Speech and Hearing Problems in India. Deafness Research Project, Christian Medical College, Vellore, India.

Kapur, Y. P. 1967. Proceedings of the Second All India Workshop on Speech and Hearing Problems in India. Deafness Research Project, Christian Medical College, Vellore, S. India.

Kapur, Y. P. 1969. Research, Training and Rehabilitation in Speech and Hearing in India. Deafness Research Project, Christian Medical College, Vellore, India.

Kapur, Y. P. 1970*a*. Hearing and Speech Services in India. Special All India Workshop, New Delhi. Deafness Research Project, Christian Medical College, Vellore, S. India.

Kapur, Y. P. 1970*b*. Needs of the Speech and Hearing Handicapped in India. Deafness Research Project, Christian Medical College, Vellore, India.

Oyer, M. J., R. Richard, R. Rajaguru, and Y. P. Kapur. 1974. Comparative visibility of four spoken languages. J. Acad. Rehab. Audio. 7(2): 42–48.

chapter 15

Communication for Hearing-handicapped People in Malaysia

Chua Tee Tee, M.A.

Malaysia is a relatively new nation, having been formed on September 16, 1963. It is physically segmented in two by about 400 miles of the South China Sea, the more populous and more developed Peninsular Malaysia of 11 states sharing a common boundary with Thailand in the north and a large eastern portion of Sabah and Sarawak of East Malaysia (Figure 1). The total area is 130,000 square miles (Federal Department of Information, 1972). This is equivalent to just under half the size of Texas.

As in many other countries, the hearing-handicapped population of Malaysia has long been neglected as far as formal organized services are concerned. No such facilities existed as late as April 1954, when the first formal class was established with an enrollment of seven hearing-impaired pupils. This late awareness of the need to provide formal educational and other allied services for those with hearing handicaps is the more striking considering the fact that formal education for handicapped children in the country began 28 years earlier with the establishment of the first school for the blind in 1926. The reasons are not difficult to find. A hearing impairment often escapes the notice of the casual observer as it does not present such a visual impact as blindness or some other more obvious physical disability. A large number of hearing-handicapped children have been attending regular schools, their disability not recognized as serious or misunderstood as dullness or mental retardation. This misconception is further perpetuated by the automatic promotion system in the country, which permits every child to proceed each year from the first to the ninth grade whether he is making any school progress or not.

With the awakening of public awareness to the existence of hearing-impaired children and the need to provide specialized services in the 1950's, the right of such children to an education adapted to their special requirements has been accepted. Both the severely and the moderately deaf can and should be educated. They need not remain deaf and dumb at

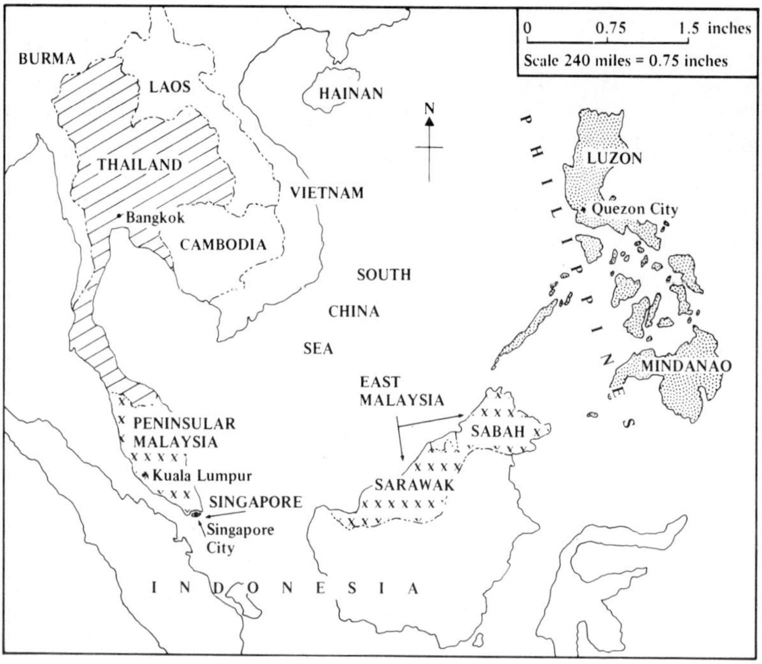

Figure 1. Location of Malaysia. (Reprinted from H. Fullard, 1962. Philips' Modern School Atlas, George Philip and Son, Ltd., London, pp. B and C.)

the same time, neither should they be isolated in "the lonely world of silence." It is now recognized that the hearing impaired can be helped and communication channels can be opened so that they can take their rightful place as worthy citizens of the country, capable of leading independent lives and contributing to the welfare and progress of the country.

DEFINITION OF AURAL REHABILITATION

A distinction is sometimes made here between aural habilitation and aural rehabilitation. The former may refer to special services for those handicapped by a hearing loss at birth or at the preschool age, while the latter is taken to mean services for those who acquire a hearing loss after speech has been developed. For the purpose of this chapter, aural habilitation and rehabilitation are used interchangeably and refer to organized special services to develop to the fullest the potentiality of each individual handicapped by a hearing loss. They imply the provision of comprehensive facilities covering both the young and the old, including "at risk" babies.

Such facilities should include early detection and diagnosis of hearing impediments, referrals, parent counseling, provision of hearing aids where necessary, special school curricular and extracurricular activities, prevocational and vocational training, job placement, and guidance and counseling throughout the life of the hearing-handicapped individual. The ultimate purpose of aural rehabilitation is to minimize the auditory handicap and optimize the potentiality of the individual so that he can become self-respecting, self-reliant, and independent.

HISTORICAL OVERVIEW

As in many other countries, formal education of the hearing handicapped in Malaysia has been pioneered by public-spirited individuals concerned with the welfare of individuals who, without special educational facilities, would be unable to receive formal education or compete successfully with normal hearing pupils. Organized concerted efforts to provide formal schooling for the hearing impaired in Malaysia have taken place in relatively recent times. In 1952, Dr. C. Elaine Field, pediatrician for the then Federation of Malaya, was concerned with the large number of deaf children without any education in the country (Chua, 1970). She referred the matter to Lady Templer, the wife of the High Commissioner and, subsequently, a meeting was called by Lady Templer in December 1952 to launch a country-wide appeal for funds, and through the generosity of many, notably the philanthropists of Penang, sufficient funds were collected to open, on an official basis, the Federation School for the Deaf in Penang, on April 1, 1954. Thus, Lady Templer became the founder member and patron of the school and, together with two other founder members, Dr. Field and Mr. R. P. Bingham, provided the initial momentum that has proved crucial in the history of deaf education in the country. In Malaysia, a person is technically deaf if he has a hearing loss of more than 60 decibels and a frequency loss from 250–4,000 cycles per second (Isa, 1972).

The special school began modestly in a converted private house at Northam Road in Penang, with an initial enrollment of seven pupils in April 1954. Seven years later, the school reached its maximum capacity of 120 pupils. The growth of the school is a good example of how both the private and public sectors can cooperate to contribute to the welfare and education of the deaf in the country. Faced with the necessity to expand educational facilities, the school successfully applied to the Social and Welfare Lotteries Board for a M $500,000.00 grant (rate of exchange: U.S. $1 = M $2.50), which was subsequently provided through the Ministry of

Rural Development, together with another M $100,000.00 from the Social and Welfare Services Board. An approach was also made to the Penang State Government for a piece of land to put up a new school. The State Government generously offered a 10-acre site facing the sea and adjacent to the Malayan Teachers' College in Glugor, Penang. Unfortunately, the site was unsuitable because of the incessant noise coming from a neighboring power station. Scouting for alternative sites subsequently focused on a 12-acre site in the Vale of Tempe belonging to a private housing developer, the Penang Realty, Ltd. The land was sold to the school at M $0.65 per square foot, with a donation of M $0.15. Together with a successful application for excision of gazetted hill-land reserve from the Penang State Government, classes at the new site began in January 1969. Until the new site was occupied, the school was beset with several administrative problems: the Northam Road school property had to be sold to pay for the new site, lessons were conducted in the afternoon session at the Shih Chung Branch School, with the school office at the former Public Trustee's Office in the Supreme Court Building; temporary classrooms were being built at the Po Leung Kuk Home; classes were carried out at the Po Leung Kuk Home, with the students residing in three different scattered places, one of which was operated by the State Welfare Department; and, finally, squatters were evicted with much difficulty (Federation School, 1970).

Enrollment at the school rose from seven in 1954 to 374 in January 1974. In the last 10 years, the absolute increase in enrollment was 260 compared to 107 in the previous decade, an almost two-and-a-half-fold increase (Table 1). This may be because of the following factors: (1) parents and guardians of deaf children have become more aware of the benefits of education and rehabilitation for the hearing impaired; (2) physical facilities in terms of classroom, accommodation, and canteen space have improved tremendously with the opening of new premises at the 12-acre site in the Vale of Tempe in 1970; and (3) there has been a steady flow of trained special education teachers of the deaf from a local teacher training institution beginning in 1962.

While the sex ratio of the deaf students at the Federation School for the Deaf was fairly well balanced in the early years of the school's history, being 50–52% female in the early 1960's, the proportion of deaf girls in recent years has dropped drastically to 38–39%. This is also reflected in the so-called normal school population in government-assisted schools where only 46.6% are girls, with only 42.4% female representation at the secondary level. This is not because of any conscious effort on the part of the Federation School to debar girls from formal education, but is related

Table 1. Enrollment at the Federation School for the Deaf, Penang from its initial establishment to the present (by sex and year)[a]

Year	Male	Female	Total	Percentage female
1954	4	3	7	42.8
1955	15	16	31	51.6
1956	31	25	56	44.6
1957	33	27	60	45.0
1958	33	27	60	45.0
1959	49	47	96	48.9
1960	57	55	112	49.1
1961	58	62	120	51.7
1962	59	61	120	50.9
1963	59	61	120	50.9
1964	59	61	120	50.9
1965	51	63	114	55.2
1966	52	63	115	54.8
1967	53	59	112	52.7
1968	69	71	140	50.7
1969	83	78	161	48.4
1970	107	90	197	45.7
1971	145	98	243	40.3
1972	178	112	290	38.6
1973	222	141	363	38.8
1974	229	145	374	38.9

[a]Collated from correspondence with Mrs. S. Yahaya Isa, Principal, Federation School for the Deaf, Penang.

to the still prevailing Asian mentality that the girl's preoccupation should be in the home and that formal education and subsequent gainful employment are more important and relevant for the male counterpart. This has been pointed out in at least three studies—by Baal (1964), Seymour (1974), and the Ministry of Education, Malaysia (1973).

Expansion of schools for the auditory impaired is not confined only to the Federation School for the Deaf in Penang. Partly in response to limited places available in the Federation School and to the scattered nature of the school-age population, the Ministry of Education took a major policy decision when it introduced the system of education of the hearing handicapped in regular schools in 1962, as a complementary service to the fully residential system at the Federation School.

Begun as two pilot classes for hearing-handicapped children in Kuala Lumpur, the nation's capital, in January 1962, such integrated classes in regular schools have grown to 65 classes in 39 primary schools in nine out of 11 states in Peninsular Malaysia. Enrollment in these special day classes has exceeded that at the Federation School as early as 1963, and now stands at 661, 77.0% more than at the special residential school. According to Hickes (1962), the first organizer for education of the deaf at the Ministry level, the obvious advantages of such integrated education are that deaf children can enjoy a normal school life, remain in close touch with the normal hearing, and be better adjusted to family life. Chua (1974) has also pointed out the pros and cons of residential special schooling and open education.

The growth of special classes for the hearing impaired in regular primary schools throughout the country can be seen in the enrollment figures as indicated in Table 2. Enrollment increased from 79 in 1962 to 661 in 1974, exceeding the number of students at the Federation School annually since 1963. This rapid expansion demonstrates, among other factors, the following: (1) there are more hearing-handicapped children that require special educational treatment than there were places available previously; (2) the financial, psychosocial, and other problems of enrolling in a distant residential special school and the limited classroom and accommodation facilities at the Federation School have seriously re-

Table 2. Enrollment of hearing-handicapped children in special classes in regular primary schools from their initial establishment to the present (by sex and year)[a]

Year	Male	Female	Total	Percentage female
1962	NA[b]	NA	79	NA
1963	NA	NA	265	NA
1964	NA	NA	340	NA
1965	267	143	410	34.9
1966	275	150	425	35.3
1967	309	170	479	35.5
1968	304	164	468	35.0
1969	224	137	361	37.9
1970	NA	NA	398	NA
1971	274	140	414	33.8
1972	306	165	471	35.0
1973	357	233	590	39.4
1974	403	258	661	39.0

[a]Collated from records in the Schools Division, Ministry of Education, Malaysia, Kuala Lumpur.

[b]NA, not available.

stricted the number of hearing-handicapped children able to receive formal education in a special school setting; (3) parents find it more convenient and advantageous to the auditory impaired children to go to nearby regular day schools with special classes; and (4) there are signs of increasing acceptance of the hearing-impaired child from parents, school principals, and teachers and normal hearing peers, instead of the negative attitude of keeping a handicapped child cloistered at home or isolating him in a segregated residential school setting.

The growth of these special classes took place initially at the national capital, Kuala Lumpur, and has now spread to 25 other towns throughout the country. These day classes cater to urban hearing-impaired dwellers, while the residential Federation School for the Deaf admits children from rural areas and others who cannot gain admission in the widely scattered special day classes.

As in the case of the enrollment at the Federation School for the Deaf, there is unequal sex distribution in the special day classes. Female hearing-handicapped pupils constituted only 33–39% of the enrollment in the last 10 years (Table 2).

Development of education for the hearing impaired in East Malaysia, comprising Sarawak and Sabah, took place rather independently, partly because these two states joined the Federation of Malaysia only recently in 1963 and one of the conditions for merger was the right to have an independent policy on matters pertaining to education, including special education. In December 1964, a school for the deaf was opened in Kuching, the state capital of Sarawak, under the Kuching Municipal Council, with an initial enrollment of 14 (Tan, 1972). Enrollment grew year by year so that it now stands at 58 students, 48.2% of whom are girls (Ghazali, 1974). There are no special schools or classes for the hearing handicapped in Sabah. These children have been sent by the State Welfare Department to Sarawak and Peninsular Malaysia for their education, fully subsidized by the Department.

The number of hearing-impaired children and youth enrolled in special schools and classes now totals 1,093, which represents only 0.04% of the primary and secondary school population. From Table 3, it can be seen that enrollment increased rapidly after 1962, with the establishment of special classes for the deaf in regular primary schools as a complementary service to the residential Federation School for the Deaf in Penang. Together with the Day School for the Deaf in Kuching, Sarawak, the total deaf school population rose significantly year by year past the thousand mark in 1974. Figure 2 shows graphically the dramatic growth of this population. It is significant to note that, before independence, under

Table 3. Enrollment of hearing-impaired students in special schools and classes in Malaysia since the initial establishment of special education programs[a]

Year	Federation School for the Deaf at Penang	Special classes in regular primary schools	Kuching School for the Deaf at Sarawak	Total
1954	7	0	0	7
1955	31	0	0	31
1956	56	0	0	56
1957	60	0	0	60
1958	60	0	0	60
1959	96	0	0	96
1960	112	0	0	112
1961	120	0	0	120
1962	120	79	0	199
1963	120	265	0	385
1964	120	340	14	474
1965	114	410	14	538
1966	115	425	17	557
1967	112	479	22	613
1968	140	468	22	630
1969	161	361	19	541
1970	197	398	21	616
1971	243	414	29	686
1972	290	471	35	796
1973	363	590	48	1001
1974	374	661	58	1093

[a]Collated from records in the Schools Division, Ministry of Education, Malaysia and the Federation School for the Deaf, Penang.

British rule in the then Federation of Malaya (now Peninsular Malaysia), very few hearing-impaired children were catered to educationally. There was a significant spurt in enrollment rate with the launching of the integrated program for deaf children in regular primary schools in 1962. The slight drop in enrollment in the school year 1969 may be accounted for by the following factors: (1) it marks the end of primary education for deaf children who began their education in special classes in regular schools in 1962, resulting in a few students terminating their school careers to assist their parents at home or seek employment outside the school and home; (2) there has been an absence of special classes in regular secondary or vocational schools for deaf and hard-of-hearing children to enable them to continue their education; (3) the number of available secondary school places at the residential Federation School for the Deaf was limited, first

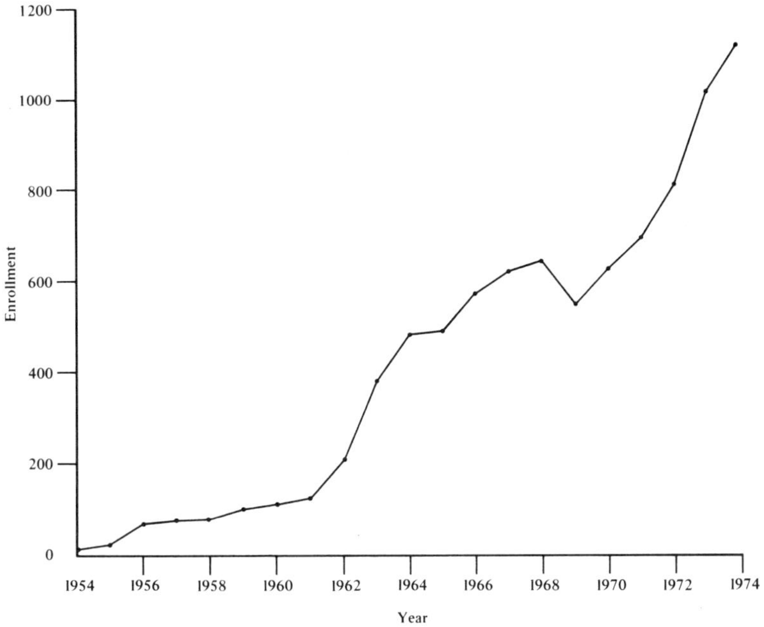

Figure 2. Enrollment of hearing-handicapped children and youth in special schools and classes in Malaysia from 1954–1974.

preference being given to their own sixth grade students and to those who have shown average or above average school performance at the primary level.

The need to cater to the increasing number of primary school graduates was partly met by the establishment of Further Education Classes for the Deaf, subsidized by the Ministry of Education. The first two classes began in 1965 in the nation's capital. They not only catered to deaf adolescents who have completed elementary education, but also to those hearing-impaired youth who have never been to school or who are too old for schooling in regular or special schools (Lee, 1968).

Public-spirited individuals have participated in initiating special classes for the deaf. The work of such individuals in the founding of the Federation School for the Deaf in Penang has been cited earlier. The National Society for the Deaf was founded in 1961, headed by a member of Parliament, the Honorable Incik Mohd. Khir Johari, former Malaysian Ambassador to the United States of America. In September 1969, this Society set up a day audiology center in Kuala Lumpur to cater to the preschool deaf children. In 1964, a Mr. Tan Yap, a pharmaceutical chemist by profession, established a special class for older deaf persons in Johor Bahru, at the southern tip of Peninsular Malaysia. When he was transferred to Kuala Lumpur in 1969, he had to close the southern class down, but he initiated special day classes for about 30 deaf children and youth in Kuala Lumpur and Port Kelang in 1969 and 1973 respectively.

GENERAL DESCRIPTION OF PRESENT PROGRAMS OF AURAL HABILITATION AND REHABILITATION

Apart from the Ministry of Education, which has direct control over special schools and classes for the hearing impaired in Malaysia, the Ministry of Welfare Services, the Ministry of Health, and four nongovernmental organizations provide some supplementary services. The Ministry of Welfare Services provides social workers who act as liaisons between the schools and the homes, carry out case studies, offer financial assistance in deserving cases, and keep a voluntary register of hearing-impaired and other handicapped people in the country. The Ministry of Health has direct control over the training and deployment of related personnel like pediatricians, doctors, ear, nose, and throat specialists, audiologists, psychologists and psychiatrists. It is concerned with diagnosis and prognosis of hearing losses and preventive aspects of deafness.

The current programs for the hearing impaired are being described under the following headings: preschool education; primary education; secondary education; postsecondary education; and problems.

Preschool Education

The Ministry of Education, which controls age limits rigidly for school admission, has laid down 6 years as the minimum age of admission into regular schools, and this has also unfortunately been applied to hearing-handicapped children, although there is increasing pressure from professional and lay bodies for the Ministry to lower the age limit for admission of deaf and other handicapped children into special schools or classes. Thus, preschool services are currently limited to a day center in Kuala Lumpur, run by the National Society for the Deaf. There are approximately 20 preschool children, there ranging in age from 2–4 years. Services include diagnostic evaluation, the supply of free or partially subsidized hearing aids, teaching speech and lipreading, and parental guidance. Parental counseling is considered an important aspect of the program. Mothers, as well as some fathers, are required to attend training sessions—both to observe, as well as to participate. There are occasional parent meetings with informal discussions, as well as talks by guest lecturers.

Primary School Education

These services are being provided at the Federation School for the Deaf in Penang and in the special classes in regular primary schools scattered throughout the country. The normal school syllabus is adopted in the main, with built-in sessions for speech and auditory training and lipreading. The current program is almost entirely oral in nature, although the Ministry of Education has indicated that there may be a place for manualism also. In 1971, some oral teachers of the deaf in the country were exposed to a 2-week exposure course on fingerspelling and sign language organized by the Ministry of Education. The American one-hand fingerspelling and the sign language used in Gallaudet College were taught at the in-service course. However, there has been no coordinated follow-up action on the extent of use and effectiveness of such teaching methods in the special classes of hearing-impaired children nor exactly how these could be integrated successfully with the oral aspects of training. Perhaps what is needed is a systematic approach to total communication involving elements of both oralism and manualism (Chua, 1974a).

The subjects covered at the primary level include: Bahasa Malaysia (the national language and medium of instruction), English, Mathematics, Science, Art and Crafts, Physical and Health Education, Local Studies (in the first three grades) and Civics, History and Geography (in the upper three grades of elementary school). The syllabus is covered in 6 years as for normal hearing children for children admitted at age 8 years. However, a 2-year bonus is permitted for children admitted at 6 years, so that the 6-year regular primary school syllabus is covered in 8 years. There is automatic promotion so that all children proceed from one standard to the next year after year. However, there are two standardized objective tests conducted in all regular and special schools by the Ministry of Education, one at grade 3 level and the other at grade 5 level. The former is semidiagnostic in nature, while the latter is basically an assessment test.

Physical facilities in almost all special classes in the regular primary school include group hearing equipment which is fixed to an arc-shaped table curved inward toward the special teacher and the chalkboard. Twelve pairs of headphones, 12 microphones, and the teacher's microphone are the standard equipment provided. Behind this long curved table are 12 portable chairs for the students. Approved class size is from 6–12 hearing-impaired pupils. Other standard electroacoustic equipment inlcudes an individual speech trainer to be shared by two or more special classes in a particular regular school. Individual hearing aids are mostly supplied on loan by the Ministry of Education, although a few pupils purchase their own individual sets. The most commonly used group hearing equipment and speech trainer is the Amplivox, although the Kamplex and the Oticon appear in some special classes. Common individual hearing aids are of the Madresco, Siemens, Daeltone, Oticon, Philips, or Danavox type.

In a recent random survey by the author of 20 sets of group hearing aids installed in 20 special classes in Peninsular Malaysia, 70% of them have been found to be in reasonably good working condition. Frequency of use varies from as low as under 2 hours per week to more than 8 hours, with 14% of the children using the equipment for less than 2 hours, 14% between 2 and 4 hours, another 14% between 4 and 6 hours, 29% from 6–8 hours, and the last 29% for more than 8 hours per week. In another random sampling of 20 individual speech trainers, 70% are estimated to be fully operational. Sixty four percent of the children sampled use the speech trainer from 1–2 hours a week, with 21% from 2–3 hours, and 15% for more than 4 hours.

Out of a random sample of 220 hearing-handicapped pupils in 21 special classes, 97% have individual hearing aids, 77% of the sets being supplied by the Ministry of Education and 23% owned by the deaf children themselves. However, out of the 214 sets, only 55% are known to be in satisfactory working condition.

Secondary School Education

After the primary level, most of the hearing-handicapped students are channeled into the postprimary streams of the Federation School for the Deaf in Penang, numbering 123 in March 1974. Secondary education is made up of 3 years of lower secondary with automatic promotion and 2 years of upper secondary. At the end of each of these two levels is a public examination, after which students may leave to seek employment. There are basically two streams at the lower secondary level, one which is academic and the other prevocational and vocational. The academic subjects include Bahasa Malaysia, English, Mathematics, Science, Art and Crafts, Physical Education and Health Education, History, and Geography. The prevocational and vocational programs comprise woodwork, tailoring, ladies' hairdressing, repair and servicing of typewriters, printing and drafting, and, more recently, poultry farming.

Postsecondary Education

There are currently no formal educational provisions for hearing-handicapped students who complete secondary education and wish to further their studies. Those few who can get along by themselves because they are partially hearing or have effective individual hearing aids compete with the so-called normal for places at the five local universities, one polytechnic, one technical college, and a number of teacher training institutions. Some have gone overseas for higher studies, as in the case of Eleanor Culas who is pursuing a degree course at Gallaudet College, Washington, D. C. on a scholarship awarded by the National Society for the Deaf, Malaysia (Berita Tulina, 1971).

Problems

One of the critical problems facing habilitation or rehabilitation of the auditory impaired is the lack of information on actual numbers of such people, together with their age, and geographical distributions, so that meaningful long-term comprehensive planning by both government and voluntary bodies can be made. The last known survey of handicapped persons in Peninsular Malaysia was conducted in 1958 and 1959 and, according to this International Labour Office report (1970), there were 8,977 deaf persons. Considering that the total population in mid-1959 was estimated at 6,815,000 (Department of Statistics, n.d.) the deaf population constituted only 0.13% of the total population, a very low percentage indeed when compared with known prevalence rates in other countries. The recent 1970 Census unfortunately does not include enumeration of deaf persons as such but includes a head count of 2,094 dumb persons (46.7% female) aged 10 and above in Peninsular Malaysia (Department of Statistics, 1973) giving a prevalence rate of 0.023% of the total population. This figure provides a very rough indication of the extent of the problem, but its usefulness is obviously limited because not all dumb people are deaf, nor are all deaf people dumb and also because persons 9 years and below who are dumb were not counted. A voluntary register kept at the Ministry of Social Welfare indicates that, on June 1, 1974, there were 2,121 deaf people listed, of whom 14.6% were aged 6 and below, 27.6% aged 7–20, and the rest (57.8%) aged 21 and above.

Another serious problem is the almost complete absence of preschool services so vital for children handicapped by a hearing loss. As pointed out earlier, the only existing facility is confined to a day center in the nation's capital, catering to a few dozen preschool hearing-impaired children and organized by a private voluntary association. The present ruling that deaf children must be between 6 and 8 years of age before they can be admitted into special schools or day classes adversely affects the early crucial development of verbal and nonverbal communication skills.

At the school level itself, the problem of which method to use–oralism, manualism, or both–has not been clearly resolved in Malaysia. All special education teachers of the deaf have been trained in the oral system of education and some have been exposed to fingerspelling and the language of signs, but there is as yet no clearly defined policy by the Ministry of Education regarding the best method of teaching the Malaysian child. The problem is compounded by the fact that the population is multiracial and multilingual, the breakdown at the 1970 census being 46.8% Malays, 34.1% Chinese, 9.0% Indians, and 10.1% belonging to other races (Department Statistics, 1972). In May 1974, the racial composition of 374 deaf students at the residential Federation School for the Deaf comprised 33.9% Malays, 54.6% Chinese, 9.6% Indians, and 1.9% other races (Isa, 1974). The relatively low Malay student population may be caused by the more rural nature of this ethnic group.

There is also unequal distribution of facilities for urban and rural deaf children. Although the country is rural in nature, with more than two-thirds of the population living in rural areas and 52.6% of the employed population engaged in agriculture (Government of Malaysia, 1973), all the day special classes in regular primary schools are located in urban areas which cater to more than 60% of the total deaf student population. Even in the residential Federation School for the Deaf which can accommodate more deaf children from nonurban areas, the proportion of deaf students from rural homes is only 43.6%. Among the causal factors are the greater inaccessibility of the rural countryside for identification of the handicap and school referrals, transportation problems to and from school for the long school holidays, demand for free labor on the farm, and conservativeness of the rural people, many of whom do not appreciate the value of formal education.

The present system of education is heavily biased toward oralism which involves the purchase of expensive electroacoustic equipment. Apart from the high cost of maintenance and related administrative difficulties, special teachers of the hearing handicapped tend to rely too much on elaborate electronic equipment to assist them in their teaching. In most cases of children who use individual hearing aids, they do not derive maximum benefit as the aids are not prescribed according to individual needs nor are ear molds made and fitted to maximize individual utilization.

There are inadequate facilities in terms of schools and diversity of choice of school subjects for the hearing handicapped who have completed primary education in Malaysia (Chua, 1974b). There should be opportunities for the many primary school graduates to proceed into regular secondary vocational schools where they can profit from a program which places emphasis on the use of the hands. At the same time, specialized instruction on speech, lipreading, and manualism could continue to be given in a special room as part of the secondary school curriculum. Related to vocational training is the problem of placement of the hearing handicapped in open employment. At present there is no provision for a placement officer even at the Federation School for the Deaf to bridge the gap between school and society. Such a person is necessary to give vocational guidance and personal counseling to the deaf person, to break down existing prejudices about employment of handicapped people, to identify specific jobs most suitable for the deaf, and to give psychological and other support for the newly employed deaf where necessary.

INTERPROFESSIONAL RELATIONSHIPS

Rehabilitation of the deaf, as for other handicapped persons, has to be treated from a multidisciplinary approach. The special education teacher in Malaysia is able to make some limited but important contact with the medical practitioner, the audiologist, the speech therapist, the ear, nose, and throat specialist, and the social worker. Before a child can be admitted into a special school or class for the hearing handicapped, he has to be examined by a medical doctor or an ear, nose, and throat specialist and it must be medically certified that he has a hearing problem. Referral to a doctor or medical specialist is done either directly by parents of a handicapped child or through the social worker attached to the State Department of Social Welfare. In addition to referrals to a medical officer, the social worker also makes a careful case study, covering social and economic aspects of a handicapped child's home life, and finally makes a referral to the relevant education authorities for special school placement. Although the special education teacher normally has no direct personal contact with the social worker or the medical officer, information on medical and socioeconomic background of a hearing-impaired child is furnished through documents for the use of special education teachers.

Special schools or classes do not have the services of full-time or even part-time speech therapists, who are attached either to government hospitals or to semigovernment bodies, such as the University Hospital in Petaling Jaya. In such circumstances, hearing-impaired children are referred to the speech therapist only minimally and only in major towns. The need to make available, on a full-time basis, such specialized personnel to special schools and classes is obvious.

The services of audiologists are in a slightly better position. In addition to a few audiologists in hospitals, the Federation School for the Deaf has two fully trained audiologists. However, in view of the fact that they are not employed as audiologists as such—one is the principal and the other a senior teacher of the school—their expertise is not fully utilized.

Moreover, the many special classes for the deaf in regular schools do not and cannot make even part-time use of these two Malaysian audiologists.

There is minimal contact among special education teachers of the deaf themselves. There is no national or state organization such as the Malaysian Guild of Educators of the Blind to keep teachers in contact with each other, to solve common problems, and to keep up with professionalism on a group basis. There is an absence of a sense of belonging to a professional group, heightened perhaps by the reluctance of the Ministry of Education to grant a special allowance to special education teachers in recognition of the special training (as is done in neighboring countries like Thailand, Indonesia, and the Philippines). There is also a lack of professional contact and leadership because, at both ministerial and state levels, the officers in charge of special education administration often do not have a background of special education training, so that teachers in the field often complain that administrators do not appreciate their real problems at the grassroots level.

There are no psychologists or psychiatrists attached to special schools or classes for the hearing handicapped even on a part-time basis. However, there are several attached to government and semigovernment hospitals and to universities. Their services are solicited from time to time, often through the intervention of the social worker, who makes known the existence of such facilities. At other times, when hearing-impaired children have serious learning or emotional problems, they may be referred by the special education teacher to the psychologist or psychiatrist in government and semigovernment hospitals. Thus, the vast majority of aurally handicapped school children or adults do not have a regular psychologist or psychiatrist to go to for any advice or assistance.

FAMILY INVOLVEMENTS

The absence of government-supported preschool programs for the hearing impaired, and the existence of only one small day center for such children in the Federal capital run by a voluntary organization, reflect the serious gap in the education of pre-elementary children. The problem is compounded by the fact that the population is multiracial and multilingual so that public parent-teacher meetings, home visits by social workers and special education teachers, have to overcome, among other aspects, the communication barrier. The scattered rural nature of the population 71.3% are in rural areas) and the relative low rate of literacy (68% are able to read and write in any language) accentuate the problem further (Treasury, 1974).

The present facilities to involve family members, particularly parents, in the total rehabilitation of their hearing-impaired children are grossly inadequate. Mention has been made of home visits by social workers while investigating their case histories. However, many are not specially trained to give parental support in terms of how to deal with the handicapped child, to recognize and accept the disability, to stimulate the child at home for maximum physical, social, emotional, and intellectual development as a necessary complementary service to formal schooling and rehabilitation. Special education teachers of the hearing impaired seldom make house calls to plan joint action for intellectual and social growth of such children.

The current family involvement, as initiated by the National Society for the Deaf in their preschool audiology center, should be expanded to cover more day centers throughout the country. Mothers, and sometimes fathers, are expected to come to the day center to observe how their children can be stimulated to communicate and speak effectively and to participate actively at the center and in the home. It cannot be overemphasized that the stress on family involvement should be in the preschool years. Smilansky and Smilansky (1967) have cited 11 reasons why the preschool period is considered crucial for intellectual, social, and physical development. Furthermore, the child spends more time at home than in a special day school or center, so that formal and informal education should be extended into the home to optimize results.

TRAINING OF PROFESSIONALS FOR THE FIELD OF REHABILITATION AUDIOLOGY

The backbone of a good rehabilitation program in any country is the competency and dedication of its professional trained staff. Malaysia is fortunate in this respect because many of the special teachers of the hearing handicapped have been trained in a number of places, enjoying a multitudinous fund of diverse professional expertise. Training institutions have included the University of Manchester in England, the University of London, Glendonald Training Centre in Melbourne, Australia, the University of Southern California, U.S.A., and a local training center at the Specialist Teachers Training Institute, Kuala Lumpur.

The bulk of the training for special education teachers has been at the local training center at the Specialist Teacher Training Institute in Kuala Lumpur, which issues a certificate on education of the deaf after successful completion of a 12 months' course. Applicants for the course must be trained teachers of so-called normal children, with a minimum of 5 years' trained teaching experience. Course work includes lectures, seminars, and tutorials on the following main topics: (1) principles of the educational treatment of hearing impairment, (2) historical survey of the education of the deaf, (3) audiology and physiology, (4) acquisition of linguistic skills, (5) development of communication skills, and (6) curriculum and specialized methods of subjects teaching in Bahasa Malaysia.

While the course is basically designed to train teachers to teach the hearing handicapped, practical experience is also provided in the assessment of deafness, parental guidance, and counseling, publicity, welfare work, and educational visits. Final assessment of the trainee's work is multifaceted, based on the standard attained in teaching and practical work in the classroom, the submission of a written thesis, the submission of a written study on two hearing-impaired children, and on a written examination on the six lecture topics mentioned above. As stated earlier, information on the development of linguistic and communication skills is almost entirely biased toward oralism, with little or no provision for sign language, fingerspelling, or even cued speech. The last-named teaching technique is passed on to Malaysian teachers trained at the Glendonald Training Centre in Melbourne.

The vast majority of Malaysian teachers of the deaf undergo a 12 months' certificated course in the training institutions mentioned earlier. A diploma in Audiology stretching over 1 academic year is also offered by the University of Manchester, which has seen the graduation of three Malaysians. This is a course of advanced study intended for qualified teachers of the deaf who have had a minimum of 2 years' experience after qualification, with emphasis placed on clinical work.

Doctors have been trained locally since the establishment of the first Faculty of Medicine at the University of Malaya in 1963. The ratio of doctors to population in Peninsular Malaysia is still relatively low, 1 to 4,562 in 1973 as compared to 1 to 7,326 in 1957. The recent introduction of compulsory government service for 2 years for newly qualified doctors as a condition for registration and the recruitment of doctors from abroad will help alleviate, to a certain extent, the medical staff shortages especially in rural areas.

The training of social and welfare workers is partly met by the establishment of Universiti Sains Malaysia in June 1969, which awards, among other degrees, the Bachelor of Social Services. Before the introduction of this course, such personnel have been trained overseas, a good number at the University of Singapore, which offers a diploma in Social Studies, which requires a mimimum period of 2 years of full-time study

(Ministry of Education, Singapore, 1972). However, the Vice-Chancellor of Universiti Sains, Malaysia, in a public address to the National Association of Professional Social Workers in early 1974, emphasized that "The graduate social scientist is not a professional social worker although he can grow into one quite comfortably with an additional year of professional training in social work" (Hamzah, 1974).

Other specialized personnel connected with hearing-handicapped children, such as pediatricians, ear, nose, and throat specialists, psychologists, and speech therapists, have to be trained overseas currently. The place of such training is usually Malaysia's former colonial master, England. There is a need to identify local needs in the Southeast Asian region and, in this respect, the University of the Philippines and the many private higher institutions of learning in the Republic of the Philippines offer possible and more relevant courses of specialization.

RESEARCH

Research on rehabilitation of the hearing impaired is confined almost entirely to the Specialist Teachers Training Institute where teachers undergo a special certificated course on education of the deaf. It is action oriented and has a practical bias. The researchers are the trainees undergoing the 1-year special training course, the research taking the form of a graduation exercise or thesis. From the available theses deposited at the Specialist Teachers Training Institute, in connection with the teacher training course on the education of the deaf, research topics cover such aspects as: (1) auditory training; (2) industrial arts for deaf children; (3) civics education for deaf children; (4) science for the deaf; (5) project education and the deaf child; (6) art for the deaf; (7) physical education for the deaf; (8) teaching music to deaf children; (9) agricultural science for the deaf; (10) playway method in mathematics for the deaf; (11) project method for the deaf; (12) deaf education in Malaysia; and (13) management of deaf children. It can be seen, therefore, that local research is almost entirely of the descriptive type and focuses largely on specific curricular areas.

Some areas that need to be researched in the rehabilitation of the hearing impaired in Malaysia include the following: (1) the incidence and prevalence rates of hearing impairment in the country; (2) causes and prevention of deafness in the local context; (3) effects of multilingualism on the education of the deaf; (4) psychosocial problems of the Malaysian deaf child; (5) the most effective way of teaching communication skills to the hearing impaired in view of special local circumstances; (6) attitudes of the hearing community toward deaf people and vice versa; and (7) employment prospects for the hearing handicapped.

The pursuit of research for its own sake is beyond the purse strings of most nations, especially in a developing one like Malaysia. Authorities funding research believe in the functional value of research and would like to see research findings translated into concrete proposals or direct application in special education or rehabilitation centers. The potential for research in the area of the hearing impaired exists at the Faculty of Education, University of Malaya, where postgraduate students may select an educational field for their M.Ed. or Ph.D. dissertation. Two faculty staff members whose areas of specialization are on the visually handicapped and the slow learner respectively may advise and supervise candidates wishing to research on deaf or other handicapped children.

ORGANIZATIONS AND ASSOCIATIONS RESPONSIBLE FOR THE HEARING HANDICAPPED

A number of lay organizations have mushroomed to look after the interests of the hearing impaired in Malaysia. The National Society for the Deaf was first formed in 1961 under the Chairmanship of a member of Parliament, the Honorable Incik Mohd. Khir Johari (former Malaysian Ambassador to the United States of America), who still holds the post of Chairman. The objectives of the Society as spelled out in its constitution are: (1) to promote, foster and deal with all aspects of the welfare services of the deaf; (2) to develop and maintain welfare services for the deaf; (3) to assist and closely cooperate with the general public and all government, voluntary, religious and philanthropic bodies concerned with, or interested in, the welfare of the deaf; (4) to provide and to assist in establishing, where necessary, schools for the deaf, or centers for training teachers of the deaf; (5) to assist existing schools or other institutions for the deaf in any manner deemed fit by the Society; (6) to disseminate information concerning the needs of the deaf and to encourage and foster an understanding of their special problems and difficulties; (7) to initiate, undertake, or assist in research in the field of deaf welfare; (8) to raise funds for the accomplishment of the above objects; and (9) to undertake such activities as may be incidental or conducive to the attainment of the objects wherein stated.

The office of the Society is sited at Loke Yew Building, Jalan Belanda, Room 601A, Kuala Lumpur. Activities have been confined largely to the national capital, Kuala Lumpur.

In September 1969, the Society set up in Kuala Lumpur a day Audiology Center which is unique as it is the only clinic in Malaysia where preschool deaf children can receive training. The services provided in the center include the following: (1) speech, language, and hearing evaluation of children who are referred by hospitals or private doctors; (2) diagnostic testing, which frequently involves various types of examination in the medical field; (3) in the event that the child is found to be deaf, services provided include fitting the child with a suitable hearing aid, enrollment in a nursery program, parent guidance (which is a major part of the program), and provision of auditory training, lipreading, speech, and building language concepts.

With the exception of two full-time staff members, all the workers teach on a voluntary basis. Volunteers consist of two teachers of the deaf, a teacher of the mentally retarded, and a few housewives, who have been generously giving their time to help the deaf. There are plans to establish a residential Audiology Center to meet the needs of the deaf from rural areas and for outstation parents of deaf children (Malay Mail, 1974).

Another lay organization concerned with rehabilitation of the hearing handicapped is the management committee of the Selangor School for the Deaf, begun in September 1969 and situated at Yoke Nam Primary School, Jalan Kelang, Kuala Lumpur. In June 1973, it started a branch school at Red Cross Building, Jalan Kereta Api, Kelang. The total number of deaf persons being served is around 30 aged 9–26 years. These two private schools, in contrast to the Ministry of Education special education programs and the National Society for the Deaf Preschool Auditory Center, teach sign language to the deaf. In addition to the language of signs, the students at the two schools are also taught the three R's. Financial support comes from both government and private sources—the salary of one full-time teacher is paid by the National Union of Plantation Workers, textbooks are supplied free by the Dewan Bahasa dan Pustaka, transportation is either paid for by the Petaling Jaya Rotary Club or provided free by the Sri Jaya Transport Company, and a small block grant is given by the Ministry of Welfare Services. Other service clubs that have given financial support are the Pudu Rotary Club and the Kuala Lumpur Inner Wheelers.

Another lay organization formed recently to look after the interests of hearing-impaired and other handicapped people is the Selangor Society for Rehabilitation of the Disabled, formally established in November 1973. It has two basic aims—to help the physically disabled and to coordinate some of the activities of several specialized societies set up to serve the deaf, the blind, and other handicapped persons (Mahmood,

1974). As the name implies, this society is only regional in nature, serving essentially the needs of handicapped people of one of 13 states which make up Malaysia. The official address of this Society is c/o University Hospital, University of Malaya, Petaling Jaya.

The last organization to be formed at the national level to look after the interests of the hearing-impaired and other handicapped people is the Malaysian Council for Rehabilitation established at the end of 1973 and sited at 12, Lengkongan Jenjarom, Batu 2½ Jalan Kelang, Kuala Lumpur. Membership is open to national voluntary organizations concerned with the welfare of physically or mentally disabled persons and state societies formed for the coordination of the rehabilitation of all categories of disabled persons within the state. Thus, the National Society for the Deaf is represented. The aims of the Council are to coordinate the efforts of voluntary organizations, government agencies, and other organizations working in the field, and to promote the establishment and development of state societies for rehabilitation. So far, two state societies for the rehabilitation of the disabled have been formed, one in Malacca and the other in Selangor. The Malaysian Council for Rehabilitation also aims to encourage or promote projects for the training of the disabled, assist in the organization of production workshops for the employment of the disabled and the resettlement of suitably trained workers into normal employment, and stimulate cooperation in the prevention of accidents and disabling diseases. The Council is affiliated with Rehabilitation International and is also a member of the Rehabilitation International Regional Committee for East Asia and the Pacific. In September 1974 it successfully organized the second annual meeting of this international organization in Kuala Lumpur, attended by representatives from Hong Kong, Australia, Japan, Philippines, Indonesia, Thailand, and Singapore.

CONCLUSION

Formalized, organized facilities for the hearing impaired in Malaysia by both government and private voluntary organizations date back only to the last two decades. Limited success has been achieved, but expansion has been bogged down by inadequate fund allocation and shortage of specialized personnel. One related causal factor in Malaysia, as in many other countries, is the nonvisibility of a hearing handicap. It does not attract public or professional attention as does blindness or an obvious crippling condition.

In the words of Isa (1971), "a deaf person looks deceptively normal and independent." Thus, the seriousness of the hearing impairment and the special needs of the deaf and hard of hearing have often been ignored. However, there are signs in Malaysia that the public and the policy makers at the ministerial level are becoming more aware of the need to rehabilitate the hearing handicapped from preschool right up to university or vocational level. It is hoped that the right of every hearing-handicapped person to develop to his full potential like any other citizen will soon be realized and necessary action taken for comprehensive rehabilitation.

RELEVANT PERIODICALS PERTAINING TO MALAYSIA

1. Asian Blind, published for Asian Affairs Committee, World Council for the Welfare of the Blind by Singapore Association for the Blind, Singapore.
2. Asian Pacific Quarterly of Cultural and Social Affairs, The Cultural and Social Centre for the Asian and Pacific Region, Seoul.
3. Asian Federation of Obstetrics and Gynaecology Journal, Singapore.
4. Bulletin, Institute for Medical Research, Kuala Lumpur.
5. Bulletin of Statistics for Asia and the Far East, Ecafe, Bangkok.
6. Bulletin of the Institute of Southeast Asia, Nanyang University, Singapore.
7. Bulletin of the Public Health Society (Malaysia), Kuala Lumpur.
8. Bulletin of the Unesco Regional Office for Education in Asia, Bangkok.
9. Development Forum, Malaysian Centre for Development Studies, Government Printers, Kuala Lumpur.
10. Dewan Masyarakat, Dewan Bahasa dan Pustaka, P.S. 803, Kuala Lumpur (in Malay).
11. Educator, National Union of Teachers, Malaysia, 321C Jalan Tuanku Abdul Rahman, Kuala Lumpur.
12. International Review of Education, Unesco Institute for Education, Hamburg.
13. Intisari, Malaysian Sociological Research Institute, 28 N. Oxley Mansions, Oxley Road, Singapore.
14. Journal, Ministry of Education, Malaysia, Federal Inspectorate of Schools, Jalan Maxwell, Kuala Lumpur.
15. Journal Pelajaran, Education Society, University of Malaya, Kuala Lumpur. (In Malay and English.)
16. Jurnal Pendidikan, Journal of Education Research, Universiti Malaya.
17. Kajian Ekonomi Malaysia, Economic Association of Malaysia, Department of Economics, University of Malaya, Kuala Lumpur.
18. Kebajikan, Ministry of Welfare Services, Kuala Lumpur. (In Malay and English.)
19. Malayan Scientist, Science Society, University of Malaya, Kuala Lumpur.
20. Malaysian Dental Journal, Malayan Dental Association, Singapore.
21. Malaysian Journal of Education, Educational Journal Press, P. O. Box 53, Kuala Lumpur.

22. Malaysian Journal of Science, Faculty of Science, University of Malaya.
23. Malaysian Scientific Directory, Malaysian Scientific Association, Kuala Lumpur.
24. Masa'alah Pendidikan, Bulletin on Education Problems, Faculty of Education, University of Malaya.
25. Mastika, Syarikat Percetakan Utusan Melayu, Jalan Chan Sow Lin, Kuala Lumpur. (In Malay.)
26. Medical Journal of Malaya, Straits Times Press (M) Ltd., River Valley Road, Singapore 9. Journal of the Malayan Medical Association.
27. Medicasia, Asian Regional Medical Student Association, Singapore.
28. New Contact, Publication of the Malaysian Guild of Educators of the Blind, 193, Jalan Abdul Samad, Kuala Lumpur.
29. Pendidek, Specialist Teachers Training Institute, Jalan Cheras, Kuala Lumpur. (In Malay and English.)
30. Psychology Echoes, Editor, 29 Ipoh Road, Kuala Lumpur, Magazine of the Kuala Lumpur Psychology Club.
31. Regional English and Language Centre Journal, a journal of English language teaching in Southeast Asia, Singapore.
32. Research Circulars, Institute for Medical Research, Kuala Lumpur.
33. Sarawak Teacher, Business Manager, City Bookstore, Wong Nai Siong Road, Sibu, Sarawak.
34. Sabah Society Journal, P.O. Box 547, Kota Kinabalu, Sabah.
35. Southeast Asian Journal of Tropical Medicine and Public Health, The Seameo Central Coordinating Board for Tropical Medicine and Public Health, Bangkok.

LITERATURE CITED

Baal, J. V. 1964. Education in non-western countries. Internat. Rev. Educ. 10: 5.

Berita Tulina. 1971. Newsletter of the National Society for the Deaf, July, p. 1, Malaysia.

Chua, T. T. 1970. Special education in Malaysia. J. Kementerian Pelajaran, Malaysia (Ministry of Education, Malaysia) 15(37): 95.

Chua, T. T. 1974. Education for exceptional children in Malaysia–Integration or Segregation? Malaysian J. Educ. 11: 26–30.

Chua, T. T. 1974a. Education of the Disadvantaged in Malaysia–An Overview. Presented at the Annual Seminar of the Malaysia Association for Education on Contemporary Issues in Malaysian Education, August 2–4, Kuala Lumpur.

Chua, T. T. 1974b. Facing New Challenges in Special Education. Presented at the Annual Methodist Head Teachers' Conference, December 1–4, Cameron Highlands.

Department of Statistics. No date. Monthly Statistical Bulletin of West Malaysia, p. 3, December 1971, Kuala Lumpur.

Department of Statistics. 1972. 1970 Population and Housing Census of Malaysia: Community Groups, March 15, p. 24, Kuala Lumpur.

Department of Statistics. 1973. Social Statistics Bulletin, Peninsular Malaysia, p. 221. 1969–1971, Kuala Lumpur.
Federal Department of Information. 1972. Ministry of Information. Malaysia 1971. Official Yearbook, pp. 2–17. Government Printer, Malaysia.
Federation School for the Deaf. 1970. The Official Opening of the Federation School for the Deaf Malaysia (Chenderamata bagi mengingati Pembukaan Rasmi Sekolah Kanak-Kanak Pekak Persekutuan Pulau Pinang Malaysia), February 28, 62 pp.
Ghazali, Y. 1974. Department of Education, Sarawak. Communication of July 26, Ref. 54/ED/AS.1398.
Government of Malaysia. 1973. Mid-Term Review of the Second Malaysia Plan 1971–75, p. 30. Government Press, Kuala Lumpur.
Hamzah, S. 1974. Education in the Social Sciences. *In* Kebajikan, Vol. 3, No. 1, p. 50. The Ministry of Welfare Services, Kuala Lumpur.
Hickes, J. M. 1962. Education of the deaf child. J. Kementerian Pelajaran Persekutuan Tanah Melayu (Ministry of Education, Federation of Malaya) 5(3): 157.
International Labour Office. 1970. Report to the Government of Malaysia on the Development of Vocational Rehabilitation Services for the Handicapped, p. 7, Geneva.
Isa, S. Y. 1971. Community service in the rehabilitation of the deaf. *In* Commun. Develop. Cent., Sabah. Report of the Seminar on Social Work and the Community. July 25–29, p. 23. Kota Kinabalu.
Isa, S. Y. 1972. In a completed questionnaire (FP 90/72) dated April 4.
Isa, S. Y. 1974. Personal communication of May 15.
Lee, E. 1968. Deaf Education in Malaysia. *In* International Society for Rehabilitation of the Disabled. Fourth Pan Pacific Rehabilitation Conference. Rehabilitation: New Talent for the Community, p. 415. September 1–7, Hong Kong.
Mahmood, M. 1974. Inaugural welcoming speech. *In* Newsletter, Selangor Society for Rehabilitation of the Disabled, No. 1, p. 2. March.
Malay Mail. 1974. November 20, p. 14. Kuala Lumpur.
Ministry of Education, Malaysia. 1973. Dropout Study (English version), p. 57. Dewan Bahasa dan Pustaka, Kuala Lumpur.
Ministry of Education, Singapore. 1972. Education in Singapore. 2nd Ed., p. 56. Educational Publications Bureau, Singapore.
Seymour, J. M. 1972. The Rural School and Rural Development Among the Iban of Sarawak, p. 328. Ph.D. dissertation, Stanford University.
Smilansky, M., and S. Smilansky. 1967. Intellectual advancement of culturally disadvantaged children: An Israel approach for research and action. *In* Internat. Rev. Educ. 13: 417–418.
Tan, M. 1972. In a completed questionnaire (FP 90/72) dated October 10.
The Treasury, Malaysia. 1974. Economic Report 1974–75, November 12, pp. 79 and lxxxv. Government Printer, Kuala Lumpur.

chapter 16

Communication for Hearing-handicapped People in Japan

Yoshitatsu Nakano, Ed.D.

According to a Ministry of Health and Welfare survey conducted in October 1970, the hearing-handicapped population of Japan was 219,200, of which 18,200 were under 18 and 201,000 were over 18. A tradition of misunderstanding and prejudice with regard to the hearing handicapped is deeply rooted in Japan, and they experience numerous social difficulties which in turn further limit the opportunities of the hearing handicapped.

The realization of the residual abilities and latent development potential of the hearing handicapped and the maximum growth of those abilities they do possess to enable them to lead as fulfilling lives as possible, in spite of their hearing handicaps, is referred to as rehabilitation. In other words, rehabilitation involves the restoration of the greatest possible degree of physical, mental, social, occupational, and economic usefulness to the hearing handicapped.

However, in the case of congenital or early acquired handicaps, *rehabilitation*—particularly the prefix *re-*—is not apt. The objectives and nature of guidance and training differ from those for persons whose handicap is acquired later. For this reason, the word *rehabilitation* is taken to include habilitation but, in more and more cases, the word habilitation can be used meaningfully to distinguish the individual and practical features of guidance and training during childhood. However, the border between rehabilitation and habilitation is not clearly defined and the two overlap in usage, nor does the author see a need to separate them. In this chapter, rehabilitation should be understood to include habilitation as well.

Rehabilitation includes: (1) psychological, (2) educational, (3) social, (4) vocational, and (5) medical rehabilitation. The effects of hearing handicaps are most directly and intensively displayed in the area of speech. The diminished ability to communicate inhibits social participation. Thus, the emphasis of rehabilitation is on improving the ability to communicate.

DEFINITION OF AURAL REHABILITATION

In the rehabilitation of the hearing handicapped, particularly in the case of congenital or severe handicaps, the stress has been on improving visual communication capacity, while auditory communication was relegated to a subordinate role and treated lightly if at all. But with the breathtaking developments in electronics, and equipment, and audiology, it was found that, if residual hearing (in the case of congenital and severe handicaps) was used systematically from the early stages, there were considerable chances for auditory communication. In the present rehabilitation of the hearing handicapped, early diagnosis and early fitting of hearing aids are a matter of course while auditory and visual communication are integrated. This is known as aural rehabilitation. In other words, aural rehabilitation is defined as the development of maximum possible communicative ability through maximum extension of auditory communicative ability to compensate for the hearing handicap, and integration of both auditory and visual communicative abilities. This involves, chiefly, training in hearing aid use, auditory training, speechreading (lipreading) training, speech conservation training supplemented by social orientation, individual counseling, etc. Aural rehabilitation for hearing-handicapped children basically seeks to have the child acquire speech and language. Hearing aid instruction and auditory training provide many stimuli through the ear and develop the disposition to acquire speech and language through the ear. Such aural rehabilitation is often termed *aural habilitation.*

In the case of people who lose their hearing after the acquisition of speech, rehabilitation involves hearing aid training, auditory and speech training if the person is sensorineural hearing handicapped (possessing residual hearing and speech ability), or speech training in the case of sudden deafness. In the case of chronic otitis media, there are hearing restorative surgery and auditory and speech training if required. In any case, treatment is individual as a rule, with counseling to supplement learning ability and social orientation.

Aural rehabilitation is carried out in speech and hearing clinics, rehabilitation centers, schools for the deaf, and special classes for the hard of hearing. Childhood rehabilitation takes place chiefly in the home. It is done by audiologists, speech therapists, speech pathologists, otologists, deaf educators, and educators for hard-of-hearing children, while parents and psychologists also play an important role.

HISTORICAL OVERVIEW

Prewar Period

Until the foundation in 1870 of the Kyoto Institution of Education for the Deaf and Blind, there was no organized educational or medical program for the hearing handicapped. Another institution was opened in Tokyo in 1880. Both relied primarily on the manual method of training with speech training in name only. Attempts were made at the Tokyo institution to utilize residual hearing. The acoustic fan, a nonelectric hearing device imported from the U.S.A., was used. This audiphone was made of a sheet of flexible vulcanite (hard rubber) in the shape of a fan with a handle. It appears to have been used only experimentally.

The Tokyo Society of Oto-rhino-laryngology was organized by Dr. Kanasugi in 1893, and studies in this field continued under the inspiration of German medicine. From the 1920's on, American and German influences, together with Japan's own work, were central, and education by the oral method became paramount.

In 1925 Dr. Hoshino developed and tested the Hoshinophone, a hearing aid using the concept of bone-conducted sound via the teeth. It did not prove practical, however. During this period there was a flood of data on the education of hearing-handicapped children from Germany and the U.S.A. In 1926 a special class for the hard of hearing was set up in the school for the deaf. In the 1930's, increased interest in the use of residual hearing led to the practical use of electric hearing devices. Audiometry was undertaken using the pure tone audiometer, and studies, which came to be used in education, were made on degree and type of hearing loss. In 1934 special training for the hard of hearing was initiated in ordinary elementary schools. Here, a simple modification of the M. Goldstein hearing aid was used.

Virtually nothing was done for adults, and their social rights were frequently not respected and they were kept at a social distance. In the war years of the 1930's, medical and educational studies on hearing handicaps and rehabilitation of those suffering from them were abandoned. Development of hearing aids lagged; they were not very effective. A lack of interest on the part of instructors and pupils meant no progress or development.

Postwar Period

After the war, seminars on the audiometer and group hearing aids were held under the auspices of Scap's Information and Education Bureau;

these rekindled interest. The Whitehurst auditory training program was also used.

In 1947 the Fundamental Law of Education and the School Education Law were enacted, and compulsory education for deaf children was set at 9 years, with implementation from 1948. The Child Welfare Law was also enacted in 1947, providing for hearing aids for the hearing-handicapped child and the nationwide establishment of homes for the deaf and mute children. In 1950 the Law for the Welfare of the Disabled was passed, providing hearing aids and a handbook of identification. Rehabilitation centers for the deaf and mute were also set up in large cities under this law and the following were initiated for the hearing handicapped: (1) medical diagnosis and treatment, (2) social adaptation therapy, (3) general educational guidance, (4) auditory and speech examinations, (5) speech and auditory therapy, and (6) occupational therapy. The Research Society on the Hard of Hearing, composed chiefly of otologists, was formed in 1950 and 5 years later became the Japan Audiological Society. Real progress in audiology began to take place.

The School Health Act was enacted in 1958, providing for health examinations and related treatments during school attendance and periodic examinations and treatment in schools. Examinations included auditory and otorhinolaryngological disorders. Beginning in the 1960's, one saw the corresponding establishment throughout the country of classes for the hard of hearing.

During the postwar era, Japanese medicine and pedagogy have been heavily influenced by developments in the U.S.A. There has been an active incorporation of American speech pathology, audiology, and educational methods which have been quite successful. International exchanges have flourished, and Japan has both held and participated in numerous international conferences. Interest in services to handicapped children has grown since 1950, and significant progress has been experienced.

GENERAL DESCRIPTION OF PRESENT PROGRAMS OF AURAL HABILITATION AND REHABILITATION

Aural Habilitation Programs for Children under 3 Years of Age

There is only a very small number of programs for children under the age of 3 years. The National Centre for Speech and Hearing Disorders (Tokyo), the Tokyo Metropolitan Rehabilitation Centre for the Physically and Mentally Handicapped, the National Institute for Special Education, and prefectural Rehabilitation Centres engage in consultation and habilitation.

There is also a number of clinics, including the Hearing Clinic for Mothers and Children by the Kobayashi Institute of Physical Research (Tokyo), the Rion Better Hearing Clinic (Osaka), the Hearing and Speech Clinic for Deaf Infants at the Ohmotoryo (Okayama), the Visual-Auditory Research Institute of the Fukuoka Medical Association (Fukuoka). These provide therapy up to the age of 6 years. Below is a description of the habilitation program at the Hearing Clinic for Mothers and Children, established in 1966, which provides the following services: (1) audiological diagnosis, (2) hearing aid selection and fitting, (3) 1-day hearing aid classes for parents, (4) 3-month auditory training for infants and young children (0–2 years) and preschool children (3–5 years). Auditory training uses portable hearing aids, but the program is parent oriented rather than client oriented. Most of the children completing this program are integrated into kindergartens or normal schools. The average hearing loss is 60 dB. Correspondence courses are available to parents in remote areas. Since opening, the clinic has conducted hearing tests on 600 children, and 200 have completed the auditory training course.

In addition, schools for the deaf conduct courses for 2-year-olds meeting from once or twice a week to once every 3 months. The only ones who can participate in these programs are those who are enthusiastic about child therapy and who have the financial resources and time available. Most children under the age of 3 years receive no particular therapy.

Habilitation and Rehabilitation Programs for Children 3–15 Years of Age

Most of the children in this age group receive training in schools for the deaf or classes for the hard of hearing. The Japanese school system under the control of the Ministry of Education provides 9 years of compulsory education for all children. Therefore, hearing-handicapped children, ranging from children with only a slight hearing loss to the totally deaf, have the same rights and obligations with regard to the 9 years of compulsory schooling as normal hearing children have. The law obliges parents to send their children to elementary school for 6 years and to lower secondary school for 3 years. The age of admission to elementary school is 6 years.

Hearing-handicapped children are placed either in a school for the deaf, special classes for the hard of hearing in ordinary schools, or are given separate individual instruction in ordinary schools. Usually, deaf children enroll in schools for the deaf. Typical schools for the deaf have programs which extend from preschool through the twelfth grade on a single campus. The program consists of preschool, elementary, lower secondary, and upper secondary school classes. Some schools have a postgraduate course with a major in a specific type of vocational training for 1 or 2 years. Day and residential pupils follow academic and vocational programs.

Table 1 shows the number of schools for the deaf in Japan and their pupils and teachers. In addition to this, there are 242 public day classes for the hard of hearing. The pupils in these classes total 1,489. The number of classes for the hard of hearing is strikingly low in proportion to the need.

Preschool Education Preschool education in Japan is voluntary. With few exceptions, these preschools are run as day schools. Children are usually accepted at age 3 or 4. A completely oral, private day school for the deaf admits deaf babies as early as possible after diagnosis. Their prime goals include parental guidance and education, as well as the education of the babies and the early fitting of hearing aids. At the preschool stage in Japanese schools for the deaf, all children are fitted with hearing aids, and auditory training occupies an important place in preschool education. In recent years, increasing numbers of these children have been integrated into normal kindergartens and elementary schools.

Elementary Education Education in the elementary grades in both schools for the deaf and in ordinary schools follows the curriculum prescribed by the Ministry of Education and seeks to provide mental, moral, physical, and esthetic education to hearing-handicapped children. The subject matter in elementary schools for the deaf includes Japanese, science, arithmetic, social studies, physical education, music, art, handicrafts, and homemaking. In addition, moral education, special activities (excursions, sports meetings, class days, homeroom activities, etc.), and special instruction are provided.

Special instruction includes hearing testing, hearing aid selection, auditory training, speech therapy and evaluation, language pronunciation and articulation training, and evaluation and various types of counseling—a systematic program of aural habilitation or rehabilitation. For first graders, this comes to 6 hours a week.

Class size is regulated, the standard size being eight pupils. In Japan, the publication of textbooks for all subjects for use in the compulsory curriculum requires the approval of the Ministry of Education. Authorized textbooks are provided free of charge to all pupils. The Ministry of Education has created a number of texts for use in schools for the deaf. Most schools use the normal textbooks for the first 3 years. Every school is provided with group hearing aids, auditory trainers, language masters, and visible speech apparatus, and most children are fitted with portable hearing aids.

Secondary Education Secondary education consists of the compulsory lower secondary school and the upper secondary school attended by

Table 1. Schools for the deaf in Japan (May 1, 1973)

Type of schools	Number of schools	Pupils					Teachers			
		Total	Kindergarten	Elementary	Lower secondary	Upper secondary	Full-time	Part-time	Dormitory personnel	Other
National	1	363	71	92	64	136	70	22	9	30
Municipal	100	14,642	2,129	5,385	3,025	4,103	4,554	170	1,027	1,458
Private	1	114	37	54	23	0	28	1	0	11
Totals	102	15,119	2,237	5,531	3,112	4,239	4,652	193	1,036	1,499

the majority of the graduates of the former. The lower secondary school has the following curriculum: required subjects–Japanese, social studies, mathematics, science, music, fine arts, health and physical education, and industrial arts or homemaking; elective subjects–English and vocational guidance. The upper secondary curriculum provides some courses in vocational training, usually printing, photography, tailoring, drafting, machine shop, laundry, hairdressing and beautician work, metal crafts, dental technician work, woodworking, and furniture design.

In both upper and lower secondary schools as in elementary schools, special instruction is provided with a planned program of auditory rehabilitation, which occupies, however, only 2 hours a week.

Postsecondary Education The deaf persons who desire an education beyond the secondary level attend either a university or a junior college for the normally hearing or a postgraduate course in the upper secondary school for the deaf. In the latter, little attention is given to the use of hearing.

Rehabilitation Programs for Persons over 16 Years of Age

There are few such programs. There are the Tokyo Metropolitan Rehabilitation Centre for the Physically and Mentally Handicapped and some prefectural centers, as well as the Rehabilitation Centres for the Deaf and Mute in Kyoto and Tokyo and the National Centre for Speech and Hearing Disorders. The Rehabilitation Centre for the Deaf and Mute is a public center which provides medical treatment, auditory training, speech training, training in fingerspelling and sign language, and other kinds of rehabilitation training as required. Training usually takes 1–1½ years. The number of people admitted at both centers is 50 a year.

At the National Centre for Speech and Hearing Disorders, the program takes 1 year and 100 people are admitted. The program includes: (1) medical diagnosis and therapy, (2) counseling and social adaptation guidance, (3) general education, (4) speech and auditory therapy–including fitting of hearing aids, enunciation training, speech training, sign language, and other communication related training, and (5) occupational therapy–printing, typing, photocomposition, cleaning, electricity, and tailoring.

Other Programs

Japan's only public broadcasting company, NHK, puts out a "TV School for the Deaf" once a week aimed at the mothers of the hearing handicapped. There is also a weekly speech therapy program. In various parts of the country, there are homes for deaf and dumb children, 21 public and

13 private, with 2,469 pupils as of November 1973. These homes are actively introducing aural rehabilitation.

To facilitate school attendance by the hearing handicapped, the government makes available various subsidies. It also funds group hearing aids and equipments for auditory training. Hearing aids are provided and repaired for possessors of the Handbook for Identification of the Physically Handicapped (see Rehabilitation Procedures).

DIAGNOSTIC PROCEDURES

The diagnosis of hearing handicaps involves the cooperation of otorhinolaryngologists, audiologists, speech therapists, clinical psychologists, teachers of the hearing handicapped, and psychiatrists. In most cases, however, diagnosis is made by otorhinolaryngologists, often with the assistance of speech therapists, psychologists, and educators. When medical treatment is possible according to otological test results, this is preferred. In any case, the case history is examined first. The case history interview covers the following: (1) birth history, (2) medical history, (3) family history, (4) developmental history, (5) sociopsychological history, (6) speech and language history, (7) auditory history, and (8) educational history and also the present situation.

In Japan, medical diagnosis is widely accepted, but educational and psychological diagnosis is not yet established. The main types of examination used in diagnosing hearing handicaps are the following:

Hearing Test

Newborn Infants In order to make early identification of neonate hearing, examinations use the auditory responses instinctive in the newborn infant as signals. These auditory responses include eye blinking or widening, turning of the head forward or away from the sound, movement of the limbs or cessation of bodily movements, rousing and sucking, or a generalized startle response known as Moro's reflex. In Japan, the Infant Audiometer TB-02 (Rion) using 1,000 Hz and 3,000 Hz warble tones is available commercially. Sounds at 40 dB and 70 dB are produced for 1–2 seconds, and the infant's responses are screened. There are problems regarding usefulness and validity, and it is used only in a small number of hospitals.

Infants In infancy, simple instinctive responses give way to learned responses. It is easier to examine responses to low intensity meaningful sounds than to high intensity sounds. The infant responds to the sounds of cups, the mother's voice, rattles, etc. The method used is SRA (startle response audiometry) in a free field.

Very Young Children During this period, from 6 months–3 years, the response to meaningful sounds increases. The orientation reflex of turning in the direction of interest in response to a sound develops more fully; SRA testing may be accompanied by COR (conditioned orientation reflex) testing or by play audiometry.

Preschool Children Play audiometry is predominant, including peep show tests, tunnel tests, number game tests, and other kinds of play audiometry. For some children, standard pure tone audiometry is possible. Results of research in this area have been particularly revealing (Figure 1).

Children Pure tone and speech audiometry are used ordinarily, as with adults. Today all audiometric results are expressed according to JIS (Japan Industrial Standard)-1956. These were established by the Japanese Standard Association in 1956. JIS-1956 is closer to ASA-1951 than to ISO-1964, and revisions are under consideration (Table 2).

In addition to the types of examination cited above, EEG audiometry, ERA, and GSR audiometry are used primarily with children who cannot or will not cooperate, the mentally retarded or malingerers. Screening tests for children over 6 may be by individual by pure tone audiometer or by whispering familiar words and numbers from a distance of 6 meters. In the case of pure tone audiometry, tones of 1,000 Hz and 4,000 Hz are produced at 20 dB, and the patient is asked if he heard them.

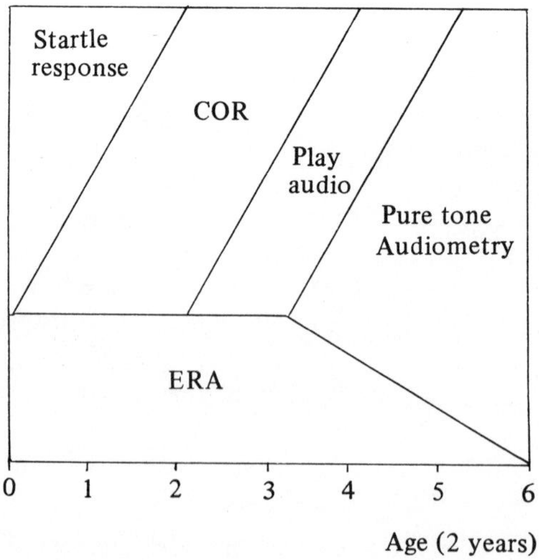

Figure 1. Age and selection of examination method (Tsuiki, 1972).

Table 2. Standard reference threshold–sound pressure levels in decibels

Hz	1951 ASA	1964 ISO	1956 JIS
125	54.5	45.5	54
250	39.5	24.5	40
500	25	11	25
1,000	16.5	6.5	17
1,500	(16.5)[a]	6.5	17
2,000	17	8.5	17
3,000	(16)[a]	7.5	16
4,000	15	9	15
6,000	(17.5)[a]	8	18
8,000	21	9.5	21

[a]The figures in parentheses are interpolations.

Intelligence Testing

There are no completely satisfactory tests in terms of reliability and validity. For children under 6 years, the WPPSI (Japanese edition), PBT (picture block test), Murayama Non-Verbal Test, the Owaki-Kohs Block Design Test, and so on are used. Development tests are often used to measure overall mental development rather than intelligence per se. These include the Tsumori Developmental Scale and the Enjoji Developmental Test. In the 6–15 age group, the WISC Performance Scale, Owaki-Kohs Block Design Test, Tanaka B-type or A-type Paper Test are used. For children 16 years of age or older, the WAIS Performance Scale or B-type and A-type Paper Test are used.

Social Maturity Scales

These include the Diagnostic Scale for Social Maturity (Suzuki), the S-M Test for Social-life Ability, etc. They are both simple, but the results vary greatly with the rater.

Other Tests

Behavioral observation techniques are often used with children and infants. Research and development of examination methods for language ability and personality assessment are in progress.

REHABILITATIVE PROCEDURES

Habilitation and rehabilitation of infants and children use primarily the oral method. Oral methods are based on speechreading (lipreading), speech, and auditory training. There is a pure oral method, which allows only minimal employment of natural gestures: anything other than oral method is excluded from the place of instruction. This method is very effective in the development of speech and thought in the hearing handicapped in early education. They can be assured of mental development equivalent to that of normal hearing persons and can communicate freely with the normally hearing. The level of achievement is frequently much higher than can be expected with persons educated by other methods. This cannot be achieved with children of all ages.

In facilities for the rehabilitation of adults, the oral method is supplemented by fingerspelling and sign language in a combined method of communication. Below is a discussion of actual training methods.

Language Training

In the case of preschool children, whose every sort of oral communication must be understood by parents and teachers, the purpose of speech training is to encourage the child to want to speak spontaneously and attempt oral communication. This means that the correction of pronunciation and enunciation is put off until the child has acquired basic speaking skills. Hearing children understand what is said to them before they begin to talk. The same development is conceivable with the hearing handicapped. Understanding precedes expression. Hearing and speech are indispensable for an understanding of language. Attempts to have the child use only his voice are futile, although they are rarely undertaken.

The utterance of speech presupposes some intricate neuromuscular coordination. The physical aspects of speech are an important key to speech acquisition in the case of the hearing-handicapped child whose auditory feedback is deficient or absent. Therefore, sensory and auditory training must be supplemented by basic training in phonation and enunciation, and various techniques have been devised.

Basic training includes: (1) games in which vocalization is easy, (2) familiarization with vibrations of various sounds and voices, (3) breathing training, (4) babbling (continuous practice in bilabial stops and bilabial nasal sounds), (5) knocking (continuous practice in dental plosives such as *t, d, n* and *r*), and (6) tongue exercises. These are practiced in game form—using paper, elastic, pingpong balls, cups, straws, pinwheels, etc.

In vocalization training, information is provided as to how various sounds are pronounced. Many attempts have been made to present pronunciation rationally. Wide use is made of diagrams showing the position of the mouth for vowels and the process of articulation for consonants. Actual teaching takes place as follows. The children are shown diagrams and the mouth of the teacher and asked to imitate and articulate while comparing their own mouths with the teacher's. For the mechanical monitoring of this process, there is the visible speech apparatus. Repetitive exercises are required in articulation training, and the child must be motivated and encouraged to continue. Enunciation is related to speech and auditory training and carried out in an atmosphere of naturalness.

Thus, language training demands the cooperation and endurance of both the teacher and the pupil, and the level of achievement at present is rather low. Generally referred to as the "9-year-old wall," achievement continues until about the third or fourth grades, after which learning stagnates and no progress is observed. The language growth of children at this time is very slow. Reading ability and progress through the stages of compulsory education lag as the years advance. Their written compositions are often monotonous and have random orders of words with incoherent portions. The style is frequently telegraphic with many grammatical mistakes. Improvements in teaching techniques underway include thorough early training in the written language and instruction of reading.

In the case of adults, speech conservation training and training to encourage language development are carried out. The level of general education is being raised, and training in reading and writing is coordinated with speech training.

Auditory Training

The training objectives during the introductory period are: (1) earliest possible fitting of hearing aids and encouragement of interest in amplified sound and speech, (2) creation of a listening attitude through provision of sounds in a normal environment, (3) creation of auditory-vocal feedback, and (4) increased speech communication ability and achievement of a general education program.

The specific sequence of training is described below. The child is fitted with hearing aids. Even if no hearing aid is fitted, the child is addressed loudly close to his ear or ordinary speech is repeated several times. Using noisemaking toys or musical instruments, he is made aware of when the noise is on or off. He is taught to respond actively to the on or off situations and to create the on state by himself. Articles which produce familiar, pleasant sound are made available, and more interesting sounds are provided. He is encouraged to take pleasure in sounds he produces himself. He is taught to orient himself quickly to noise sources and to discriminate environmental and musical sounds of sufficient loudness. He is then taught to recognize speech patterns and reproduce voice intonations. He is taught to pick out the essential words in short sentences and then to enunciate these words himself. Two- or three-word sentences are spoken and acted out to teach him to understand them. Emphasis is not on natural gestures as much as on meaningful vocal expression so that he will come to be able to express his own desires and commands to others. He is taught to see simple utterances as a key to understanding situations. He, thus, gradually learns to understand longer utterances. During the first introductory stage, the unisensory method predominates, but, depending on the child, the multisensory method may be used instead or together.

Instruction of school-age children is essentially the same as the introductory stage. Individual and group instruction is given using tape recorders, pitch indicators, visible speech apparatus, auditory trainers, language masters, videocorders, etc.

In adult auditory training, it must first be diagnosed by an otologist or other specialist that hearing loss does not respond to medical treatment. Then training proceeds in accordance with the following considerations: (1) coordination with psychological and social counseling, (2) training on the basis of individual vocational and economic needs, (3) training usually linked to speech training, and (4) concern for language conservation training. Training is begun only after an individual has been judged capable of profiting from it in proportion to the time spent.

Suitable valid standards for measurement of auditory training effectiveness have not yet been established. Training effectiveness is assessed arbitrarily and may run to excesses of praise and confidence in both directions.

Specialists in auditory training are extremely few. The work is tackled enthusiastically in schools for the deaf and in classes for the hard of hearing, but it is sustained by a small number of people. Services to adults are hampered by limited space and personnel.

Speechreading (Lipreading)

The word lipreading is gradually falling into disuse in Japan, in favor of speechreading. Speechreading is taught along with pronunciation and auditory training. The most important thing in teaching speechreading is to get the pupil to watch the speaker's face carefully. In the introductory stage of child habilitation, the child is taught to associate lip movements with toys, animals, and other interesting objects and to become able to identify things from mouth shapes. Instruction begins with easily recognizable mouth shapes and names of such familiar objects as parts of the body. Speechreading of questions, imperative forms, and ordinary phrases occurs in natural situations. As in ordinary language education, speechreading training is based on repeated practice with syllables, then words and sentences. There is also a whole method whereby single sentences are introduced from the outset. In practice, both are used together. In both methods, frequent repetition is fundamental. As the child grows older, his vocabulary may be expanded by written instruction. Serious thought should be given to the use of films, television, video tape recorders, etc., in speechreading training.

Unlike listening, speechreading requires concentration and proves fatiguing after long periods. Short periods continued daily are preferred.

In the case of severe hearing handicaps, one cannot expect to utilize auditory function. Comprehension of phonetic language must depend on visually grasping (speechreading) the message. This is highly abnormal and poses many difficulties. Only very few people would attempt to understand abstract concepts and complex semantic concepts through speechreading alone.

Speechreading training is applied to only a few of those who have lost their hearing after language acquisition. They are fitted with hearing aids and taught to speechread familiar words and sentences and news material. Training centers on the daily use of words and phrases. As progress occurs, training involves difficult materials that can be deduced from context.

Sign Language and Fingerspelling

The standard fingerspelling used in Japan is based on the system used in the U.S.A. Sign language is a graphic, meaning-oriented method of expression. It does not correspond, in a fixed manner, to the system of Japanese language. While it does follows the grammar of the written language, it has its own grammar. It uses hand motions and their rich expressive powers to communicate a small number of semantic concepts. Sign language is usually prohibited in school education, and it usually varies considerably from area to area. Recently, a sign language dictionary was published (Japanese Federation of Associations of the Deaf and Mute, 1969) and further consistency is expected. Children begin to learn sign language as soon as they enter the elementary course in the school for the deaf. It is not taught as such—the younger children pick it up from the older ones.

Training in fingerspelling and sign language for the hearing handicapped is given only at the National Centre for Speech and Hearing Disorders and a few other places and most people receive no systematic, thorough training at all. Nevertheless, many know and use this communication system.

In a survey the author participated in (Shimura et al., 1973), it was found that 953 pupils (aged 15–19) of schools for the deaf and 580 deaf adults said they did not understand sign language (below 5% in both groups). Fewer than 20% did not know fingerspelling. The adults showed a higher incidence of not knowing fingerspelling than the students, particularly women. The greatest number used both oral and sign language to communicate with other deaf or mutes. The figures were 70% for students 40% for adult women, and 30% for adult men. Many adults used sign language and fingerspelling, with more than 40% not using oral language in conjunction. For communication with ordinary people, most use oral language and writing. It seems strange that, while sign language is widely used in adult society, no systematic education in it is available.

There are programs to train sign language interpreters in the various cities and prefectures but, almost without exception, the participants are students and others with hearing. The trend is to use a sign language which follows Japanese syntax, and sign language used in conjunction with oral language is spreading gradually. Sign language and fingerspelling are indispensable in the lives of the hearing handicapped, and it is hoped very much that it will be disseminated properly. At present, sign language training is aimed at those with a basic grasp of language. Begining with names and words for familiar things, it proceeds to the expression of more complex ideas. The objective is to get hearing handicapped to understand first, then express.

Total Communication

Systematic instruction takes place only at one school, the Tochigi School for the Deaf, and rehabilitation centers for adults. They use the Tochigi simultaneous method, based on the simultaneous method used at Gallaudet College (Washington, D.C.) and the Soviet neo-oralism. The children begin with oral speech and fingerspelling, and sign language is added later. It is a special method used at that school and has not spread to other schools.

Hearing Aids

Hearing handicapped who have received a Handbook for the Identification of Disabled Persons under the Child Welfare Law or the Law for the Welfare of Disabled Persons are eligible to receive free hearing aids. According to a 1970 Ministry of Health and Welfare survey, 5,900 persons under 18 and 105,000 over 18 have received these free hearing aids. They have received the advice and guidance of specialists on selection and fitting in clinics, schools for the deaf, classes for the hard of hearing, etc. However, adults—particularly the hard-of-hearing aged—ordinarily receive almost no advice or training regarding selection and fitting. It is estimated that one-third of those who purchase them do not use them. According to one study, 3,400,000 need hearing aids, of which 2,600,000 know about them but do not wear one, 600,000 wear one, and 800,000 do not know about them. In Japan, an estimated 20,000 hearing aids are manufactured annually by National, Rion, Sony, Trio, Cortitone, etc.

Many are imported from Danabox, Siemens, Zenith, Dahlberg, Omniton, and Omikron. About three imported hearing aids are used to every 10 Japanese ones. Japanese hearing aids are exported to Europe and Southeast Asia. Compared with foreign hearing aids, the Japanese products are characterized as cheaper in value and worse in efficiency.

INTERPROFESSIONAL RELATIONSHIPS

If rehabilitation of the hearing handicapped is to develop in a desirable direction, interdisciplinary cooperation and a combined effort will be required in the related sciences. This has often been stated but, unfortunately with a few exceptions, has not been put into practice.

Fully qualified audiologists and speech pathologists are few and are unable to meet the demand. The number of physicians interested in rehabilitation is also small, and few psychologists are ready to deal with hearing handicaps. However, the number of applications is gradually spreading, and it is expected that interprofessional relations will improve as rehabilitation grows, leading to close cooperation.

FAMILY INVOLVEMENTS

Any child has already been subjected to influences from various quarters related to his personality and educational development by the time he reaches school age. In the case of a child born with a hearing handicap or acquiring one in his infancy, the first years of his life are a most important period, which may permanently determine the rest of his life. The child with normal hearing and no handicap affecting his communication ability will hear his own voice and the voices of others around him during these years and learn to talk. Without effort, he can acquire the ability to use the structure of language naturally. If the hearing-handicapped child wants to acquire speech and language, he will require special assistance from the early stages of his life.

Therefore, the family and particularly his parents play an important role. Their accurate knowledge and love are the most important things to the handicapped child. But ordinarily parents are disturbed and let down to find that their very own child has an incurable handicap. This is frequently a real bolt out of the blue to parents confronted with a hearing handicap whose etiology is not understood. Society's tolerance of the distorted speech brought on by handicapped hearing has historically been lower than its tolerance of other handicaps, such as visual handicaps. This mental anguish is lasting and profound.

To these parents, otorhinolaryngologists, speech therapists, psychologists, and teachers provide various forms of counseling and guidance. In some hospitals and clinics, and in most schools for the deaf, there are planned, systematic programs of parent education.

The principles of parent guidance, stated generally, are: (1) the parents must properly understand the child's problem and accept the child; (2) planned, systematic guidance; (3) understanding examination results and training content; (4) allocation of parental responsibilities in training; and (5) suggestions for home training.

Actual examples of parent education programs include training services with visits by specialists to the home. These services and correspondence courses have just begun in Japan. Generally from age 3 years, children in schools for the deaf are taught in the preschool sections and the parents are asked to attend and are given guidance as well. To show them how the children are taught and to let them assist the instructors, the parents are required to attend sessions over long periods in many schools for the deaf. When possible, parents are asked to spend 3 years in the preschool and 3 years in the elementary division (transportation for this is covered by the government). But this is a problem. In many schools for the deaf, children from age 2 up are trained one or two times a week, once monthly or once quarterly, with parent education too.

Table 3. Parent class program at heaing clinic for mothers and children

Meeting[a]	Topic
1	Orientation
2	Nature of hearing and causes of handicaps
3	How the handicapped child hears and countermeasures
4	Desirable development of auditory function
5	Desirable mental and physical development in the child
6	Desirable development of speech and language
7	Desirable family situation
8	Recent trends of education for the hearing-handicapped children
9	Psychodrama
10	Final discussion

From Kahashi et al. (1971).

[a]Two hours a week for 9 weeks.

Table 3 shows the parent education program used by the Hearing Clinic for Mothers and Children, sponsored by the Kobayashi Institute of Physical Research (Tokyo).

Parent education by television is flourishing in Japan. The nationwide network of NHK puts out "The TV School for the Deaf" and "Classroom for Speech Handicapped Children" once weekly for the speech- and hearing-handicapped child's education in the home. These are used by many parents. This may be a unique approach in the world.

Many books and pamphlets aimed at parents are distributed too. There are translations and discussions of *Your Deaf Child* (Myklebust, 1950) and the John Tracy Clinic Correspondence Course for Parents of Little Deaf Children.

TRAINING OF PROFESSIONALS FOR THE FIELD OF REHABILITATIVE AUDIOLOGY

The only serious training of specialists in this field is carried out by the Training Centre for Speech and Hearing Specialists attached to the National Centre of Speech and Hearing Disorders under the Ministry of Health and Welfare. There is also a short course for audiometrists held by the Japan Audiological Society.

Specialized knowledge and techniques in educational audiology are available through training courses for teachers of the hearing handicapped at six national universities and The National Institute for Special Education's Department of Speech and Hearing Handicapped, Research Institute of Rehabilitative Education, attached to Tokyo University of Education.

The Training Centre for Speech and Hearing Specialists attached to The National Center of Speech and Hearing Disorders (1 Toyama-cho, Shinjuku-ku, Tokyo) is described as follows: (1) purpose: to train speech and hearing specialists engaged in the rehabilitation of the speech and hearing handicapped; (2) date of establishment: April 1, 1971; (3) enrollment: 20; (4) length of course: 1 year; (5) condition of admission: graduation from 4-year college or university and less than 30 years old; (6) entrance examination: examination of scholastic ability, interview, and health examination; (7) others: there is no admission charge or tuition and no dormitory facilities are available. See Table 4 for the curriculum (the standard courses and hours offered at this training center during the 1-year training period).

Graduates are engaged in the following work at various social welfare institutions or hospitals: (1) examination and evaluation concerning speech, language, and hearing functions (this includes examination and

Table 4. Curriculum of the training center for speech and hearing specialists

Courses	Number of hours
Basic	
Introduction to Speech Pathology	15
Voice and Speech Science	150
Anatomy and Physiology	120
Statistics	30
Psychology	195
General Medical Science	90
Introduction to Social Welfare	30
Subtotal	630
Clinical	
Introductory courses[a]	315
Courses related to specific disorders	600
Subtotal	600
Total	1,545

[a]Introduction to Audiology, Introduction to Logopedics and Phoniatrics, Development and Education of Hearing Handicapped Children, Hearing Aids, Teaching of Language to the Hearing Handicapped, Measurement of Hearing, etc.

evaluation of hearing and speechreading abilities and examination and evaluation of speech and language abilities); (2) therapy, training, and guidance (including auditory training, speechreading training, planning and execution of speech and language therapy, prognostic evaluation; hearing aid evaluation and training in its adjustment; prediction of aggravated hearing loss and its prevention; planning and execution of speech and language therapy for various communication disorders, i.e., cleft palate speech, articulation disorders, delayed development of speech and language, stuttering, speech and language disorders related to cerebral palsy and aphasia, as well as their prognostic evaluation, and counseling of the family and patient). The Teacher Training Course of Hearing Handicapped is offered at six national universities: Kanazawa University, Tokyo Gakugei University, Osaka Kyoiku University, Hiroshima University, Ehime University, Fukuoka University of Education. Admission requirements include upper secondary school graduation and being under 18 years of age. The course length is 4 years. Fifteen students are admitted at each school per year. The curriculum includes: general education, foreign language, and physical education, as well as elementary or middle school teaching. Also included are special subjects related to education of the hearing handicapped. Those taught at Hiroshima are: (1) fundamentals: Education of Exceptional Children, Psychology of Exceptional Children, Brain Physiology, Clinical Psychology of Handicapped Children, History of Education for Handicapped Children, Theory and Practice of Psychological Testing, Social Psychological Problems of the Handicapped, Welfare for the Handicapped Children, and Research Methods of Handicapped. Each is a 30-hour elective subject; and (2) special: History, Education, and Guidance of the Hearing Handicapped; Theory and Method of Teaching to the Hearing Handicapped, Auditory Training, Education of the Speech Disorders, the Teaching of Speech and Language to the Hearing Handicapped, Special Problems of Teaching Speech and Language to the Hearing Handicapped, Psychology of the Hearing Handicapped, Special Problems in Psychology of the Hearing Handicapped, Hearing Tests and Other Testing, Physiology of Speech and Hearing, Pathology of Speech and Hearing, and Hearing Theory. These are 30-hour courses, most at which are required. There are also Observation and Practicum. Because of the nonexistent demand for highly competent specialists, only few exist. Opinions about the basic qualifications for audiologists differ. The Ministry of Health and Welfare is now considering a bill on recognized qualifications for audiologists and speech therapists. According to this bill, audiologists would be required to perform paramedic duties under doctors' supervision. The basic qualification of 3 years of special training after graduation from high school is strongly opposed, as competence is considered very low. An increasing number of voices are preferring that graduate education be required.

RESEARCH

Research in this field is carried on by physicians, speech therapists, speech pathologists, social workers, etc., working in the areas of audiology, psychology, deaf education, and otology. And the results of their researches are published in their respective professional society journals. Let us take a look at the most important of these, the Japan Audiological Society. A look at the papers published in the 1974 issues and the papers presented at the annual general meeting can be divided into seven categories: (1) general–1; (2) anatomy, physiology, and pathology of the ear–33; (3) psychology of hearing–6; (4) audiometry–73; (5) hard of hearing–48; (6) rehabilitation–26; and (7) others–2. In the area of audiometry, there were numerous papers on malingering, electrocochleographic examination, auditory brain stem response, infantile audiometry, EEG audiometry, ERA audiometry, Békésy audiometry, etc. Papers on the hard of hearing concentrated on variations in hearing ability. Under rehabilitation, as always, there are reports on problems related to hearing aid fitting, training and habilitation of hearing-handicapped children, integration of the hearing-handicapped child, etc. However, because of the membership make-up, most research seems to center on audiometry and variations in hearing capacity of the hard of hearing from a medical standpoint, while the number of studies on rehabilitation is increasing year by year, although it remains small. It is hoped that research in this area will develop further in the future. This situation reflects the fact that there are very few physicians with an interest in education and rehabilitation and psychologists ready to deal with hearing handicaps.

In Japan there have been excellent pioneering studies in this field, but the number of researchers remains small and the studies made are educational and smack of piecemeal work. This fact has also been spurred by the lack of a central research organization for the accumulation and exchange of research data. The few comprehensive studies that may be mentioned are Audiometric Test for Young Children (Goto, 1964) and Study of Hearing Handicapped Young Children (Suzuki, T., 1969).

In view of this situation, there is a real need for comprehensive (interdisciplinary) longitudinal research on all fields of rehabilitation.

PROFESSIONAL AND LAY ORGANIZATIONS AND ASSOCIATIONS RESPONSIBLE FOR THE HEARING HANDICAPPED

The Japn Audiological Society (Oto-rhino-laryngological Seminar, Faculty of Medicine, Tokyo University, 7 Hongo, Bunkyo-ku, Tokyo), formerly the Research Society on the Hard of Hearing, founded in 1955, is a professional society with membership confined to otolaryngologists, educators of the deaf, physiologists, psychologists, and technicians. Two-thirds of the 1,500 members are otolaryngologists. The Society holds: (1) a meeting for the presentation of papers on research topics, (2) a lecture meeting, (3) research meetings, (4) study of otological inspection, and (5) short training courses for audiometrists. In addition to these, it engages in investigations on hearing and the hard of hearing and in diffusion of knowledge on hearing and the hard of hearing. The Society's official organ *Audiology Japan* is the most important journal on audiology and related sciences.

The Oto-rhino-laryngological Society of Japan (c/o Château Takanawa, 3-33 Takanawa, Minato-ku, Tokyo), founded in 1893, is an academic organization engaged in research related to otorhinolaryngology. The Society holds an annual meeting for the presentation of papers and publishes the *Journal of Otolaryngology of Japan*. It has regional branches which meet 3–12 times a year.

Research Society for the Education of the Deaf in Japan (c/o Osaka Prefecture Sakai School for the Deaf, 1-70 Higashi-Uenoshiba, Sakai City, Osaka) was founded in 1959. The purpose of the organization is to carry on basic scientific research on the education of the hearing handicapped. It holds an annual conference and publishes *Soundless World.* It also publishes monographs. The 1,100 members include educators, physicians, psychologists, teachers, and welfare workers.

National Council of Teachers of Special Classes for Speech and Hearing Handicapped Children (c/o Nishimachi Elementary School, 2-23-17, Taito-ku, Tokyo), founded in 1971, has a membership of 1,000 and is comprised of the teachers of special classes for the hard of hearing and speech disorders at 400 schools. It holds an annual meeting, and its activities include information exchanges, research reports, studies, and attempts to raise the quality of education.

All Japan Conference of Teachers of the Deaf (Yokohama Municipal School for the Deaf, 144 Tokiwadai, Hodogaya-ku, Yokohama City, Kanagawa Prefecture), founded in 1966, is an organization for teachers of schools for the deaf. The Conference consists of nine subordinate organizations that serve at the local level. In 1974 there were 4,004 members. It holds an annual general meeting on the education of the deaf, symposium, a lecture meeting, and discussion meetings. It has assisted in stimulating and supporting research projects and the dissemination of research information. Its publications are the annual research papers and newsletters.

The Japanese Society of Education and Welfare for the Auditory Handicapped (c/o Sakurauchi Office, Japan Trust Bank Bldg., 2-3 Shiba-Tamura-cho, Minato-ku, Tokyo), founded in 1942, has a membership of 15,000. Its activities include: (1) promotion of education for the hearing handicapped, (2) studies and guidance on vocations for the hearing-handicapped, (3) publications of books and periodicals on hearing handicap education, (4) sponsorship of discussion meetings, (5) early education for 0–3-year-olds and parent guidance. Subsidiaries include: (1) Parent Association of Hard of Hearing Children (c/o S. Okahashi, 4-28 Komae High Town, 179 Koashidachi, Komae City, Tokyo) and (2) National Association of Parents of Speech and Hearing Handicapped Children (c/o 1-2-2 Horifune, Kita-ku, Tokyo).

Japan Society for Speech Pathology and Audiology (c/o H. Torii, 5-24-3, Minamimagome, Ota-ku, Tokyo), founded in 1972, carries on scientific research on topics related to auditory training and education of the hearing and speech handicapped and seeks to raise the standards of professionals working in the field. Activities are: (1) general and discussion meetings once or twice a year; (2) research meetings once a month; (3) discussion meetings; and (4) publication of a society journal. Three hundred-fifty people, primarily educators, comprise the membership.

The Japanese Federation of Associations of the Deaf and Dumb (110 Waseda-Tsurumaki-cho, Shinjuku-ku, Tokyo) is a national organization of deaf adults. As subordinate organizations, 62 local associations of deaf and dumb persons were formed all over Japan with a membership of about 10,000. The federation is one of the most innovative of all organizations of handicapped people. It publishes several books and pamphlets. The federation is dedicated to: (1) the defense of the rights and lives of all handicapped persons, (2) the acquisition of the right of the deaf and dumb to apply for driver's licenses, (3) the inclusion of a sign language interpreter in all public offices, and (4) the immediate establishment of welfare centers for the hearing handicapped, etc.

PERIODICALS ON HEARING PUBLISHED IN JAPAN

1. Audiology Japan (bimonthly), The Japan Audiological Society, c/o Otorhinolaryngological Seminar, Faculty of Medicine, Tokyo University, 7 Hongo, Bunkyo-ku, Tokyo.
2. Auditory Disorders (monthly), National Education Association of Auditory Disorders, c/o National School for the Deaf, attached to Tokyo University of Education, 2-2 Konodai, Ichikawa City, Chiba Prefecture.
3. Communication Disorder Research (quarterly), Publication Office of Communication Disorder Research, c/o The Research Institute for the Education of Exceptional Children, Tokyo Gakugei University, 4-780 Nukui-Kitamachi, Koganei City, Tokyo.
4. Japan Journal of Logopedics and Phoniatrics (three times annually), The Japan Society of Logopedics and Phoniatrics, c/o Research Institute of Logopedics and Phoniatrics, Faculty of Medicine, Tokyo University, 7 Hongo, Bunkyo-ku, Tokyo.
5. Soundless World–The Japanese Journal of Research of the Deaf (quarterly), Research Society of the Education of the Deaf in Japan, c/o Osaka Prefectural Sakai School for the Deaf, 1-70 Higashi-Uenoshiba, Sakai City, Osaka.
6. Journal of Otolaryngology of Japan (monthly), The Oto-rhino-laryngological Society of Japan, c/o Château Takanawa, 3-33 Takanawa, Minato-ku, Tokyo.

LITERATURE CITED

Committee of Study on Sign Language Method. 1969–1972. Our Sign Language. Vols. I, II, and III. Japanese Federation of Association of the Deaf and Mute, Tokyo. 192 p., 223 p., 204 p.

Goto, S. (ed.). 1964. Audiometric Test of Young Children. Maruzen, Nagoya. 170 p.

Goto, S. (ed.). 1972. The Hearing Handicapped. Ishiyaku Publishers, Tokyo. 480 p.

Hattori, H. 1971. A longterm observation of the hearing of children wearing hearing aids. Audiol. Jap. 14: 65–69.

Imai, H., and T. Hoshi. 1963. Auditory education for young deaf children. Bull. Faculty Educ. Tokyo Univ. Educ. 9: 141–151.

Iwaguchi, H., and T. Yokoyama. 1972. The efficiency of hearing aid use of hearing impaired children in special class. Audiot. Jap. 15: 585–592.

Kohashi, Y., C. Kanayama, N. Hayashi, I. Ito, and H. Imai. 1971. Hearing clinic for mothers and children of Kobayashi Institute of Physical Research. Audiol. Jap. 14: 180–188.

Kojima, Y. 1971. Rehabilitation for the Handicapped in Japan. The Japanese Society for Rehabilitation of the Disabled, Inc., Tokyo. 106 p.

Ministry of Education. 1970. Understanding and Instruction of Young Hearing Handicapped Children. Printing Office, Ministry of Finance, Tokyo. 247 p.

Ministry of Education 1973. Handbook of Auditory Training. Higashiyama Shobo, Kyoto. 370 p.

Nakano, Y. 1960–1961. A study on the factors which influence lipreading of deaf children. Bull. Faculty Educ. Tokyo Univ. Educ. 6: 141–146; 7: 315–342.

Nakano, Y. 1967 and 1970. Visual communication. Bull. Faculty Educ. Tokyo Univ. Educ. 13: 157–168; 14: 119–131; 16: 153–163.

Nakano, Y. 1968a. Speechreading performance and cue of their material. Jap. J. Spec. Educ. 5(2): 22–31.

Nakano, Y. 1968b. A study on relationships between speechreading ability and personality. Psychol. Educ. Except. Child. 72–86.

Nakano, Y. 1970. Psychology of hearing impaired children. *In* T. Sonohara et al.(eds.), Lectures on Child Psychology, 10, pp. 115–179. Kaneko Shobo, Tokyo.

Nakano, Y. (ed.). 1971–1972. Fundamentals of Auditory Education. Parts I–IV. Research Society of Education for Hearing Handicapped. Tokyo University of Education, Tokyo. 131 p., 146 p., 120 p., 124 p.

Ojima, S., and Y. Nakano. 1961–1963. An experimental study of lipreading practice. Parts I, II, III. Bull. Faculty Educ. Tokyo Univ. Educ. 7: 243–287; 8: 91–120; 9: 163–167.

Okamoto, M., H. Shono, S. Sakamoto, T. Ozawa, and K. Fukuyama. 1972. A new system for the individual fitting of hearing aid. Audiol. Jap. 15: 604–613.

Owada, K., and Y. Nakanishi. 1972. Introduction to Hearing and Speech Disorders. 2nd Ed. Igaku Shoin, Tokyo. 368 p.

Research Society of the Education of the Deaf in Japan (ed.). 1972–1974. Fundamentals of Auditory Education. Parts V, VI. 122 p., 64 p.

Seki, I. 1972. A study on speechreading training in hearing impaired adults. Bull. Natl. Center Speech Hear. Disord. 1970: 11–20.

Shimura, H. et al. 1973. Research survey on communication of deaf. Bull. Natl. Center Speech Hear. Disord. 1971: 41–60.

Suzuki, T. 1967. The Hard of Hearing. Kanehara Publishers, Tokyo. 236 p.

Suzuki, T. (ed.). 1969. Study of Young Hard of Hearing Children. Jap. J. Otol. (Suppl. 5). 160 p.

Suzuki, H. 1973. Oral communication in special environment: Some problems on diver communication and educational technology of severe hard of hearing. *In* S. Hiki (ed.), Speech Information Processing, pp. 276–302. University of Tokyo Press, Tokyo.

Tanaka, Y., M. Shindo, and T. Motomiya. 1973. A speechreading test using a television and communication ability in the hearing-impaired. Audiol. Jap. 16: 109–119.

Tanaka, Y., H. Ishida, and M. Shindo. 1974. Environmental problems concerning integration of young hearing-impaired children into kindergartens or nursery schools. Audiol. Jap. 17: 282–288.

Tsuiki, T. 1972. Hearing Test. Nankodo, Tokyo. 193 p.

Yasuno, T., S. Ibata, S. Ohyama, K. Kawamura, K. Veda, K. Hataguchi, and C. Nirei. 1974. The factors of auditory training for the deaf children. Audiol. Jap. 17: 246–252.

Yoshino, T. 1974. Trials of integration resulting from early educational program—A case of severe hearing handicapped children. Jap. J. Spec. Educ. 11(3): 48–61.

PART III
Summary

chapter 17
Summary Comments

Herbert J. Oyer, Ph.D.

As one might assume, there are observable similarities among the authors of the preceding chapters as regards the manner in which they define the concept of habilitation-rehabilitation of hearing-handicapped persons. The common thread running throughout is the primary emphasis placed upon the development of language as a means by which the hearing-handicapped person can facilitate his self-adjustment and his adjustment to society as well. Not all agree that the language must be totally oral in form, but all would concede to the fact that a blend of oral and manual has something to offer too.

The basic pattern of development of programs throughout the various countries has been highly similar. The first concern seems to have been for the profoundly deaf and, as a result, programs and schools have emerged to take care of this segment of the hearing-handicapped group. Later, attention has been directed toward those who sustain less severe losses of hearing. Emphasis seems to have been placed, in all instances, upon programs for children. Later, the adults were brought into the picture, but it can be said that even today the care of hearing-handicapped adults lags in most countries.

Descriptions of programs for hearing-handicapped persons having disorders of communication throughout the various countries, as reported in this book, vary substantially. In some countries, there appears to be a full spectrum of services rendered as regards diagnosis and habilitation-rehabilitation, for both children and adults, whereas, in others, the focus is primarily on the educational assessment, description of performance, and achievement of children. In some countries, both private and public support are given to programs serving the hearing handicapped, whereas in other countries, the source of financial support is the state. Programs also vary according to the type of professional training of persons who provide the leadership. Much of the early and current leadership has come from individuals trained in the field of medicine. The United States is a notable exception, with leadership being rendered principally by those trained specifically as teachers and clinicians.

The diagnostic procedures employed in programs as described by the authors of the foregoing chapters all aim toward determination of hearing level. Pure tone as well as speech audiometric tests are applied by all to determine the hearing status of both children and adults. In numerous instances, conditioning procedures are employed. Greater reliance is shown by some than by others on the advanced audiometric tests, depending upon the general level of audiological development in the country and whether or not the program is under principally medical, audiological, or educational leadership. As one might expect, the more advanced clinical tests are used in medical and audiological clinics. One area of diagnosis which shows up as in need of development in all countries is that of "diagnosis of handicap." Inasmuch as this writer can determine, there has been, and is, too little development in the realm of diagnosis which specifies the handicapping effects as related to the organic auditory deficit.

In programs focusing specifically upon the profoundly deaf, the great emphasis seems to be upon language development. There is not, by any stretch of the imagination, agreement among writers as to the relative importance of lipreading or signing and fingerspelling as supportive techniques in the language-building process. One contributor suggests that we can no longer ignore the beneficial effects of a total communication approach. Another contributor suggests that a multisensory approach cannot be upheld in light of neurophysiological research findings. Thus, patterns of procedures vary among clinicians.

Hearing aid usage is universally reported by writers from the various countries. It is of interest to note, however, that there is an apparent variance of some magnitude as to the handling of the aids and their application to the ear(s) of the hearing handicapped. Some report highly refined approaches to the analysis of hearing aid characteristics as related to the fitting of them to individuals. Others allude to the problems of importing good hearing aids to their countries and the struggles involved in the domestic development of hearing aids. Not only do some countries have the problem of getting good hearing aids, but they also are virtually without any support system to keep the aids in good working condition.

It probably comes as no surprise to the reader that the professional training and responsibilities of those working with the hearing handicapped are highly diverse among the countries. In programs from countries reported upon, with the exception of Great Britain, Ireland, Canada, and the United States, the professional person in charge of programs is often trained as a physician. He or she may be a medical audiologist, a phoniatrist, an orthophonist, or an otolaryngologist. The supportive personnel are teachers, logopedists, audiometric technicians, engineers, and, in some instances, psychologists. In Great Britain, Ireland, Canada, and the United States, the teacher of the deaf, audiologist, and speech pathologist are in management roles as regards clinical and educational programs for the hearing handicapped with communication disorders. Of course, there is a close liaison with specialists in medicine (principally the otologist), the psychologist, and, frequently, the social worker. Irrespective of titles and backgrounds of those who manage programs and those who support in this effort, the most crucial element to be considered is the multiple input so necessary in the complex task of habilitating-rehabilitating hearing-handicapped persons with related communication problems. One might speculate that, in the future, depending upon the success of electrode implants in the cochlea, the neurophysiologist and bioengineer will also play professional roles in the habilitation-rehabilitation process.

The picture is mixed concerning family involvements as stimulated by directors of services for the hearing handicapped. Rather elaborate programs of education concerning causes and effects of hearing loss and individual counseling of parents, siblings, and spouses are carried on in some settings. In other settings, this does not seem to be a point of great emphasis, except perhaps with parents of the profoundly deaf child.

Training of professionals for the field of rehabilitative audiology has, except for a few countries, meant the training of teachers of the deaf, the special training of physicians following their graduation from schools of medicine, and the training on a short-term basis of technicians to serve as logopedists or hearing aid assistants. In England, there is now specific training of audiologists. In the United States, the training of the audiologist must be through the master's degree, followed by a clinical fellowship year after which a national board examination is taken for purposes of achieving the Certificate of Clinical Competence from the American Speech and Hearing Association. Additionally, there is a growing list of states that have enacted legislation requiring licensure of audiologists.

There is considerable research taking place in the countries from which reports were made. At the risk of over-generalizing, it appears as though the research can be classified as falling within two categories, namely *descriptive studies* of the number of profoundly deaf in the country, their schools, vocational placement and needs, and *studies of causes of deafness* and the medical and surgical means of handling hearing loss. Amplification via group aids and individual hearing aids has also been the subject of some study. Noticeably lacking are in-depth studies of the extent to which individuals are handicapped by hearing loss in psychosocial and educational areas.

The majority of the countries reported upon have well developed professional and lay organizations that focus attention upon the handicapping conditions associated with hearing impairment. Efforts of both kinds of organizations are directed toward preparing hearing-handicapped people to enter a society in which they can be productive citizens or, in the case of adults, helping them to remain in the mainstream of society or returning to it successfully. In each country, there have been concerned individuals who have aggressively dedicated their energies toward making life more meaningful for the hearing handicapped. In order to communicate among themselves and to the larger society, journals and magazines have been developed which cover a variety of topics ranging from experimental research in hearing science to clinical and educational programing to the education and counseling of parent groups. They all serve distinct purposes and are useful in their own particular way to advance the quality of clinical treatment and education of persons suffering communication problems associated with hearing loss.

It is the sincere hope of this writer that this comparative presentation of philosophies, programs, procedures, and research in the area of hearing handicap will provide keener insights into the problems of hearing handicap and deeper appreciation of the efforts being made to claim or reclaim the human potential that could so easily be lost to society through handicaps associated with hearing impairment.

Index